The Cementless Fixation of Hip Endoprostheses

Edited by E. Morscher

With 230 Figures

Springer-Verlag
Berlin Heidelberg New York Tokyo 1984

Prof. Dr. Erwin Morscher
Orthopädische Universitätsklinik
Felix-Platter-Spital, Burgfelderstr. 101
4001 Basel/Switzerland

ISBN-13: 978-3-642-69008-2 e-ISBN-13: 978-3-642-69006-8
DOI: 10.1007/ 978-3-642-69006-8

Softcover reprint of the hardcover 1st edition 1984

2124/3140-543210

Preface

The main problem with regard to alloplastic joints is the loosening of the implant. Twenty years ago, Charnley first introduced bone cement to hip surgery, enabling total hip replacement to be practised on a larger scale. There is no question, however, that new approaches must be found to solving the problems of implant loosening, either by developing a new type of cement or by directly anchoring the implant without using cement. Much research has been done in this direction in recent years.

The methods which have already been tested or are currently being tested were presented and discussed at a symposium on Cementless Fixation of Endoprostheses organized by the Orthopaedic Clinic of the University of Basel and held on 24–26 June 1982. Various possible approaches which might be realized in practice were discussed in a relaxed atmosphere. In addition to the biomechanical bases of cementless fixation of endoprostheses, the various models were discussed, with special regard to their biocompatibility, physical characteristics, design, clinical applicability, and previous clinical experience. This book contains the papers delivered at this symposium.

June 1983 E. Morscher, Basel

Table of Contents

List of Contributors

Dr. K. Bläsius, Orthopädische Abteilung der Universitätsklinik, Hugstetterstraße 55, D-7800 Freiburg

Prof. Dr. Renato Bombelli, Via Lampugnani, I-20025 Legnano (Milano)

Dr. N. Böhler, Labor für Knochenforschung, Histologisch-Embryologisches Institut, Schwarzspanierstraße 17, A-1090 Wien

Dr. F. Bornand, Avenue Eglantine 5, CH-1006 Lausanne

Prof. Dr. G. Bousquet, F-St. Etienne

Dr. K. E. Brinkmann, Leitender Arzt der Orthopädie-Traumatologie, Rehabilitations-Krankenhaus, D-7516 Karlsbad-Langensteinbach

Dr. G. H. Buchhorn, Orthopädische Universitätsklinik, Robert-Koch-Straße 46, D-3400 Göttingen

Dr. P. De Meester, Department of Metallurgy and Division of Orthopaedic Surgery, Katholieke Universiteit, B-3030 Leuven

Dr. W. Dick, Kinderspital, CH-4058 Basel

Dr. K. und Y. Draenert, Histo-Morphologische Arbeitsgruppe der Orthopädischen Klinik Rechts der Isar der Technischen Universität, Alte Landstraße 26, D-8012 Ottobrunn

Prof. Dr. P. Ducheyne, Department of Metallurgy and Division of Orthopaedic Surgery, Katholieke Universiteit, B-3030 Leuven

Dr. K. H. Elsner, Orthopädische Abteilung des Krankenhauses der Augustinerinnen, Jakobstraße 27, D-5000 Köln 1

Prof. Dr. F. Endler, ehemals Primarius der Orthopädischen Station der KFA und des Gottfried-von-Preyerschen-Kinderspitales, Wiedner Hauptstraße 36, A-1040 Wien

Doz. Dr. M. Endler jun., Wiedner Hauptstraße 36, A-1040 Wien

Dr. A. Engelhardt, Facharzt für Orthopädie, Donnersbergstraße 42, D-6000 Frankfurt/M.

Dr. P. Frank, Orthopädisches Krankenhaus Wien-Gersthof, Wielemansgasse 28, A-1180 Wien

Dr. E. Gabriel, Orthopädische Klinik der Universität, Brettreichstraße 11, D-8700 Würzburg

Prof. Dr. J. Galante, Rush-Presbyterian-St. Luke's Medical Center, 1753 W. Congress Parkway, Chicago, IL 60612/USA

Priv.-Doz. Dr. A. Gächter, Orthopädische Universitätsklinik, Kantonsspital, CH-4031 Basel

Prof. Dr. R. Ganz, Direktor der Klinik und Poliklinik für Orthop. Chirurgie, Inselspital, CH-3010 Bern

Priv.-Doz. Dr. P. Griss, Oberarzt, Orthopädische Klinik Lindenhof, D-6800 Mannheim

Dr. F. Grundschober, Labor für Knochenforschung, Histologisch-Embryologisches Institut, Schwarzspanierstraße 17, A-1090 Wien

Prof. Dr. J. Harms, Leitender Arzt, Orthopädie-Traumatologie I, Rehabilitationskrankenhaus, D-7516 Karlsbad-Langensteinbach

Dr. W. W. Herrmann, Anatomisches Institut, Abteilung für Systematische Anatomie, Bühlstraße 26, CH-3012 Bern

Prof. Dr. G. Hierholzer, Ärztlicher Direktor, BG-Unfallklinik, Grossenbaumer Allee 250, D-4100 Duisburg 28

Dr. Ch. A. Homsy, Direktor Prosthesis Research Labor, Fondren Orthopedic Center, The Methodist Hospital, 6560 Fannin, Houston, Texas 77030/USA

Prof. Dr. K. J. Hüttinger, Institut für Chemische Technik der Universität, Kaiserstraße 12, D-7500 Karlsruhe 1

Dr. W. Hüttner, c/o Fa. Schunk & Ebe GmbH, Postfach 64, D-6300 Gießen

Prof. Dr. A. Huggler, Leitender Arzt der Orthopädischen Klinik, Kantonsspital, Loestraße 170, CH-7000 Chur

Dr. H. A. C. Jacob, Klinik Balgrist, Forchstraße 240, CH-8008 Zürich

Dr. H. Jenny, Orthopädische Universitätsklinik, Felix-Platter-Spital, CH-4055 Basel

Doz. Dr. K. Knahr, Orthopädisches Krankenhaus Wien-Gersthof, Wielemansgasse 28, A-1180 Wien

Prof. Dr. W. Küsswetter, Orthopädische Klinik der Universität, Brettreichstraße 11, D-8700 Würzburg

Dr. M. Martens, Department of Metallurgy and Division of Orthopaedic Surgery, Katholieke Universiteit, B-3030 Leuven

Dr. h.c. R. Mathys und R. Mathys jun., Fabrik für Chirurgie-Instrumente, CH-2544 Bettlach

Prof. Dr. E. Mäusle, Institut für Pathologie der Universität des Saarlandes, D-6650 Homburg/Saar

Prof. Dr. H. Mittelmeier, Direktor der Orthopädischen Universitätsklinik und Poliklinik, D-6650 Homburg/Saar

Dr. W. Mönch, Stadtkrankenhaus, Chirurgische Abteilung, D-8940 Memmingen

Prof. Dr. E. Morscher, Vorsteher der Orthopädischen Universitätsklinik, Felix-Platter-Spital, CH-4055 Basel

Dr. J. C. Mulier, Department of Metallurgy and Division of Orthopaedic Surgery, Katholike Universiteit, B-3030 Leuven

Dr. R. Parhofer, Chefarzt, Chirurgische Abteilung Stadtkrankenhaus, Bismarckstraße, D-8940 Memmingen

Dr. D. Parpan, Klinik für Orthopädie, Inselspital, CH-3010 Bern

Prof. Dr. Sr. M. Perren, M. E. Müller-Institut für Biomechanik der Universität, Murtenstraße 35, CH-3008 Bern

Univ.-Doz. Dr. H. Plenk jun., Labor für Knochenforschung, Histologisch-Embryologisches Institut, Schwarzspanierstraße 17, A-1090 Wien

Dr. G. Pflüger, Labor für Knochenforschung, Histologisch-Embryologisches Institut, Schwarzspanierstraße 17, A-1090 Wien

Dr. W. Pommer, Universitätsklinik für Chirurgie, Landeskrankenhaus, Auenbruggerplatz, A-8036 Graz

Prof. Dr. A. Reichelt, Direktor der Orthopädischen Abteilung, Universitätsklinik, Hugstetterstraße 55, D-7800 Freiburg

Prof. Dr. H. Rettig, Direktor der Orthopädischen Universitätsklinik, Klinikum der Justus-Liebig-Universität, Freiligrathstraße 2, D-6300 Gießen

Prim. Dr. G. Rupp, A.ö. Landeskrankenhaus, Unfallabteilung, A-4840 Vöcklabruck

Prof. Dr. M. Salzer, Vorsteher des Orthopädischen Krankenhauses Wien-Gersthof, Wielemansgasse 28, A-1180 Wien

Dr. R. F. Santore, Via Lampugnani, I-20025 Legnano (Milano)

Dr. V. Santner, Universitätsklinik für Chirurgie, Landeskrankenhaus, Auenbruggerplatz, A-8036 Graz

Dipl.-Chem. H. Scharbach, c/o Pfaudler-Werke AG, Scheffelstraße 55, D-6830 Schwetzingen

Prof. R. Schenk, Anatomisches Institut, Abteilung für Systematische Anatomie, Bühlstraße 26, CH-3012 Bern

Dr. S. Schider, Labor für Knochenforschung, Histologisch-Embryologisches Institut, Schwarzspanierstraße 17, A-1090 Wien

Prof. Dr. D. Schöllner, Chefarzt der Orthopädischen Abteilung, Krankenhaus der Augustinerinnen, Jakobstraße 27, D-5000 Köln 1

Prof. Dr. A. Schreiber, Direktor der Orthopädischen Universitätsklinik, Balgrist, Forchstraße 340, CH-8008 Zürich

Dr. H. Seidel, Chefarzt der Chirurgischen Abteilung, Hafenkrankenhaus, Zirkusweg 11, D-2000 Hamburg 4

Dr. M. Semlitsch, c/o Gebr. Sulzer AG, CH-8401 Winterthur

Priv.-Doz. Dr. Y. Suezawa, Klinik Balgrist, Forchstraße 340, CH-8008 Zürich

Dr. O. Stampfel, Oberarzt, Universitätsklinik für Chirurgie, Landeskrankenhaus, Auenbruggerplatz, A-8036 Graz

Dr. B. Störmer, BG-Unfallklinik, Grossenbaumer Allee 250, D-4100 Duisburg

Dr. T. Stuhler, Orthopädische Klinik der Universität, Brettreichstraße 11, D-8700 Würzburg

Dr. L. Töpfer, Orthopädische Klinik der Universität, Brettreichstraße 11, D-8700 Würzburg

Dr. R. Trauner, Universitätsklinik für Chirurgie, Landeskrankenhaus, Auenbruggerplatz, A-8036 Graz

Prof. Dr. K. Walcher, Chefarzt der Chirurgischen Klinik II der Städt. Krankenanstalten, Kulmbacher Straße 23, D-8580 Bayreuth

Priv.-Doz. Dr. U. Weber, Facharzt für Chirurgie, Oberarzt der Orthopädischen Universitätsklinik, Freiligrathstraße 2, D-6300 Gießen

Prof. Dr. H.-G. Willert, Direktor der Orthopädischen Universitätsklinik, Robert-Koch-Straße 46, D-3400 Göttingen

Dr. A. Zeibig, Rosenthal Stemag Technische Keramik AG, D-8560 Lauf an der Pegnitz

Dr. P. Zoephel, BafB, Ostend 29, D-6103 Griesheim b. Darmstadt

Doz. K. Zweymüller, Orthopädische Universitätsklinik, Allgemeines Krankenhaus, Garnisonsgasse 13, A-1090 Wien

Introduction I

E. Morscher

Nowadays when we speak of cementless fixation of hip endoprostheses, we are actually returning to the early days of hip arthroplasty. This is not to say, however, that the use of bone cement is a thing of the past.

Polymethyl methacrylate, a well-known dental cement, was first used in hip surgery by Haboush [9] in 1951. In 1957 Wiltse et al. [41] actually introduced self-polymerizing polymethyl methacrylate to orthopedic surgery as a fixation material. In 1960 Charnley [3] made definitive use of this cement for the implantation of his total hip replacement.

There is no question that the introduction of methyl methacrylate cement to hip surgery has enabled total hip replacements to be practiced on the wide scale that we know today. However, it is equally true that the use of bone cement entails a number of disadvantages, the major one being the inability of bone cement (in its present form, at least) to ensure the stable, permanent fixation of an implant. This problem has led to a reawakening of interest in techniques of cementless prosthesis fixation.

At the start it must be acknowledged that the primary results of cemented arthroplasties are entirely satisfactory. It is only the long-term results that need improving. Generally, 5 years of follow-up are needed for femoral prostheses, and 8–10 years for acetabular components, before an assessment can be made as to the superiority of one fixation method over another.

The main long-term problem in hip arthroplasty is loosening of the implant and the consequent need for revision. Statistics at our clinic, for example, indicate that while the number of primary hip arthroplasties has remained fairly constant since 1973, with a rate of about 300 per year, the incidence of revisions has steadily increased from year to year (Fig. 1). This is not altered by the fact that only about two-thirds of the reoperated patients had their primary arthroplasty performed at our clinic.

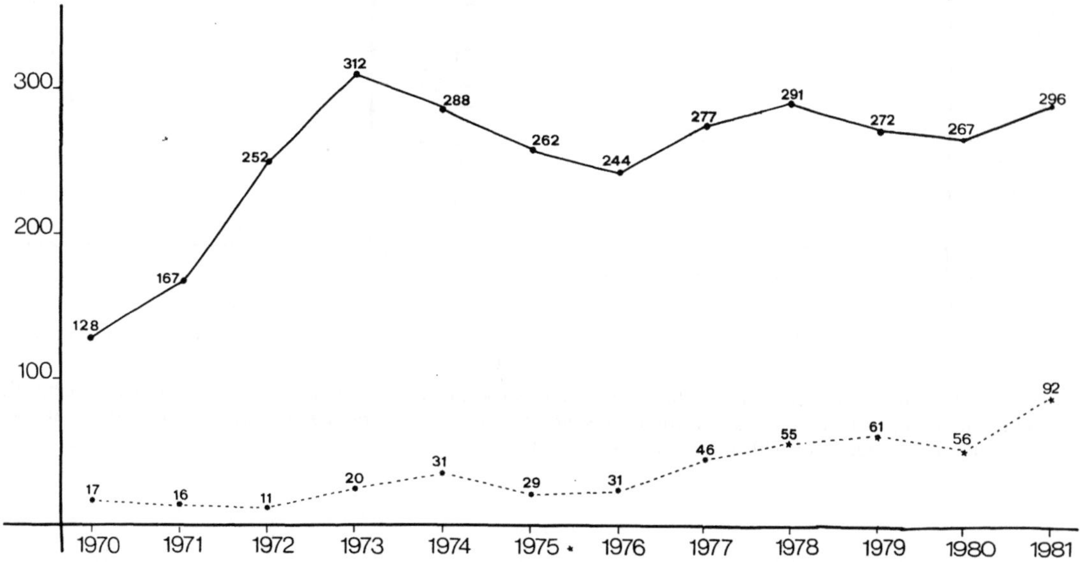

Fig. 1. Statistics on total hip arthroplasties and revision arthroplasties performed at the Orthopedic Clinic of the University of Basel, Switzerland, from 1970 to 1981 (— primary operations, --- reoperations)

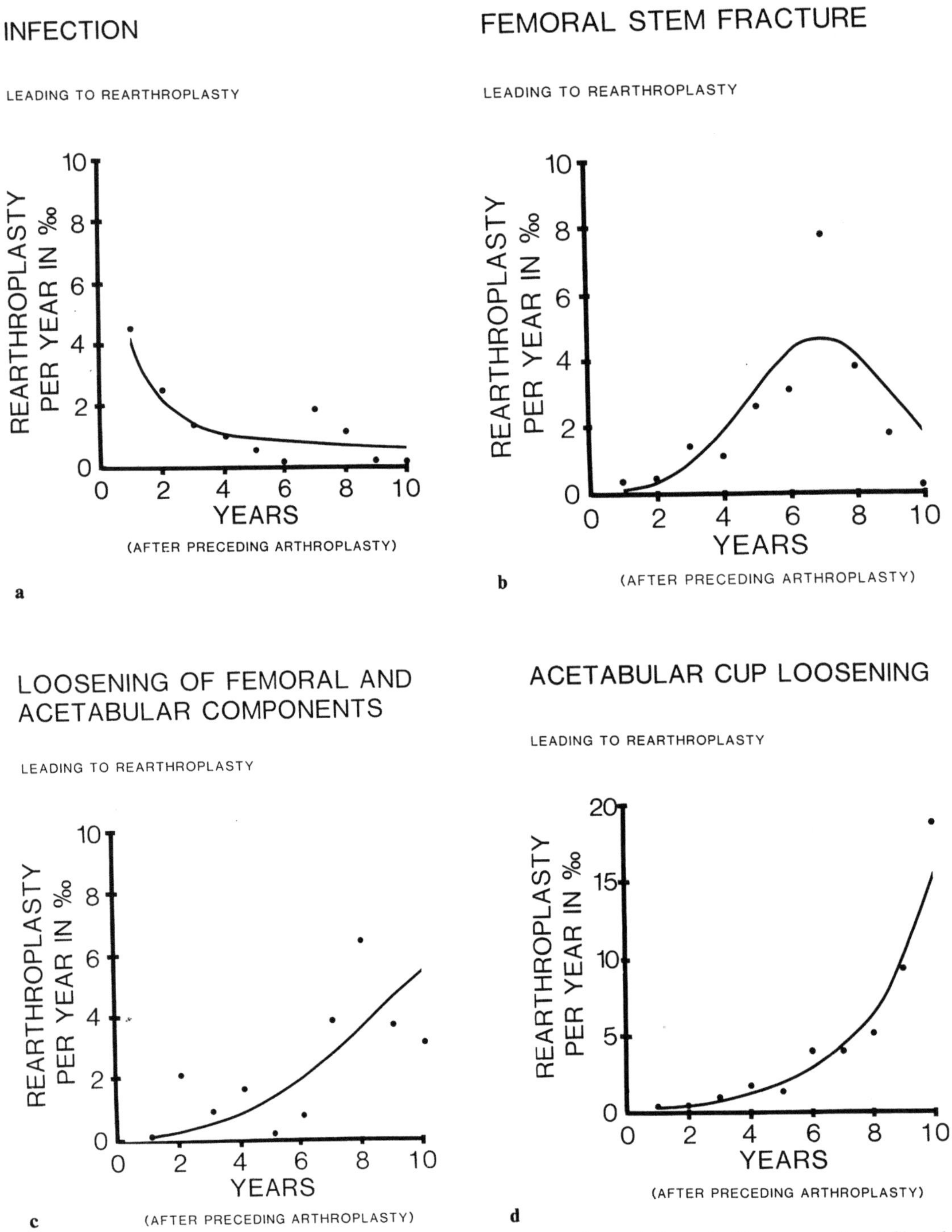

Fig. 2 a–d. Time of reoperation as a function of the cause of primary failure. 1–10 year results of Charnley Müller total hip arthroplasty. **a** infection; **b** stem fracture of femoral component; **c** loose stem; **d** loose acetabular component. N = 320 (10 years) – 2456 (1 year)

In an effort to detect trends in the area of revisional total hip arthroplasty, we constructed a mathematical model based on 2669 Charnley-Müller arthroplasties and 141 revisions (5.3%) performed during the period from November 1970 to February 1982 (mean observation time = 5.4 years). During the same period an additional 235 revisions were performed for other types of arthroplasty (McKee, Wagner double cup, Isoelastic TP, etc.) and on patients referred from outside. Our findings may be summarized briefly as follows:

- The incidence of reoperations due to infection declines sharply after the 2nd postoperative year.
- The incidence of stem fractures of the femoral component increases from the 5th to 7th postoperative year and then declines.
- The incidence of stem loosening increases fairly constantly with each year.
- Loosening of the acetabular component is relatively rare prior to the 5th postoperative year, but its incidence rises exponentially after 8 years. This shows clearly that loosening of the acetabular component is the major long-term problem in hip arthroplasty.

The cementless fixation of hip endoprostheses can be rated superior to cement fixation only if its results surpass those currently available for cement fixation, bearing in mind, of course, the progress made in recent years owing to technical improvements in prosthetic materials, design, and operating technique. In particular, it must be noted that improvements in cementing techniques have already enabled a better prosthetic attachment to be realized, and that the development of new bone cements might well bring improvements in long-term results.

An example of progress in this area is the new "bioactive bone cement" [37] having the following composition: 30 wt.% polymethyl methacrylate, 60 wt.% glass ceramic with a grain size of 80–180 μ, 10 wt.% silanized glass fibers 3 mm long and 10 μ in diameter. The impact and bending strength of this cement are inferior to that of Palacos-R, but the cement shows substantial improvement in terms of elasticity modulus, which is 3 times higher than that of Palacos-R and thus more closely approximates that of natural bone.

In addition, the maximum exothermal temperature of the bioactive glass ceramic is reduced by about 10 °C. Carbon-reinforced acrylate cement is also of interest in this connection owing to its 4-times-higher fatigue strength, as pointed out by Mittelmeier et al. [23].

Moreover, despite our enthusiasm for cementless prosthetic fixation, we must recognize that there will always be cases, as in tumor surgery, where the use of bone cement cannot be dispensed with.

The goal of this monograph is to determine how far research has progressed in the area of cementless fixation, the extent to which this method offers a practical alternative to cement fixation, and, above all, the direction in which further research in this area should proceed.

It might be well at this point to review briefly the history of total hip replacement arthroplasty, bearing in mind the admonition of the philosopher Santayana that "those who do not remember the past are condemned to repeat it." We might also recall a remark made by a distant predecessor of mine, Dr. Hans Debrunner [5], who also was a Professor of Orthopedics in Basel: "The history of hip arthroplasty offers a splendid example of human behavior and confirms Gehlen's thesis of man as an active being. Man's ambition compels him to actively meet the challenges of life, and it is this active intervention that enables man, who lacks instincts, to survive. However, this behavior also takes man again and again to the very limits of what can be achieved and compels him to examine the results of his actions after these actions have already been carried out."

The first interposition arthroplasty in general was probably performed in the early 1930s by Rehn [28] in Freiburg/Germany. Smith-Petersen [36] subsequently adopted and popularized this technique.

The first total hip replacement was implanted in 1938 by Philipp Wiles in London. It consisted of two steel components. The first published case in which a metal prosthesis was anchored by insertion into the intramedullary canal is from Moore and Bohlman in 1943 [25]. The case involved the replacement of a tumor by a specially constructed metal prosthesis. The operation took place on September 28, 1940.

Before it was generally recognized that only a total hip replacement that included an acetabular component could ensure long-term success, a decade and a half passed in which hemiarthroplasties were performed almost exclusively. Recall the unprecedented "boom" in arthroplasty that the Judet brothers [16] of Paris triggered after the Second World War with their spherical plexiglass prosthesis for the femoral head. In the U.S., the metal prostheses of Moore [24], Thompson [38], Leinbach (1982, personal communication) and others were widely used and enjoyed great popularity for some years. All these prostheses were implanted without cement and had recesses and cavities that enhanced the fixation through bony ingrowth.

Early on, McKee [17, 18] attempted to develop a total hip replacement consisting of two metal components. His first model was developed in 1940 but was never tested clinically, and the second was implanted in three patients in 1951. It consisted of a metal acetabular component that was screwed into the pelvis and a metal head that was attached by a screw driven into the femoral neck. McKee's third model consisted of a metal cup that also was screwed into the pelvis, but the femoral head was replaced with a Thompson prosthesis inserted into the medullary cavity. The results of these metal combinations were poor, however, until the advent of bone cement. As McKee wrote in 1970 [17], "In 1960 methyl methacrylate was used as a cement and immediately the success rate was greatly improved and is now over 90 per cent. This is due to the fact that it spreads the load over a wide area of bone, whereas the use of a screw tends to concentrate the load at one point." With this, McKee touched upon what is perhaps the key problem of prosthetic fixation in general: the distribution of forces at the interface between prosthesis and bone.

The cementless metallic total hip replacement that has exhibited the best long-term success rate to date is probably that of Ring [30], in which the acetabular component is screwed to the pelvis and the femoral head is replaced with a Moore-like prosthesis anchored by insertion into the medullary cavity. The first model was implanted in 1964. The Ring prosthesis is still in use today, although the author himself has since abandoned the metal cup in favor of a cementless polyethylene cup.

Because bone cement was not approved by the Food and Drug Administration for general use in the United States until the early 1970s, uncemented prostheses were used almost exclusively during the 1960s, such as the combination of the Urist hip socket with a Moore or Leinbach prosthesis.

Siwash [35] of the Soviet Union developed his own prosthesis in the early 1960s that was widely used primarily in Eastern countries. It is very similar to the Rumanian "Etropal" prosthesis, which is fabricated from titanium (Ti Al 6V4) and can be attached with or without cement. The Siwash prosthesis was also used at our clinic by my predecessor, Prof. G. Chapchal, who implanted it in 15 patients. Most of these prostheses had to be replaced because of loosening.

If an arthroplasty is to be permanent, it is essential that a state of biological and mechanical equilibrium be established between the implant and the surrounding bone. The processes that take place between the implant and bone are comparable to those that occur when a fracture is immobilized by internal fixation. The essential difference is that in the latter case, the function of the implant is gradually assumed by the healing bone. In arthroplasty, on the other hand, the implant must continue to function permanently and at maximum capacity. This is possible only if a permanent biomechanical integration of the implant is achieved. This integration is chiefly a function of interfacial conditions between the implant and bone. To achieve a biomechanically harmonious equilibrium, certain conditions must be satisfied such as biocompatibility, corrosion resistance, strength, fatigue resistance, sterilizability, good primary fixation, and a design (shape) suitable to ensure that stresses will be transmitted from the implant to the bone and vice-versa principally in the form of compressive forces, so that relative movements will not occur at the interface. In addition, a prosthesis should be simple to insert *and* relatively simple to remove in case revision is necessary.

The importance of these factors is reflected in the observable dependence of success and failure rates of hip arthroplasties on the degree to which these conditions are satisfied.

Tissue compatibility, meaning the biochemical and cytological reactions to an implant material, must of course be tested in experimental animals. However, the history of endoprosthetics has demonstrated time and again how the behavior of implants under clinical use can differ significantly from that shown experimentally, sometimes with catastrophic results. Thus, Teflon, polyester and polyacetal have had to be abandoned in conditions where these materials must perform a gliding function under loads. Even high-density polyethylene, which has proved most effective to date, is subject to frictional wear, and the resulting wear debris can provoke massive osteolysis. The "soft-top" prosthesis [39] illustrates this problem particularly well. In this prosthesis, which was designed for hemiarthroplastic use, a small metal head moves within a larger polyethylene head, which in turn moves against the cartilage of the acetabulum. This can cause a large degree of frictional wear leading to extensive bone resorption.

The forces acting on an artificial hip joint have also been underestimated in terms of corrosion resistance, strength and fatigue resistance. Too little attention has been given to the fact that a prosthesis must have chemical as well as mechanical stability in order to ensure longevity.

Because the permanent biomechanical integration of an implant relies largely on conditions at its interface with living bone, it is little wonder that the properties of the implant surface play a central role. To ensure a harmonious transmission of forces, this surface must conform to the bone, and the contact areas through which forces are transmitted should be as large as possible in order to avoid "stress concentrations." These requirements must be reflected in the surface characteristics of the implant, its physical properties, and its overall design.

Mittelmeier [22], for example, developed his "supporting rib" design for the purpose of maximizing the surface area of the implant to improve stress distribution and thus reduce pressure.

The Judet brothers achieved a similar effect by using metal implants with a porous surface ("porometal") [15]. Due to initial failures, however, various modifications had to be made by altering the design of the prosthesis, improving its metallurgy, and using screws to enhance the fixation of the acetabular component.

Lord has reported excellent clinical results with his cementless "madreporic" prosthesis [20].

However, the increase in implant surface area achieved with macroscopic perforations and recesses is relatively minor compared with the possibilities offered by microporosity. The idea is to provide a surface with chemically-stable pores having diameters greater than 20 μ that are receptive to bony ingrowth [12, 13]. Pore diameters in excess of 100 μ permit calcification of the osteons. A pore size of 20–300 μ, with a volume porosity of 40–80%, is considered ideal. Enlarging the pores and increasing the volume porosity promotes the ingrowth of bone tissue.

Recognizing that the stabilization of an implant is dependent upon four key parameters – the "chemistry" of the implant, its surface area, surface geometry and dynamic characteristics – Homsy developed "Proplast" for use in the coating of metallic prostheses. Proplast has a pore size of 100–500 μ and a volume porosity of 75%. The interpore connections are 200 μ wide. Chemically, the material consists of polytetrafluoroethylene polymer and glassy carbon fibers. Proplast-coated femoral-head prostheses were first used here in Basel in the mid-1970s in patients with femoral neck fractures. The results of these operations were somewhat disappointing, however. Analogous observations have been made by Sadr and Arden [31].

Galante et al. [7] reported in the early 1970s on the first attempts to increase implant surface area by the use of "fiber metal," a sintered titanium wire mesh.

Important contributions to the problem of surface microporosity were later made by the Toronto research group of Pilliar et al. [27], who sintered Co–Cr–Mo coatings with a 20–100 μ pore size and 35–45% porosity onto the prosthetic surface.

We must also mention the work of Ducheyne [6] and his group in Belgium, who applied porous coatings of stainless steel (AISI 316 L) with a 50–100 μ pore size and 42–48% porosity to the prostheses.

Boutin of France was the first, in 1969, to use porous ceramic ("alumine frittée") for attaching a prosthetic cup directly to the acetabular bone; he also used the first titanium femoral prosthesis in 1975 [1, 2].

In the German-speaking countries, Mittelmeier [22], Griss [8] and the Viennese group of Salzer [32, 33] gathered the largest volume of research data and practical experience on the use of ceramics for bone implantation.

A prerequisite for direct bonding between the implant and bone is the absence of relative motion at the interface, i.e., mechanical rest [29]. This requires good primary fixation of the implant, as well as measures to eliminate secondary relative movements. The selection of a material with suitable physical properties and a good prosthetic design are crucial in this regard.

One means of achieving mechanical rest is – for instance – by using a rigid implant that stiffens the entire bone-implant system. This raises the question of whether "stress protection," known from the use of rigid implants in fracture management, will be a problem. Jackson-Burrows [14] was among the first to state that femoral endoprostheses which remove too much pressure from the bone lead to bony atrophic changes. On the other hand, in an artificial joint all forces are transmitted from the implant to the bone, or vice-versa, regardless of the elasticity of the implant or bone. A change in elasticity mainly leads to a change in stress distribution and thus in the pattern of force transmission. The sum of forces in a prosthesis is always 100%, in contrast to implants used for internal fracture fixation. In an attempt to normalize the stresses between the prosthesis and surrounding bone, or between the contact surface of the fixation material and a reconstructed bony surface, and thus normalize the associated changes in the lines of weight-bearing, the late Hoffmann-Daimler [10] suggested in 1972 the use of specially-shaped elastic elements that would surround the endoprosthesis in weight-bearing areas of the acetabulum and head. He claimed that this substitute for biological elasticity would be able to neutralize the harmful components of compressive forces while splitting up the altered pattern of weight-bearing into specific vectoral forces.

A further question is whether a sizable difference between the elasticity moduli of the implant and bone will necessarily cause relative movements between them, as Homsy [12] and Sarmiento [34] assume. Obviously this depends largely on the nature of the forces. Under compressive forces, differences in elasticity will be of minor importance. Under bending forces, on the other hand, the implant, which transmits the forces to the bone, obviously must be more rigid than the bone. This rigidity, of course, depends not just on the elastic modulus of the prosthetic material, but also on the design of the prosthesis. From this standpoint, a marked difference exists between the forces occurring between an acetabular cup and the pelvis, and those occurring between a prosthetic stem and the femoral bone. In the case of the acetabular cup, a spherical design is best for ensuring that stresses will be transmitted from the pelvis to the acetabulum largely in the form of compressive forces. The femoral shaft, however, is exposed to sizable bending and rotational forces. The latter are made up of both compressive and tensile stresses, which is why the implant must be relatively rigid at least in areas where the greatest forces are transmitted from implant to bone, i.e., in the proximal part of the shaft. This will prevent significant deformation with the development of potentially damaging compressive and tensile forces. A femoral prosthesis that is not considerably more resistant to deformation in the neck area than the femoral bone that contains it will inevitably loosen [26].

The interrelationship between prosthetic elasticity and design, individual anatomy, and patient activity and body weight is vividly demonstrated by our 9 years of experience with the "isoelastic" prosthesis.

The problems that face us today in hip-joint arthroplasty can scarcely be understood in their full scope. They require the applied knowledge of orthopedic surgeons, engineers, technicians, biomechanics experts and physiologists, and above all a free exchange of information among these specialties. In years to come, increasing attention will also be given to the voice of the financier (whoever that may be in the health-care industry) and of the patients themselves. Today the development of new technologies is inconceivable without close cooperation between medicine and industry. True science must be free, of course, and must be able to develop and progress in an atmosphere that is, to a certain extent, unencumbered by financial and other constraints. This attitude can only be carried so far, however, and in recent years the limits have very nearly been reached and with them the limits of potential growth: While the possibilities of what is theoretically possible are expanding almost exponentially, the curve of available resources is leveling off, and that of the cost-benefit ratio is becoming asymptotic. A mutual dialogue among different specialities and professions will help to improve the quality of information exchange, so that each expert will be able to pursue his speciality on a more efficient, goal-directed basis, and perhaps recognize and avoid blind alleys.

References

1. Boutin P (1972) Arthroplastie totale de la hanche par prothèse en alumine frittée. Rev Chir Orthop 58:229–246
2. Boutin P (1974) Les prothèses totales de la hanche en alumine. L'ancrage direct sans ciment dans 50 cas. Rev Chir Orthop 60:233–245
3. Charnley J (1960) Anchorage of the femoral head prosthesis to the shaft of the femur. J Bone Joint Surg [Br] 42:28
4. Charnley J (1970) Editorial comment. Clin Orthop 72:2
5. Debrunner H (1969) Gedanken zur Hüftarthroplastik. In: Rütt (Hrsg) Die Therapie der Coxarthrose. Thieme, Stuttgart
6. Ducheyne P, Aernoudt E, de Meester P (1978) The mechanical behaviour of porous austenitic stainless steel fibre structures. J Mat Sci 13:2650–2658
7. Galante J, Rostoker W, Lueck R, Ray RD (1971) Sintered fiber metal composite as a basis for attachment of implants to bone. J Bone Joint Surg [Am] 53:101–114
8. Griss P, Andrian-Wehrburg von, Heimke G, Krempien B, Reipa S, Hartung HJ, Lauterbach HJ (1975) Ergebnisse der experimentellen Prüfung und klinischen Anwendungsmöglichkeiten der Aluminiumoxydkeramik in der Alloarthroplastik. Z Orthop 113:756–759
9. Haboush EJ (1953) A new operation for arthroplasty of the hip. Bull Hosp Joint Dis 14:242
10. Hoffmann-Daimler S (1975) Mechanische Faktoren der Implantatlockerung und Möglichkeiten ihrer Beseitigung. Symposium Arbeitskreis Biomechanik zur 59. Tagung der DGOT Berlin 1972. Med Orthop Tech 95:4–5
11. (see 13)
12. Homsy CA (1973) Implant stabilization, chemical and biomechanical considerations. Orthop Clin North Am 4:295–311
13. Homsy CA, Cain TE, Kessler FB, Anderson MS, King JM (1972) Porous implant systems for prosthesis stabilization. Clin Orthop 89:220–235
14. Jackson-Burrows H (1971) Replacement of tumors affecting the bone by major internal prosthesis. Biomedical engineering and its clinical application in orthopaedic surgery. British Council, London
15. Judet R (1975) Total-Hüftendoprothesen aus Porometall ohne Zementverankerung. Z Orthop 113:828–829
16. Judet J, Judet R (1950) The use of artificial femoral head for arthroplasty of the hip joint. J Bone Joint Surg [Br] 32:166–173
17. McKee GK (1970) Development of total prosthetic replacement of the hip. Clin Orthop 72:85–103
18. McKee GK, Watson-Farrar J (1966) Replacement of arthritic hips by the McKee-Farrar prosthesis. J Bone Joint Surg [Br] 42:245–259
19. Leinbach, IS (1982) Pers. comm.
20. Lord G, Marotte HH, Blanchard JP, Guillamon JL, Gory M (1978) Etude expérimentale de l'ancrage des arthroplasties totales madréporiques de hanche. Rev Chir Orthop 64:459–470
21. Lyman-Smith (1963) Ceramic-plastic material as a bone substitute. Arch Surg 87:653–661
22. Mittelmeier H (1974) Zementlose Verankerung von Endoprothesen nach dem Tragrippenprinzip. Z Orthop 112:27–33
23. Mittelmeier H, Harms J, Hanser U (1980) PMMA cement with carbon fibre reinforcement and apatite ingredients: Mechanical properties and tissue reaction in animal tests. 1. World Biomaterials Congress, Baden/Austria
24. Moore AT (1952) A metal hip joint, a new self-locking vitallium prosthesis. South Med J 45:1015–1019
25. Moore AT, Bohlman HR (1943) Metal hip joint. J Bone Joint Surg 25:668
26. Morscher E, Mathys R (1975) Erste Erfahrungen mit einer zementlosen isoelastischen Totalprothese der Hüfte. Z Orthop 113:745–749
27. Pilliar RM, Cameron HU, Macnab I (1975) Porous surfaced layered prosthetic devices. Biomed Eng 10:126
28. Rehn E (1934) Zur Wiederherstellungschirurgie der Gelenke. Arch Klin Chir 180:395–400
29. Rhinelander FW (1977) A flexible composite as a coating for metallic implants, microvascular and histological studies. Int Orthop 1:7786
30. Ring PA (1968) Complete replacement arthroplasty of the hip by the ring prosthesis. J Bone Joint Surg [Br] 50:720–731
31. Sadr BG, Arden P (1976) A comparison of the stability of proplastcoated and cemented Thompson prostheses in the treatment of subcapital fractures. Injury 8:234–237
32. Salzer M, Zweymüller K, Plenk H, Punzet G (1975) Erste Erfahrungen mit einer Hüftendoprothese aus Biokeramik. Med Orthop Tech 6:162
33. Salzer M, Knahr K, Locke H, Stärk N (1978) Cementfree bioceramic double-cup endoprosthesis of the hip-joint. Clin Orthop 134:80–86
34. Sarmiento A (1972) Austin Moore prosthesis in the arthritic hip. Clin Orthop 82:14–23
35. Siwash KM (1969) The development of a total metal prosthesis for the hip joint from a partial joint replacement. Reconstr Surg Traumatol 11:53–62
36. Smith-Petersen MN (1939) Arthroplasty of the hip. A new method. J Bone Joint Surg 21:269
37. Strunz V, Gross UM, Maenner K, Zuehlke H, Deutscher K, Broemer H, Ege W (1979) Gewebsreaktionen auf bioaktiven Knochenzement. Vortrag Arbeitsgemeinschaft für Kieferchirurgie der Deutschen Gesellschaft für Zahn-, Mund- und Kieferheilkunde, Mai 1979, Bad Homburg
38. Thompson FR (1954) Two and half years' experience with a vitallium intramedullary hip prosthesis. J Bone Joint Surg [Am] 36:489

39. Wegg PJ, Wright KWJ, Winter GD (1980) The monk "soft top" endoprosthesis. J Bone Joint Surg [Br] 62:174–179
40. Wilson JN, Scales JT (1970) Loosening of total hip replacements with cement fixation. Clin Orthop 72:145–160
41. Wiltse LL, Hall RH, Stenehjem JC (1957) Experimental studies regarding the possible use of self-curing acrylic in orthopaedic surgery. J Bone Joint Surg [Am] 29:961–972

Introduction II
Hip Joint Prostheotoplasty

I. S. Leinbach

Many surgeons deserve credit for their pioneer work in the development of "Interposition arthroplasty" of the hip joint. From 1827, with the work of John Rhea Barton in Philadelphia, and the contribution of Smith-Petersen of Boston in 1923, the object of arthroplasty was to establish movement in the ankylosed joint by osteotomy or by the remaking of bone surfaces. The early use of "replacement arthroplasty" of the hip joint is credited to Hey-Groves of England, Moore of the United States and the Judet brothers of France, while the development of the concept of total hip replacement arthroplasty has been credited to Gluck, Wiles and Haboush [1].

Much of our understanding of the entire scope of total hip replacement, as well as its successful use in clinical practice and research, is the result of the work of Sir John Charnley of England and of such pioneers as McKee, Ring, Müller and Buchholz and others who advanced the clinical application of total hip replacement.

The first case report of a metal hip joint replacement in the American literature appeared in the American edition of the Journal of Bone and Joint Surgery, Volume XXV, No. 3, July 1943, by Austin T. Moore, M. D. and Harold R. Bohlman, M. D.

In 1938, Philip Wiles of London designed a stainless steel femoral head and acetabulum ground so as to fit accurately. The femoral head was secured by a bolt passing down the neck of the femur and the acetabulum stabilized by three projecting loops secured with screws. Six operations were performed in patients with Still's disease with some degree of success but the records were lost during the war. Although this pioneer work was the forerunner of the era of total replacement arthroplasty, none of these were fully successful. It was in 1951, that McKee first carried out an operation in three patients shown at the meeting of the British Orthopaedic Association, in Cambridge. One of them in which cobalt-chrome alloy was used most successfully: "The first ever successful case of total hip joint replacement" [2].

The major factor holding back development of this type of surgery in the United States was doubts regarding the safety of the acrylic cement. In 1967, the American Food and Drug Administration in Washington, D. C., permitted reputable and qualified orthopaedic surgeons to receive a special license to allow them to assess the clinical value of the available methods under properly controlled conditions.

The value and/or the necessity for the use of acrylic cement was questioned by many of our early investigators. Peter A. Ring, F.R.C.S. of England, stated in 1968, "There is no indication that the use of bone cement significantly lowers the risk of loosening, nor is there any indication that there is any special group of patients in whom loosening is prone to occur and in whom the use of bone cement might diminish the risk" [3].

This Symposium will provide a survey of methods and trends and introduce the current interest in Cementless Fixation of Hip Endoprostheses. Professor Morscher and his colleagues are to be congratulated for their superb organization, for enlightening us as to what alternative procedures are available to the hip surgeon and for stimulating discussion and encouraging research for the ultimate improvement in the care of our patients.

I was highly honored when Professor Erwin Morscher asked me to speak before this distinguished group of world renowned surgeons. It is with a keen feeling of friendship that I stand before this audience, for I have known many of you since my formal acceptance of membership as one of the founders of the A-O. It has been my pleasure to have shared your intellectual companionship. I thank you.

Irwin S. Leinbach, M. D.*
A.A.O.S., F.A.C.S.,
F.I.C.S., DSc.

---

* Presented by Invitation. Symposium for Cementless Fixation of Hip Prostheses. Kantonsspital, Basel, Switzerland, June 24, 25, 26, 1982

References

1. Haboush EJ: A New Operation for Arthroplasty of the Hip. Bull. Hosp. for Joint Dis. 14:242, 1953
2. McKee GK: Personal communication, March 1981
3. Ring PA: Complete Replacement Arthroplasty of the Hip. Jour. B & J. Surg., Vol. 50B 720, 1968
4. Leinbach IS: Prostheotoplasty for Treatment of Arthritis of the Human Hip Joint. Jour. Western Pacific Orthop. Asso. VI 2, 1969

The Bone Cement Cuff in Hip Endoprostheses: Results of 80 Postmortem Studies

A. Gächter

Introduction

Despite increasing interest in the cementless fixation of implants, bone cement still has an important place in hip replacement surgery. Indeed, polymethylmethacrylate (PMMA) has been largely responsible for the growing clinical interest in total hip replacements.

Nevertheless, the loosening of implants cemented with PMMA remains a serious problem. Many factors have been incriminated in these loosenings. Besides possible flaws in the implant and technical errors during implantation, these include cement breakage, induction of bone resorption by wear debris, elasticity discrepancies between implant and bone, infection, trauma, allergy, and many others. This prompted us to examine the cement bed of stem prostheses in femurs removed at autopsy in an effort to discover to what extent the cement fixation method per se, can be held responsible for the loosening of stem prostheses, and to evaluate the causal significance of the bone cement itself.

Materials and Methods

In all hip prosthesis patients that were autopsied at the Institute of Pathology of the University of Basel during the period from 1977 to 1979, the proximal part of the femur bearing the endoprosthesis was removed for study. The femurs were carefully dissected free of soft tissues and then radiographed in two planes. After careful extraction of the prosthetic stem from the cement sheath, the specimens were stored in deepfreeze until needed. Over 2800 autopsies were performed during the period indicated, and a total of 84 hip prostheses were removed. Four of these had been implanted without cement, and so a total of 80 specimens had a cement mantle that could be studied. The 84 prostheses were obtained from 69 women and 15 men. Fifty were hemiarthroplasties with femoral head prostheses, and 34 were total hip replacements. Three of the arthroplasties were revisionary; six were done for pathologic fractures secondary to tumor metastasis. Osteoporotic fractures constituted the main indication for arthroplasty in the autopsy material examined. Osteoarthritis and unknown indications were found in 31 cases.

The age at implantation ranged from 40 to 93 years. The duration of implantation (time between last implantation and death) was between 0 days and 13 years. Twenty-one patients died within 3 months after surgery, and 47 survived longer than 1 year. Two revision patients survived one year, and one survived two years. Age at death was between 48 and 98 years.

The first study of the cement sheath involved a gross evaluation of the specimens. (Our histologic assessment will be reported at a later time.) The macroscopic evaluation was supplemented with contact radiographs made in the AP and lateral projections. These radiographs were more accurate than *in vivo* films owing to the absence of intervening soft tissue.

Each femur was sectioned as accurately as possible in the frontal plane through the center of the lumen of the cement sheath. Of the 80 cemented implants, 63 could be sawed perfectly through the center of the lumen. The others sustained dome degree of damage during extraction or sawing. Because the cement cuff could not be accurately assessed in these cases, these specimens were excluded from the study. The cement sheaths were examined grossly for defects, cracks, cement distribution, blood contamination and evidence of corrosion. The color of the cement was documented photographically. The stems were arbitrarily divided longitudinally into a proximal, middle and distal zone, and any defects noted were listed according to zone (Fig. 1). The medical histories of the

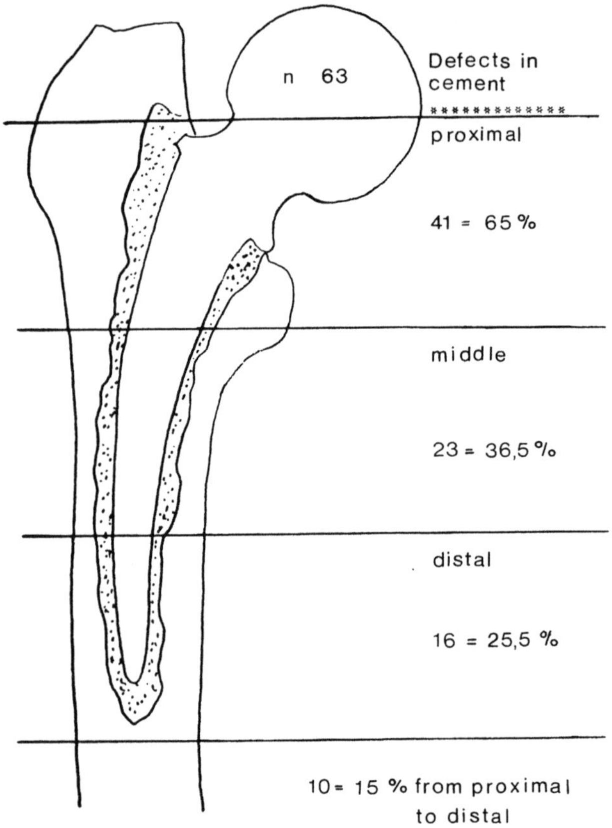

Fig. 1. Division of autopsy specimens into 3 zones. Cement defects are most common in the proximal third

patients were available to us for making an overall evaluation.

Results

Among the 84 prosthetic stems examined, we observed no stem fractures or grossly visible cracks. Among the 80 cemented stems, the radiographs showed that 24 were in a varus position, 38 in a neutral position, and 18 in a marked valgus position. The lateral films showed that, owing to the antecurvation of the femur, most of the stems had been inserted in a slight anterior-to-posterior orientation, i.e., the tips of the stems pointed toward the posterior cortex of the femoral shaft. A definite, general stem loosening could be diagnosed in only three cases from the presence of a broad osteolytic seam. The remaining x-rays showed no evidence of loosening.

Osteolysis, atrophy or rarefaction of the calcar area was witnessed in 25 cases (31%) [4]. The calcar changes were seen in 10 of the varus implants, 11 of the neutral implants and 4 of the valgus implants. A marked reactive thickening of the distal cortex was seen in six cases. Five of these showed concurrent resorptive changes in the calcar. The cortical thickening was especially marked around a collarless, straight-stem prosthesis that had been in the body for 10 years (Fig. 3).

On examining the cement sheaths, we quickly observed that the color of the cement changed with time. The cement from relatively recent implantations was whitish with a tinge of green (Fig. 2). In prostheses implanted for several years, the cement showed a light- to dark-brown discoloration and usually was more brittle than the more recent specimens (Fig. 3). In two cases black discolorations were additionally seen at the distal tip of the cement. In one case these metal corrosion products had their source in an unstable trochanteric cerclage wire (revision), and in the other they resulted from corrosion of the prosthetic stem (steel prosthesis).

On examining the cut surface of the cement sheaths for defects, we found that only 11 of the 63 specimens examined had a cement sheath that was grossly intact throughout (17.5%). All others showed defects (82.5%). The defects, or cracks, were distributed as follows according to the segment of the cement sheath (proximal, middle or distal) involved:

Proximal to distal, 10; proximal only, 23; proximal and middle, 8; proximal and distal, 0; middle only, 5; middle and distal, 4; distal only, 2 (Fig. 1).

In the great majority of cases, then, the cement sheath becomes damaged in its proximal portion. Damage confined to the distal third is very rare. These observations also show that some cracks run through the entire cement sheath, while others involve only portions of it.

The cause of the defects could not be determined in all cases. In some cases the prosthesis was in direct contact with the bone tissue, creating a gap in the cement sheath. In other specimens true cracks had formed that could be explained only by a bursting effect exerted by the prosthetic stem. Several defects resulted from the presence of blood within the cement, which interfered with local polymerization. As could be deduced from the medical histories, this occurred mainly when the cement had been packed manually into the femoral shaft. Other defects could be attributed to extraction of the suction drain from the medullary cavity or directional changes during insertion of the prosthesis.

The *contact radiographs* revealed differences in bone structure as a function of implantation

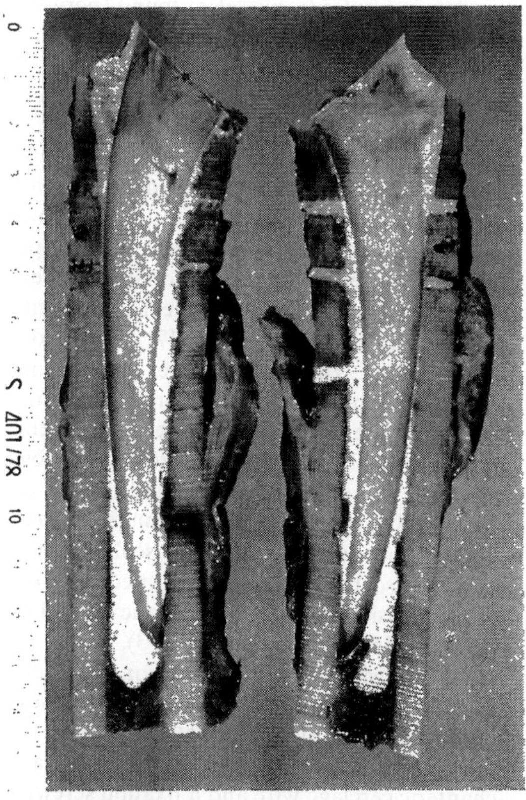

Fig. 2. Cut-away specimen of a proximal femur obtained at autopsy. A Charnley-Mueller total prothesis had been implanted 3 months before autopsy. Prior to that, internal fixation had been done to immobilize a pertrochanteric fracture. Note the grossly intact (albeit thin) cement cuff. The bone cement has penetrated into the transverse screw holes. The cement is pale-green in color

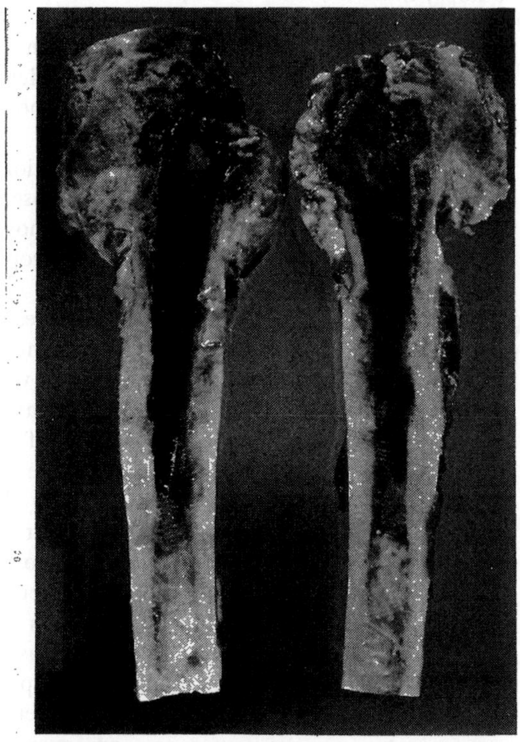

Fig. 3. In contrast to Fig. 2, the bone cement shows brownish discoloration and is brittle. A collarless, straight-stem prosthesis had been implanted 12 years prior to autopsy. Corrosion products from the steel prosthesis can be seen in the middle and distal zones of the cement sheath. Note the resorption in the calcar region and the distal thicking of the cortex

time. As expected, femurs in which the stems had been implanted for only a short time showed no appreciable change in bony structure. With the long-term implants (3 years or more), a change of trabecular structure often was apparent in the trochanteric region, consisting of horizontal zones of increased density. It is possible, however, that a portion of the forces acting on the trochanter are transmitted to the bone cement via trabecular structures [3].

Discussion

Ideally, of course, the bone cement should completely fill all voids between the implant and bone. This will create a strong mechanical interlock between the cement and the surrounding bony trabeculae. The bone cement additionally serves to transmit and distribute forces between the implant and bone. In the present autopsy material, most of the prostheses were of the Charnley-Mueller type (tapered stem). In theory, then, the endoprosthesis should remain permanently anchored if conditions are ideal. Loosening could occur only as a result of bone resorption or cement breakage.

There are many theories and observations concerning the possible causes of such loosenings. The present investigation clearly shows that most cement sheaths exhibit macroscopic defects on the very day of the operation. Additional weak spots in the cement may result from such factors as poor mixing of the cement, air inclusions, and inadequate molecular wetting [12]. The cement sheath is subjected mainly to shear, bending and torsional stresses. If the sheath already is defective on the day of the implantation, preexisting cracks can readily develop into true cement fractures during service [11]. In osteoporotic bone with a thinned cortex and rarefied trabeculae, full circumferential contact between the cement and bone is impaired. Moreover, with prostheses that are available in only *one* stem width, the relationship between the cortex, sheath and prosthetic stem is apt to be unsatisfactory, i.e., an excessive amount of cement would have to be used to stabilize the implant. This would result in excessive heat generation and extensive bone necrosis.

There is still much debate concerning the etiology of calcar resorption [3, 4, 5]. Excessive stresses, stress shielding, the deposition of wear debris with osteolysis, and vascular lesions have all been postulated. Sarmiento [8] found a low incidence of calcar resorption when relatively heavy stresses were placed upon the calcar (3%). When the calcar was shielded from stresses, the incidence of calcar atrophy rose to 13%. The stress effect was also implant-dependent. With titanium stems it was 30% less and with steel stems 21% less than in the normal femur. Ling [6] ruled out stress shielding, devascularization by osteotomy, thermal injury and monomeric toxicity as causes of calcar resorption, while emphasizing the causal importance of infection, polyethylene wear debris and microinstability between the cement and bone. In our material, calcar resorption was commonly associated with a thickening of the distal shaft, suggesting that the resorption was related to a bypassing of the calcar by lines of stress transmission. In several long-term implants we also found periosteal new bone, especially in the dorsal part of the shaft, that obviously did not represent the linea aspera and had to be interpreted as a reactive change. In two Minneapolis-type prostheses with a horizontal collar seating, the bone beneath the collar showed a considerable density increase on the medial side, and apposition of cortical bone was found even in the peritrochanteric region. It is questionable, however, whether this observation alone is sufficient to validate the theories of Lord [7] on horizontal collar seating. The color changes in the cement cuffs were obviously a function of wear time. Generally the discolorations were homogenous and so probably were not caused by corrosion products. In some cases we found typical local changes due to frictional corrosion (steel stems). Besides showing a brownish discoloration, the cement also had become embrittled. The obvious conclusion is that an enzymatic degradation of the PMMA was involved (Fig. 3).

It is possible for the corrosion products to migrate along the femoral shaft. In two cases we found dark corrosion material at the distal tip of the cement stemming from corrosion of a trochanteric cerclage wire and a fixation screw.

On examining the cement sheaths for defects, we found that some ⅔ of all defects were situated in the proximal third. This observation assumes particular importance when it is considered that most loosenings have their start in the proximal part of the stem (Fig. 4 and 5). The

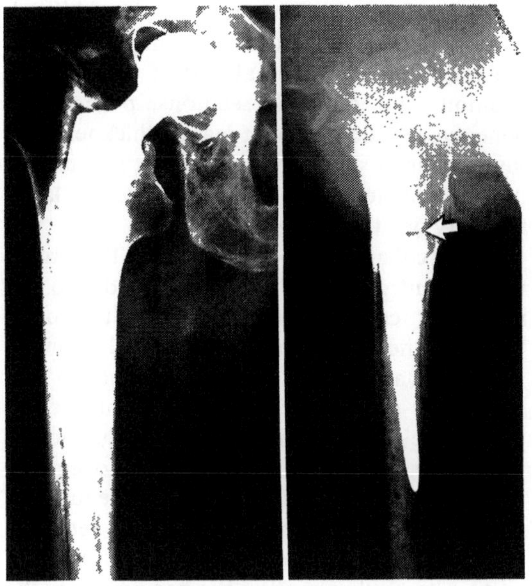

a b

Fig. 4 a, b. Secondary cement fracture (*arrow*). The stem prostesis is completely loose only 2 years after implantation (operative finding). **b** The cement distribution is poor, and the prosthetic stem is too narrow for this femur a straight-stem prosthesis of Mueller

distal part of the stem tends to be solidly anchored to the surrounding bone. The relative micromovements that develop between the proximal cement and bone, create a "pump" mechanism which causes wear debris and corrosion products to become insinuated between the cement and bone. Willert [10] states that some of the wear debris may be removed via the blood and lymph. But as soon as the wear particles exceed a certain size, they start to accumulate at the cement-bone interface in an infiltrative process that proceeds centrifugally from the capsule and is most pronounced in the intertrochanteric region. In animal experiments with polyethylene-carbon acetabular sockets, we were able to show that the abrasion products (which in this case are black in color) infiltrate the calcar region from the capsule. As loosening progresses, these products may be found throughout the femoral and acetabular region (cf. Fig. 6). The occurrence of stem fatigue fractures between the distal, securely anchored part of the stem and the proximal, loose portion provides further evidence that loosening has its start in the proximal part of the implant. This lends a special significance to the cement defects commonly found in this region, for weak spots in that area could very well accelerate the loosening process. When we compared the radiographs with the sectioned specimens, moreover, we found that the cement distribution often may appear favorable on x-ray when in reality it is not. Even larger cracks and defects may not be visualized.

In recent years increased effort has been devoted to the improvement of cement filling techniques (e.g., Weber [9]). The use of bony, plastic or cement plugs at the tip of the prosthesis makes it possible to achieve higher pressures within the femoral shaft, as it ensures better containment of the cement distally. However, as Charnley [5] points out, this tends to enhance filling primarily in the distal part of the cavity,

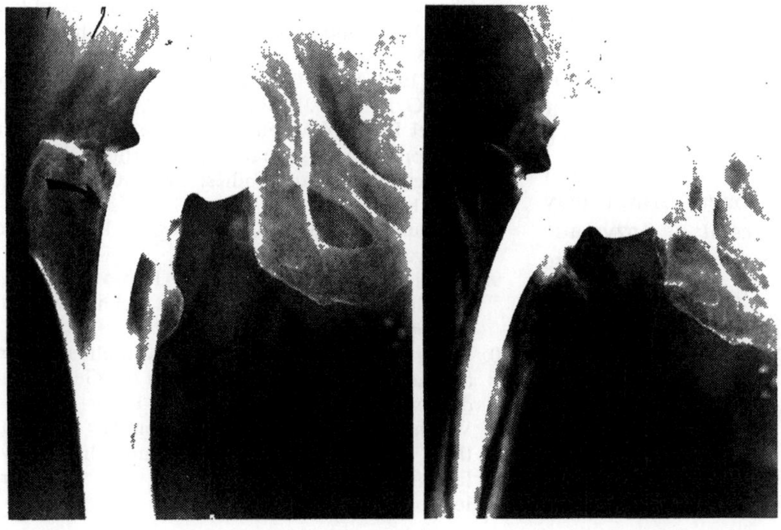

a b

Fig. 5 a, b. Unusually poor cement distribution (visible even in x-ray) around a femoral head prosthesis. **a** After only 5 weeks the stem has acquired a varus malposition (*arrow*). **b** After 16 months the prosthesis is completely loose

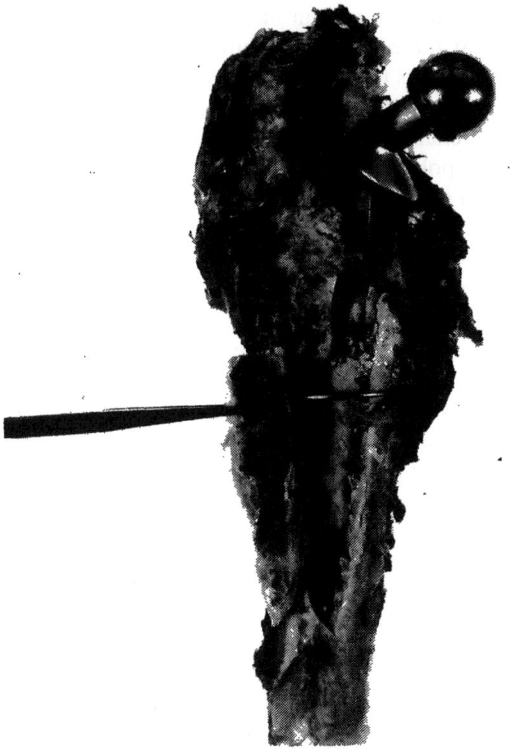

Fig. 6. Specimen 10 months after implantation of a total prosthesis in a dog femur. Due to a primary preexisting instability (cerclage for shaft fracture), the polyethylene-carbon wear particles have worked down to the tip of the cement mantle. The distal, ventral bone flap has been reflected laterally, and the underlying cement sheath is visible

where anchorage is generally good. The goal should be to optimize anchorage in the proximal region. Even today, the pattern of cement distribution is all too often left to chance (Fig. 5).

In the short term, bone cement can be considered a true cause of loosening only if it damages the bone irreversibly through excessive heat generation, toxic effects, or the induction of an allergic response. In the longer term, it may deteriorate and fail as a result of enzymatic degradation. Ideally the cement will stabilize the implant from the first day on. Prosthetic loosening is "preordained" by poor cement distribution and by the presence of defects and cracks, especially in the proximal third of the cement mantle. Additional factors such as wear debris, osteolysis, infections secondary to instability, etc. tend to accelerate the loosening process.

A significant improvement can be achieved only by adopting a good cementing technique, especially for the proximal part of the stem. In addition, an optimal relationship between bone cross-section, cement mantle thickness and stem diameter should be strived for. This means that several stem sizes must be made available for every prosthetic model.

With collarless prosthetic stems, the proximal cement generally must be packed into the medullary cavity manually by digital force. With prostheses that have a broad collar, proximal filling appears to be less of a problem owing to the proximal containment, which compresses the cement and drives it forcibly into the trabeculae. The prevention of micromovements in the proximal part of the stem will reduce the buildup of wear debris, thereby also reducing the risk of premature loosening. In our estimation, too little attention has been given to the prosthetic collar as a "pressurizer" for enhancing proximal cement distribution.

References

1. Bayne SC, Lautenschlager EP, Compere CL, Wildes R (1975) Degree of Polymerization of acrylic bone cement. J Biomed Mater Res 9:27–34
2. Beaumont PWR, Young RJ (1977) Strength and fracture of acrylic bone cement and cement-metalinterfaces. Plastics and Rubber: Materials and Applications (Febr. 1977)
3. Bertini G, Calderale PM, Dettoni A, Gallinaro P, Corenzo GL (1980) Cortical bone changes after hip replacement: radiographic study. Acta Orthop Belg 46:735
4. Blacker GJ, Charnley J (1978) Changes in the upper femur after low friction arthroplasty. Clin Orthop 137:15
5. Charnley J (1979) Low friction arthroplasty of the hip. Theory and practice. Springer, Berlin Heidelberg New York
6. Ling (1981) SICOT-Kongress 1981, Rio de Janeiro
7. Lord G, Marotte JH, Blanchard JP, Guillamon JL, Bancel P (1980) Valeur de l'assise horizontale et de l'appui diaphysaire dans la répartition des contraintes du fémur prothésé. Rev Chir Orthop 66:141–156
8. Sarmiento A (1981) SICOT-Kongress 1981, Rio de Janeiro
9. Weber BG, Stühmer G (1979) Improvements in total hip prosthesis implantation technique. Arch Orthop Trauma Surg 93:185–189
10. Willert HG, Semlitsch M (1975) Kapselreaktionen auf Kunststoff-und Metall-Abrieb bei Gelenksendoprothesen. Techn Rundschau 2:1
11. Wright TM, Burstein AH, Robinson RP (1982) Fatigue crack propagation in Polymethylmethacrylate. Transactions, 28th Annual ORS, New Orleans, 1982

Remodeling of the Femur in Conventionally-Implanted Hip Prostheses

H. Küsswetter, E. Gabriel, T. Stuhler and L. Töpfer

In recent years numerous clinical and experimental studies have dealt with the problem of aseptic loosening of conventionally-implanted hip prostheses.

Jäger and associates investigated the experimental torsional loosening of hip prostheses that had been implanted with methylmethacrylate by various techniques. Münzenberg and Dennert, examining the problem of aseptic loosening as it relates to age-dependent bone remodeling, investigated the histomorphologic changes occurring at implant surfaces. In 1971 Rütt drew attention to the remodeling of the bone in aseptic loosening. In 1972 Willert and Puls performed histomorphologic studies on postmortem and biopsy material in the interfacial zone of femoral and acetablular implants, and were able to prove that remodeling had taken place in the compact bone. These observations were confirmed by Mach (1982) in serial x-rays of cemented and uncemented Siwash-type endoprostheses. Until now no quantitative histologic investigations of this phenomenon had been carried out.

Materials and Methods

We examined a total of 12 femurs removed at postmortem from patients who had had no problems with their hip prostheses prior to death. All implants were metal stem prostheses of the Mueller-Charnley type that had been conventionally implanted with methylmethacrylate. Manual examination showed the prostheses to be securely anchored in all specimens.

Seven specimens were subjected to microradiographic analysis. The prostheses had been in the body for periods ranging from 2 to 7 years (average 4½ years). The average age of the patients was 71. The cause of death was unrelated to the hip prostheses, and the patients had not been bedridden for a significant time before death.

The seven specimens with implanted prosthetic stems were sectioned in three planes with a special saw. The planes were located in the proximal, middle and distal thirds of the stem (Fig. 1). After the specimens had been embedded in synthetic resin, cross-sections of bone 120–160 μm thick were prepared.

Microradiographs of these sections were obtained and then evaluated on a Quantimet image analyzer. In the cortical area, the proportion of compact bone tissue to voids in the bone was determined for the medial, lateral, anterior and posterior quadrants of each cross-section. The ratio of the two areas, which provides a measure of the porosity of the cortical bone, decreases as bone substance is lost, i.e., as porosity increases.

Using the same technique, cross-sections of bone were taken from the femur of a 75-year-old donor without a prosthesis for purposes of

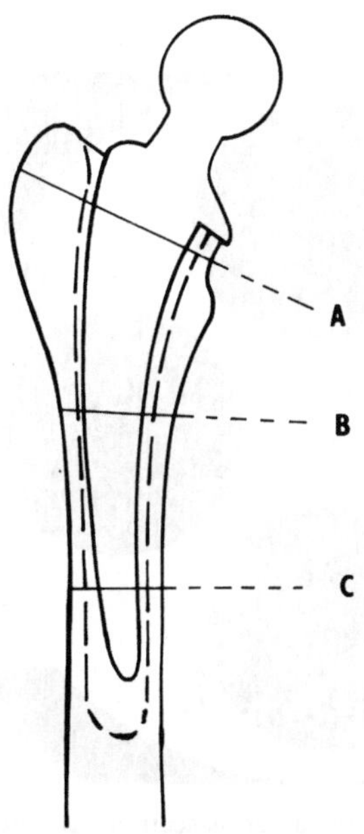

Fig. 1. Location of the femoral cross-sections at the collar of the prosthesis (*A*), the midportion of the stem (*B*), and the distal end of the stem (*C*)

comparison. An analogous determination of bone porosity was made, and results were checked planimetrically.

To complete the study, we examined an additional series of macroscopic cross-sections of five femurs removed from donors in the same age group. The sections were taken from the implant area and distal to it. The prostheses had been in the body for periods ranging from a month to 10 years.

Results

Microradiographs

The microradiographs of the implant-containing sections showed a high degree of cortical porosity. In contrast to the implant-free sections, this porosity was grossly visible and was apparent at all levels (Fig. 2). Image analysis and planimetric results confirmed this observation. While the average bone/void ratio was between 0.21 and 0.76 in bones with implants, it was between 3.2 and 17.4 in sections without implants. As the radiographs clearly indicate, the porosity of the implant-containing sections was markedly greater than that of the implant-free sections.

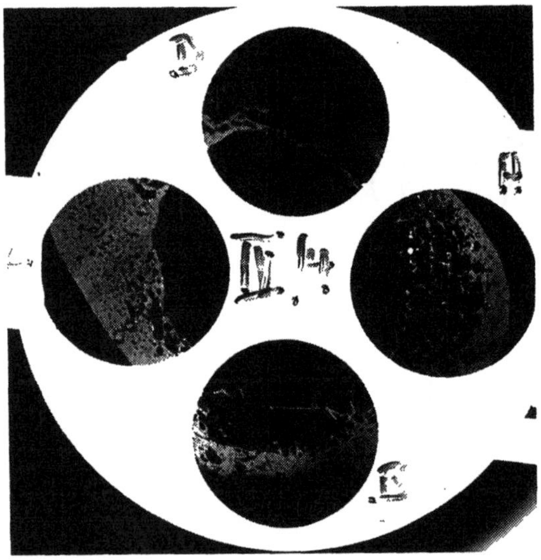

Fig. 2. Microradiograph of a cross-section at the middle of the stem (73 years; 5 years postimplantation). Considerable cortical porosity is evident in all parts of the femoral wall

We also found that the distribution of porosity varied appreciably with the level of the section. In the specimens with implants, the distal and middle sections were least porous in the lateral quadrant, while the proximal section was least porous in medial quadrant. The anterior and posterior porosities were comparable at all three levels (Fig. 3a).

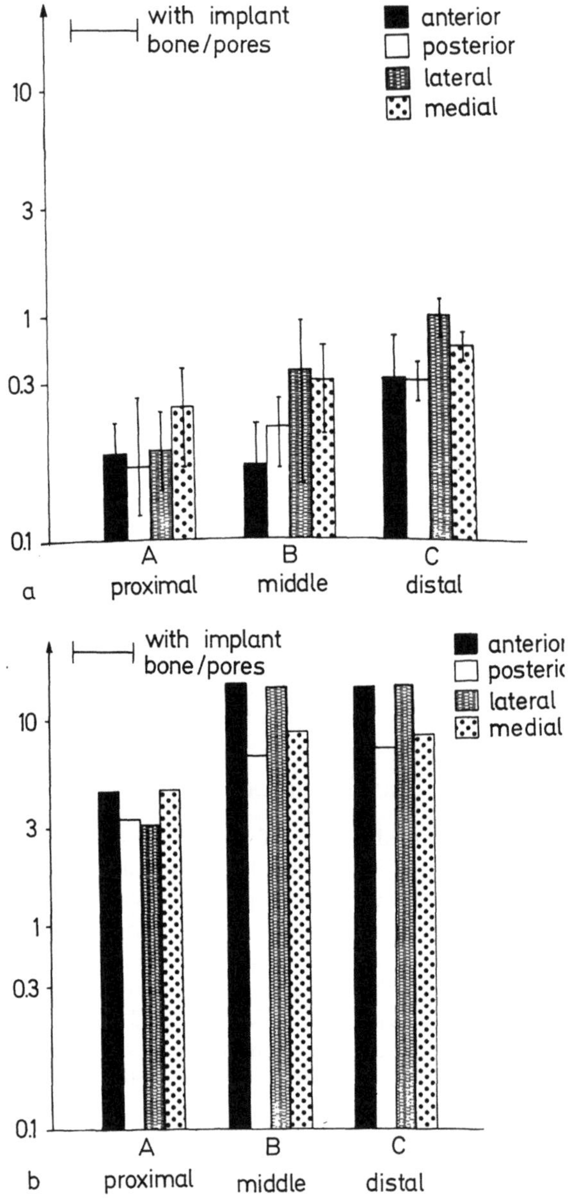

Fig. 3a, b. Quantitative assessment of the bone/pore ratio (logarithmic plots). **a** Specimens with implants. **b** Specimens without implants

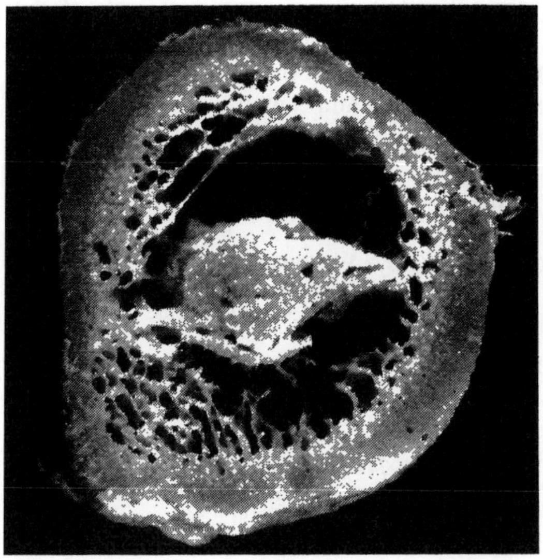

Fig. 4. Macroscopic cross-section of the femur below the distal end of the prosthesis (71 years; 6 years postimplantation). Note the porosity of the cortical bone; large cavities surround the cement plug

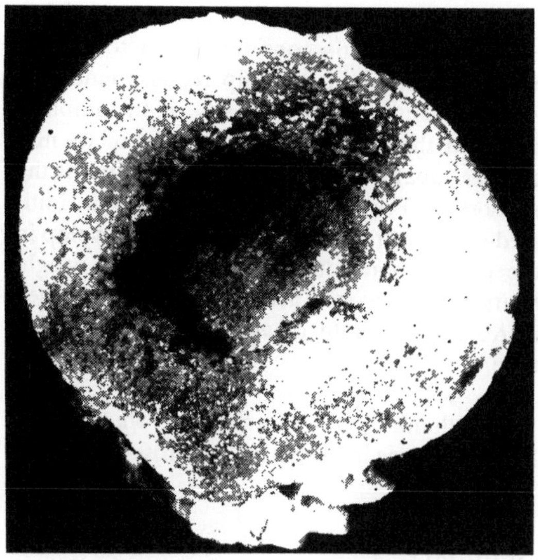

Fig. 5. Macroscopic cross-section of the femur below the distal end of the prosthesis (85 years; 4 weeks postimplantation). There is close apposition between cement and bone. Cortical porosity is negligible compared to that in Fig. 4

In the specimens without implants, the middle and distal sections were least porous in the lateral and anterior quadrants, and the proximal sections in the medial and anterior quadrants (Fig. 3 b).

In the sections with implants as well as those without, the porosity diminished in a proximal-to-distal direction.

Series of Cross-Sections

Our series of cross-sections, which we had not been able to evaluate quantitatively until now, showed heavy gross porosity in the area of the cement plug below the prosthesis. A further attenuation of the cortex is apparent 2 cm below the distal end of the prosthesis; 8 cm distal to the implant, an increase in cortical thickness and density are observed (Fig. 4).

In the case of one 85-year-old patient who died of a pulmonary embolism 4 weeks after the prosthesis was implanted, the macroscopic series of cross-sections distal to the prosthesis showed a thick, dense cortex with no evidence of unusual porosity (Fig. 5).

Discussion

The results of our investigation may be summarized as follows:

1. The cortex surrounding a femoral endoprosthesis undergoes a remodeling which can lead to porosity of the compact bone.
2. The porosity is apparent in all parts of the cortex and increases with time.
3. The density of the bone increases again distal to the implant and cement.

Our investigations confirmed the histologic and x-ray observations that remodeling, in the form of porosity increase, occurs in the bone adjacent to femoral endoprostheses. This involves the entire cross-section of the femoral cortex, the degree of porosity varying somewhat from one quadrant to the next. Our findings are similar to those of Gordes et al., who in 1974 demonstrated morphologic changes in the bone surrounding internal compression plates. On comparing femoral sections with implants and without, we found that the bone density is up to 20 times higher in specimens without an endoprosthesis. The increasing weakness of the implant area with time is explained by the increasing porosity in this area. This porosity, which we attribute to the elasticity difference between the implant-cement complex and the bone itself, must be considered a factor in the aseptic loosening of total hip replacements. Inevitably, the observed porosity in the implant area and the resulting deterioration of its mechanical quality will hamper the stability of the anchorage. Presumably the loosening is initiated by microfractures that gradually develop in the porous bone during the course of weight bearing. This would account for the observed increase in the rate of aseptic loosenings with time.

We thank T. Oesman and M. Volk for their kind assistance in preparing the cross-sections.

Summary

Twelve postmortem femoral specimens with implanted femoral endoprostheses were investigated. Cross-sections were prepared, and the porosity of the cortical bone was evaluated.

1. The cortex surrounding a femoral endoprosthesis undergoes a remodeling which can lead to porosity of the compact bone tissue.
2. The porosity is apparent in all parts of the cortex and increases with time.
3. The density of the bone increases again distal to the implant and cement.

References

Gördes W, Kossyk W, Bödefeld P (1975) Versuche zur Kalksalzbestimmung an der osteotomierten und stabilisierten Tibia des Kaninchens. Arch Orthop Unfallchir 81:125

Jäger M, Ungethüm M (1976) Korrelation klinischer und technischer Aspekte zur Frage der Endoprothesenlockerung. Orthop Praxis 12:578

Jäger M, Küsswetter W, Rütt J, Ungethüm M, Burkhardt R (1974) Experimentelle Torsionslockerung technisch verschieden implantierter Hüftendoprothesenpfannen. Z Orthop 112:34

Mach J (1982) Zum Problem der Spongiosierung nach Hüftarthrodesen und Hüftgelenksendoprothesenplastiken nach Siwash. Beitr Orthop Traumatol 29:240

Münzenberg KJ, Dennert R (1975) Pfannenlockerung bei Hüftgelenkstotalendoprothese infolge altersabhängigem Knochensubstanzverlust. Z Orthop 113:947

Willert HD, Puls P (1972) Die Reaktion des Knochens auf Knochenzement bei der Alloarthroplastik der Hüfte. Arch Orthop Unfallchir 73:33

Causal Histogenesis (Pauwels, Kummer) and Related Biomechanical Discoveries as a Basis for the Cementless Fixation of Hip Endoprostheses

A. Engelhardt

The structural makeup of an organ is a product of functional adaptation. An implant that is inserted to replace a skeletal defect must conform to the prevailing scheme. In this way disruptive effects can be avoided, and, because the implant is surrounded by living and thus reactive tissue, proprioceptive stimuli can be preserved. These are necessary as control signals, especially for the cell and its dependent functions, because metabolic feedback is crucial in ensuring that tissues develop and are maintained in accordance with the functions they perform. The "master program" is the genetic code. The functional stimuli associated with static and dynamic loads provide a kind of trigger impulse of varying magnitude and quality which initiates processes, either directly or indirectly, that carry out the adaptation to loads within genetic constraints.

When an artificial part is introduced into this system, the primary requisite is that it be anchored solidly and permanently owing to an accurate geometric fit or, even better, by virtue of its material composition. Three steps must be carried out in every implantation:

1. repair of the operative defect,
2. maintenance of the fixation,
3. establishment of a permanent tissue bed that is capable of absorbing the forces transmitted by the implant and transferring them as impulses to other skeletal members.

A number of nineteenth-century authors (v. Meyer, 1867, 1882; Culmann, 1866; Wolff, 1892; Roux, 1885) laid the groundwork upon which Pauwels (1954) and later Kummer (1978) formulated the theory of causal histogenesis. This theory has found confirmation in many areas, most notably in the results of operative and nonoperative fracture management. More recent findings are supplementing and expanding the theory as it relates to fracture treatment and are providing an impetus for the development of improved implants.

When dealing with a bone-implant system, however, we find certain deficiencies in Pauwels' simplified model of osteogenesis stimulated by hydrostatic pressure produced either by external forces acting on mesenchymal tissue or by "internal forces created when a volume increase in the tissue caused by swelling or a mass increase acts against a resistance on all sides" (Pauwels, 1954).

A mechanism of this type would require a closed space filled with a medium that behaves as a pure fluid. An intact periosteal sheath would also be required in order to contain the hypothetical fluid. Ultimately the cells would have to assume a spherical shape, which is conceivable in vesicular cartilage or in the nuclei of mesenchymal cells but cannot be assumed for all developmental stages in this simplified scheme.

The theory of shape distortion, which according to Pauwels leads to connective tissue formation because the "strain" provides a mechanical stimulus to which the cells and especially the surrounding intercellular substance respond with the synthesis of collagen fibrils, is a further indication that the hypothesis is incomplete as stated.

When Perren and his colleagues (1972) studied fracture surfaces immobilized with well-fitting, prestressed compression plates, they did not find the series of intermediate preosseous cell stages that generally is assumed to be present under conditions of fracture healing. Knese (1979) describes the formation of collagen precursors in mesenchymal cells, while Becker and Murray (1979), expanding on the work of Fung (1972), state that an electric field (piezoelectricity) may be responsible for the activation of protein-synthesizing organelles in osteogenic cells.

Various mechanisms have been reported by which electrical signals can be generated in bone (Bassett, 1972, in Bourne), e.g., by standing potentials, by stress-generated potentials, by ferromagnetic potentials, and by intercellular electrolytes.

When we further consider the results of reparative processes following experimental fractures in chicken embryos, the following picture emerges: Hours after a fracture, preosseous mesenchymal cells migrate into the fracture exudate and become oriented along lines of force that can be visualized by optical stress analysis techniques. These cells are the most dense in the region where the fragments are closest together, and they are aligned in the direction of the field lines.

It would appear that bioelectric potentials align the molecules in the exudate and thus define the initial tissue orientation. The signal may be generated by mechanical stresses within the bone, by muscular contractions, by injury potentials, or by chemical or physicochemical processes (Becker et al., 1963). It is also significant that osteons subjected to bending stresses become electropositive on the convex side and electronegative on the concave side. This leads to processes of synthesis and lysis, which continue until the anatomical axes and the stress lines coincide as a result of remodeling.

These discoveries show that increased attention must be given to the cell, fiber structure and intercellular substance, and they demonstrate the special importance of the fibrillary component as a crystalline material. It is known that collagen, and not apatit, is a generator of piezoelectric signals *in vivo*.

Thus, it becomes necessary to consider a tissue-implant composite differently from a fracture line. A physiological, bioelectrical or biochemical impulse cannot be expected to arise spontaneously from an implant surface. Hence, the function of "tight junctions", which are credited not only with enhancing mechanical anchorage but also with the transfer of information, terminates at the tissue-implant interface or is at best a one-way process. Perhaps the signal pattern in the adjacent tissue is incomplete or the impulse sub-threshold. In any case, it is clear that interference with normal patterns of stress transfer has adverse effects on tissue development, possibly leading to impaired tissue maturation, a delay in the development of tissue structure, and/or an unfavorable balance between synthesis and lysis.

In the light of these facts, we may list several requirements that must be met by a biological implant fixation system:

1. As little bone as possible should be resected at operation in order to minimize disruptions of the bony architecture that might interfere with normal patterns of impulse and stress transfer.
2. The implant should have close circumferential contact with the bone to minimize the "repair volume."
3. The implant geometry should conform to specifications in 3 dimensions, rather than just 2, so that unphysiologic stresses, such as relative motion, can be kept to a minimum even in the micro-range.
4. Damage to adjacent structures from physical and chemical influences should be avoided (temperature, monomers).
5. Progressive, controlled weight-bearing should be initiated postoperatively to provide the stimulus necessary for the development of a load-bearing implant bed, while avoiding excessive loads that would hamper the formation of a strong bone-implant bond during the reparative period and predispose to relative motion and consequent fibrous tissue proliferation.

Our own findings in the femoral neck of a cortisone-treated patient, confirmed by the discussions of Huggler and Schreiber (1978), demonstrate that it can take up to a year for a fully stress-competent bond to develop between the implant and bone. Placing the plane of resection perpendicular to the axis of the osteons inflicts the maximum degree of "structural insult," which can be largely avoided with the use of an anchoring screw and shell.

Given the remodeling capability of the tissue, the secure primary fixation of an implant by no means guarantees a permanent, stress-competent anchorage. Fatigue fractures in intact bones show that unphysiologic loads must lead to resorptive processes, and thus to loosening, in accordance with biomechanical laws. It must be remembered that bone is an active material that is constantly changing from a structural standpoint. A stable implant fixation can be maintained only if reparative processes are not outstripped by lytic processes, and the bone and implant materials behave similarly under loading. Once loading is initiated, the bone should not be forced to undergo structural changes by altering the patterns of force transmission.

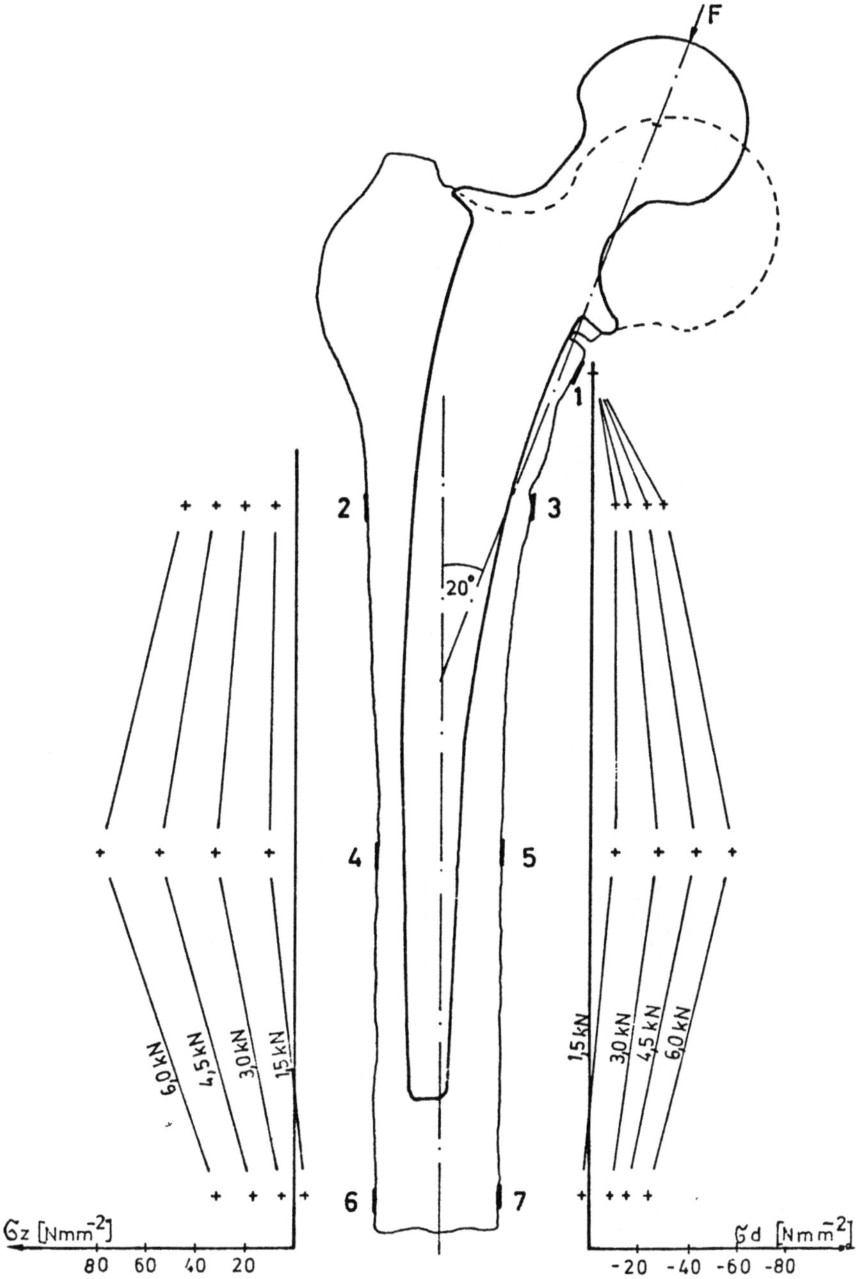

Fig. 1. Longitudinal stresses in the femur with a conventional prosthesis. Measurements were made with strain gauges under various loads (outline drawing and x-ray)

We conducted studies in this area based upon plane and 3-dimensional computations as well as experiments with strain gauges and photoelastic films (Figs. 1–4). Our specimens consisted of implant-containing bones that had been removed at autopsy. The contralateral femur also was examined for reference purposes.

The following results were obtained:

1. Gross inspection showed that none of the implants was in full contact with the cut surface of the femur. We attribute this to the broad

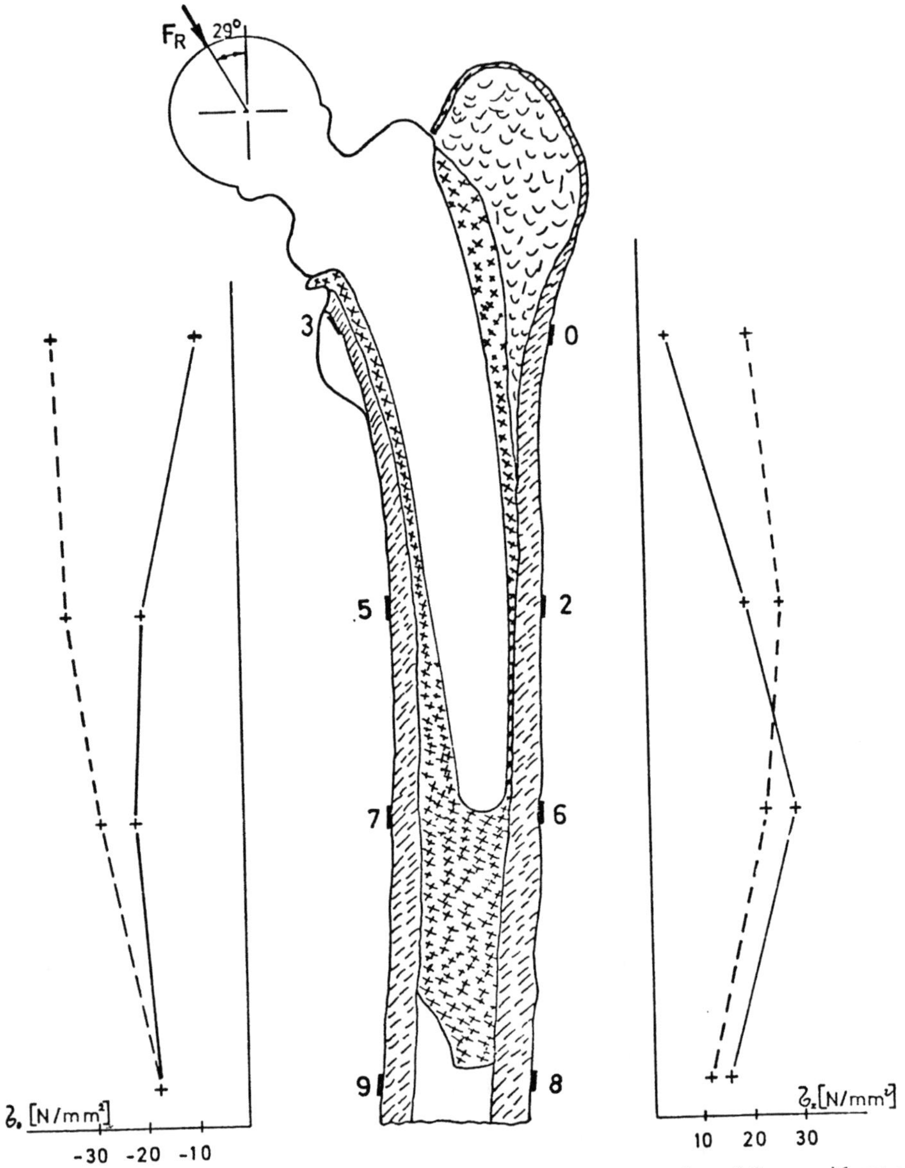

Fig. 2. Stress measurements in a femur with an implant and the contralateral femur without an endoprosthesis. Longitudinal stresses for $F_R = 1.75$ kN; — with prosthesis; - - - - without prosthesis

fixation of the rigid implant within the femoral shaft, which shielded the calcar area from stresses. Thus, surgically-induced resorption of the defective cells in the area of the resection leads to the development of a gap that remains unfilled due to an absence of physiologic loading. The result is disuse osteoporosis.

2. Plane analysis reveals the presence of two force components, one of which impacts the implant into the femoral canal, while the other rotates the proximal part of the implant in a medial direction. Depending on the fixation (e.g., with cement), the alternating loads that arise during gait can have various effects:
   - The stem of the implant comes under a bending stress that may lead to fatigue fracture.
   - Depending on the configuration of the distal part of the implant (cement sheath or stem)

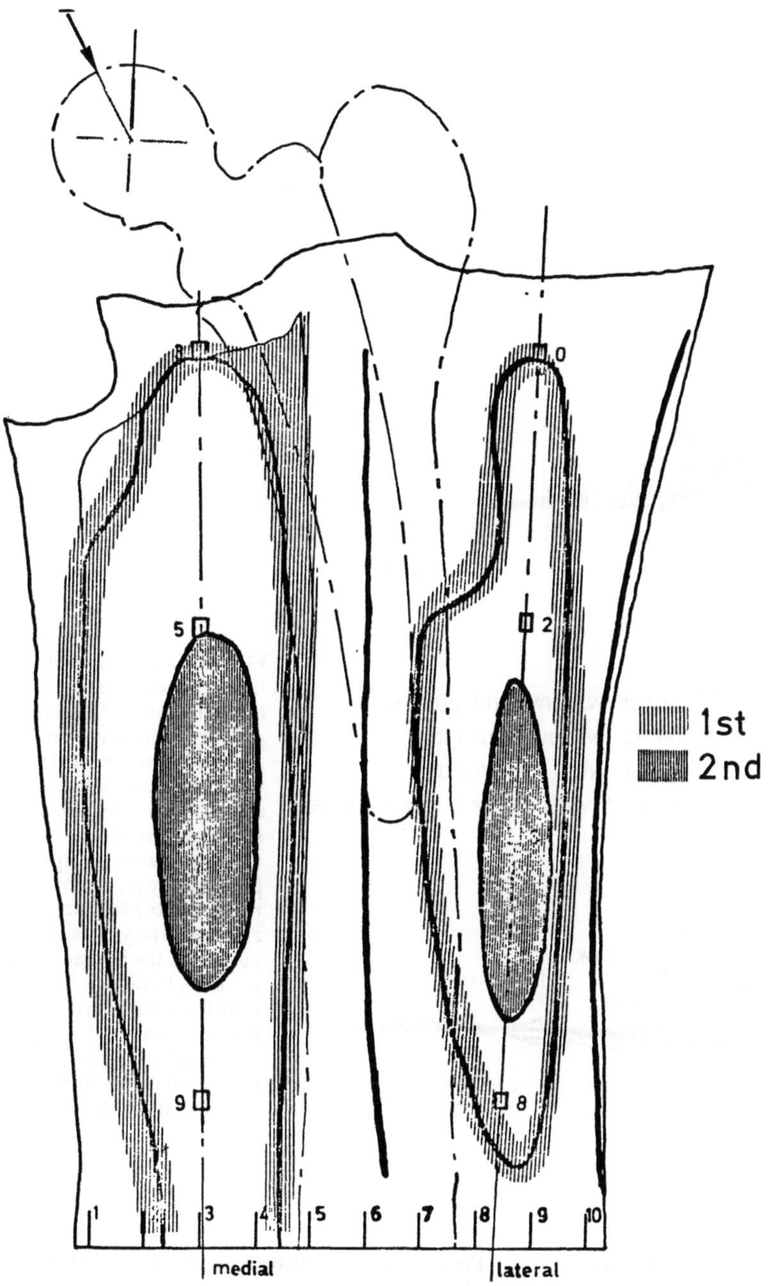

Fig. 3. Visual representation of superficial stresses in a femur with implant (see Fig. 2 for control)

and its contact with the bone, interfacial stress concentrations may form, leading to fractures of the bone cement or resorption of the bone.

- While the proximal part deviates medially, the distal part may be displaced laterally. Depending on the frequency and magnitude of the load, this can either lead to fatigue fracture of the bone or cause the distal end of the implant to penetrate the lateral femoral cortex.
- Because the implant is loosened by all the processes listed above and is not supported by the atrophic femoral neck, the axial force (and perhaps others) will cause impaction of the prosthetic stem into the

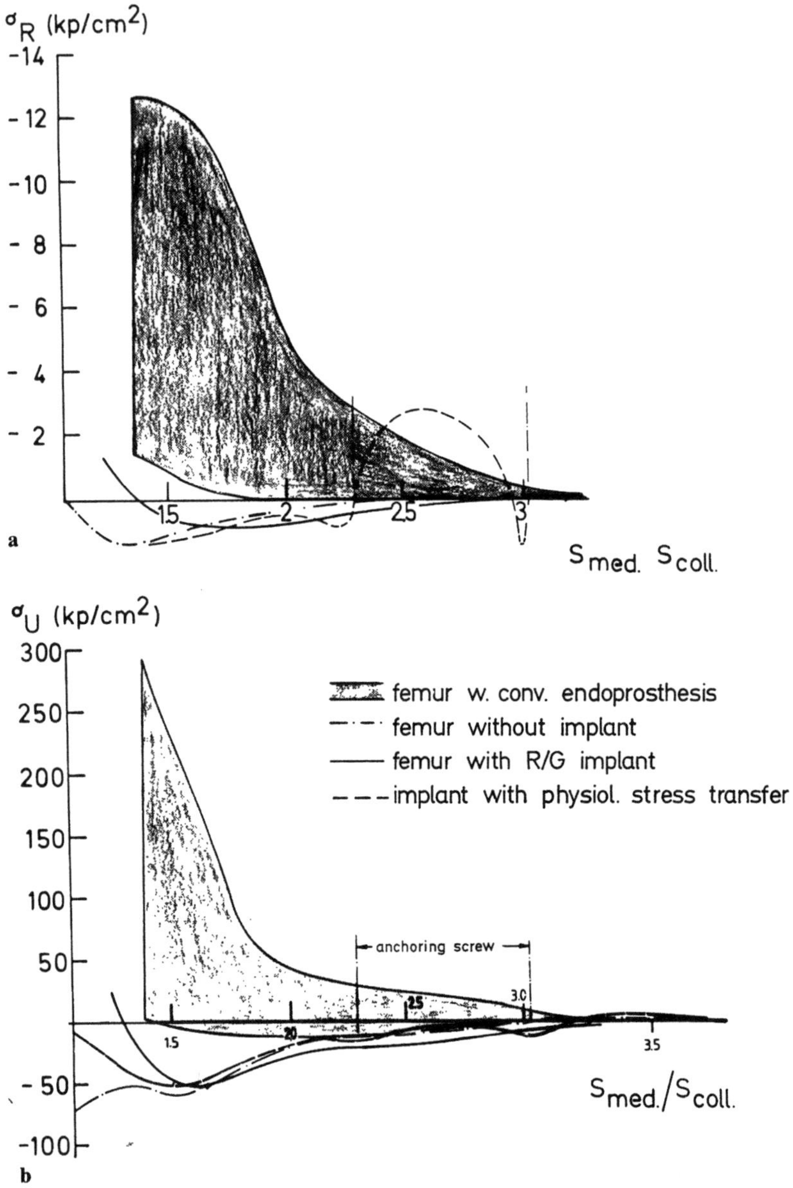

Fig. 4a, b. Partial results of finite element analysis (Cosa Dornier). The comparative representation of stress patterns for various types of endoprostheses shows the unphysiologic stress pattern of conventional implants, the approximately physiologic pattern of the R/G implant, and the largely physiologic pattern of the implant with a quasi-physiologic stress transfer. **a** Radial stresses in the inner wall of the medial cortex. **b** Circumferential stresses in the outer wall of the medial cortex

medullary cavity. This process can occur repeatedly unless the load is reduced.

The 3-dimensional calculation based upon a finite element analysis confirms the results described. It shows considerable departures from normal stress patterns, in some cases with a change of sine.

Our results may be summarized as follows as they relate to the primary and secondary fixation of endoprostheses:

1. Skeletal elements have a structural organization which corresponds to their function. Processes of synthesis and lysis within the physiologic setting, modulated by the genetic code, enable both a genotypic and phenotypic adaptation to prevailing mechanical loads. This adaptation becomes a master plan which initiates and regulates pertinent biological processes.
2. The pioneering theories of Wolff (1892), Roux (1895), Pauwels (1948, 1954), Kummer (1978) and others are still a valid basis for the development and maintenance of bony tissue and thus for the biological fixation of implants.

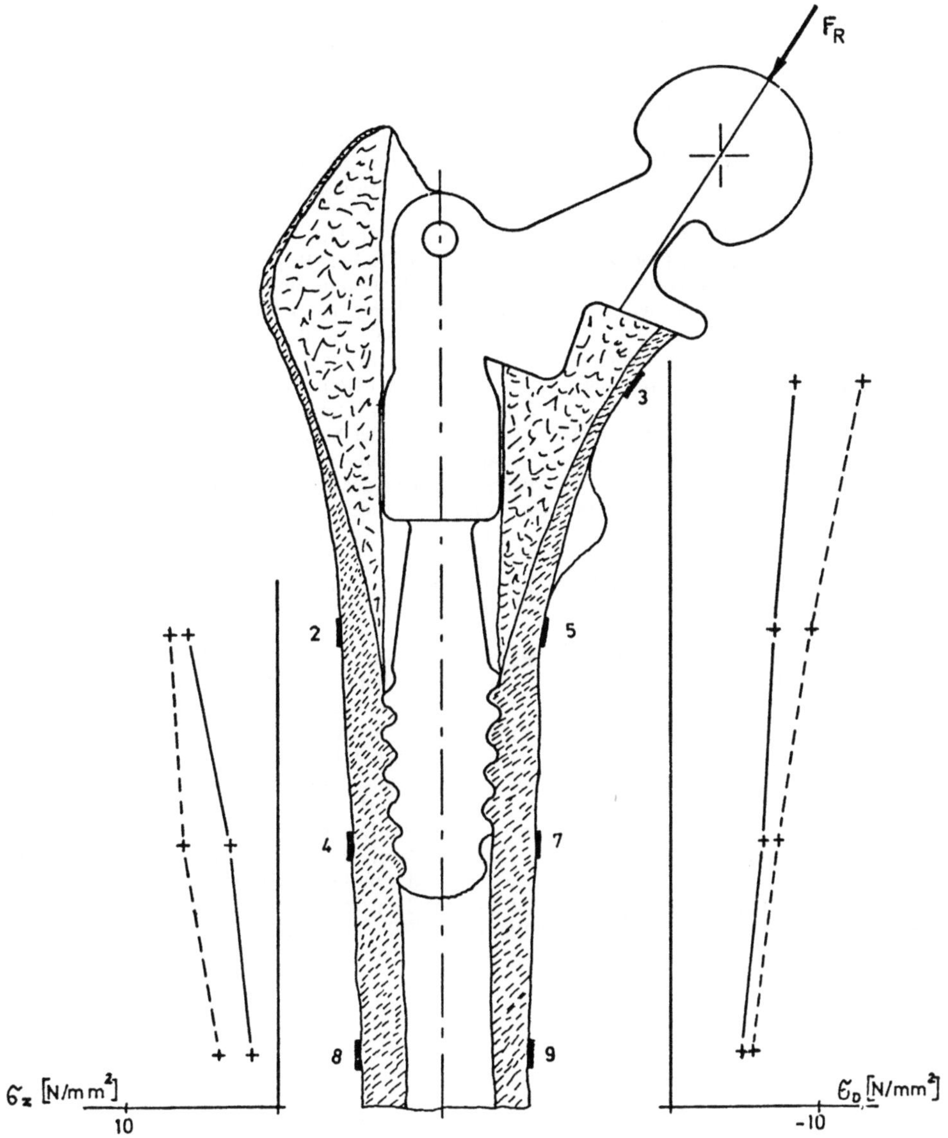

Fig. 5. Check of calculations (finite element method) by strain gauge experiments. Longitudinal stresses with $F_R = 1.75$ kN; — with prosthesis; - - - - without prosthesis

Their expanded interpretation in terms of signals and control processes may be viewed as a partial confirmation of the basic biomechanical concept. While noting that, unlike fractures, the implantation of an endoprosthesis places a nonbiological material in contact with biologic tissue, it may still be said that the principle of causal histogenesis remains an important guideline for the primary and secondary anchorage of endoprostheses.

The obvious conclusion is that the implant should be designed and constructed, and the patient managed, in such a way that the processes of causal histogenesis that underlie functional adaptation are disturbed as little as possible. The forces acting across the endoprosthesis-bone interface are of primary interest in this regard (see Fig. 5). These premises formed the basis for new implants which reproduce the normal patterns of stress transfer, and which have enabled a permanent, cement-free endoprosthetic anchorage to be achieved even in young patients.

References

Bassett AL (1966) Electromechanical factors regulating bone architecture. In: Fleisch H, Blackwood HJJ, Owen M (eds) Calcified tissues 1965, Proc. Eur. Symp. 3rd, 1965. Springer, Berlin Heidelberg New York, pp 78–89

Bassett AL (1968) Biologic significance of piezoelectricity. Calcif Tissue Res 1:252–272

Becker RO, Bassett CAL, Bachmann CH (1963) In: Bone biodynamics. Frost H (ed) Bioelectrical factors controlling bone structure. Little, Brown, Boston, pp 209–231

Becker RO, Murray DG (1980) The electrical control system regulating fracture healing in amphibiens. Clin Orthop & Rel Res 73, pp 169–198. In: Fung YC (1981) Biomechanics – mechanichal properties of living tissue, Springer, Berlin Heidelberg New York

Bourne H (1971/72/76) "The Biochemistry and Physiology of Bone", Bd 1–4, Academic Press, New York

Culmann K (1866/1873) Die graphische Statik, Bd 1, 1. Aufl (1866); 2. Aufl (1873). Zürich

Engelhardt A, Flemming M, Scholten R et al. (1972) Kraftflußberechnungen in Knochenstrukturen und Prothesen. Bundesminist. für Bildung und Wiss., Forschungsber.

Engelhardt A, Grell H, Scharbach H et al. (1977) Reasons for loosenings of hip endoprostheses and their consequences for new hip implant designs. S Afr Mech Eng 28:6

Fung YC (1981) "Biomechanics – Mechanical Properties of Living Tissue", Springer Berlin Heidelberg New York

Huggler AH, Schreiber A (1968) Die Alloarthroplastik des Hüftgelenkes mit Femurschaft- und Totalendoprothesen, 2. Aufl. Thieme, Stuttgart

Huggler AH, Schreiber A (1978) Alloarthroplastik des Hüftgelenkes, 2. überarb. und erweiterte Auflage. Georg Thieme Verlag Stuttgart

Knese KH (1979) Handbuch der mikroskopischen Anatomie des Menschen, Bd 2, Teil 5. Springer, Berlin Heidelberg New York

Kummer B (1978) Mechanische Beanspruchung und funktionelle Anpassung des Knochens. Verh Anat Ges 72

Meyer Hv (1867) Die Architektur der Spongiosa. – Reichert, Du Bois-Reymond's Arch 615

Meyer Hv (1882) Statik und Mechanik des menschlichen Knochengerüstes. Cotta, Stuttgart

Pauwels F (1948) Die Bedeutung der Bauprinzipien des Stütz- und Bewegungsapparates für die Beanspruchung der Röhrenknochen. Z Anat 129–166

Pauwels F (1954) Eine neue Theorie über die kausale Histogenese der Stützsubstanzen. Vortrag 52, Vers Anat Ges, Münster

Perren SM, Huggler A, Russenberger M et al (1969a) A method of measuring the change in compression applied to living cortical bone. Acta Orthop Scand [Suppl] 125:7

Perren SM, Huggler A, Russenberger et al. (1969b) A dynamic compression plate. Acta Orthop Scand [Suppl] 125:29

Perren SM, Ganz R, Rüter A (1972) Mechanical induction of bone resorption. 4th Int. Osteological Symp. Prag (contribution)

Rittmann WW, Perren SM (1974) Corticale Knochenheilung nach Osteosynthese und Infektion. Biomechanik und Biologie. Springer, Berlin Heidelberg New York

Roux W (1895) Der züchtende Kampf der Teile oder die „Teilauslese“ im Organismus, zugleich eine Theorie der funktionellen Anpassung. Ges Abh Bd I und II, Leipzig

Wolff J (1892) Das Gesetz der Transformation der Knochen. Hirschwald, Berlin

Biocompatibility of Endoprosthetic Materials

H.-G. Willert and G. H. Buchhorn

Requirements of Implant Materials

Biostability and biocompatibility are the most important *biological* requirements that a material must satisfy in order to make a suitable implant material.

A material is *biostable* in an ideal sense if exposure to the corrosive physiologic milieu effects no change in its chemical and physical properties. This requirement is most readily satisfied by metals in a stable, passive state (e.g., with a strongly adherent oxide film) and by polymeric materials that have a minimal fluid uptake.

A material is *biocompatible* if neither the material itself nor any substances released from it (breakdown or corrosion products, wear debris, additives, etc.) in any way harm the tissue of the implant recipient. At the very least, products released by the material must not exceed the tolerance limit of the tissue. A "peaceful coexistence" must be established between the implant and tissue [4].

Another factor essential to irritation-free tolerance of the implant by the host tissue is a complete *absence of motion* at the tissue-implant interface.

Other essential prerequisites for implant materials are a high, permanent *mechanical strength* and *resistance to wear.*

Unfortunately, none of the materials that are currently available (nor, in all likelihood, any that will be developed in the future) satisfy all these requirements in an ideal fashion. Therefore, the process of implant material selection is one of trade-offs and compromises, in each case choosing the material that is best suited for a given application.

Testing of Implant Materials

The suitability testing of a new implant material begins with the *testing of its physical properties.* This involves a battery of standard mechanical tests in which standard specimens are tested for their resistance to tension, bending, notch impact bending, torsion and compression. Materials intended to provide articulating surfaces are additionally tested for their tribologic properties (friction, lubrication).

The corrosion resistance of metallic materials can be tested by *electrochemical methods.*

Following these technical tests, *biological tests* are conducted to evaluate biostability and tissue compatibility.

The Biomaterials Group of the DGOT has set up procedural guidelines for the testing of implant materials and implants intended for use in orthopedic surgery [40]. According to these recommendations, implant materials should be tested according to a specified sequence, and the results at each stage should be evaluated in terms of known materials. Inhibition-zone, cell and tissue cultures (*in vitro* tests), various animal tissues corresponding to the proposed site of implantation, such as the subcutaneous tissue, muscle, bone and joints (*in vivo* tests), and finally the proposed implantation site in humans (clinical tests) constitute the *test milieu.*

Granules of varying sizes, fracture particles, test specimens of simple geometry, and specimens with an application-oriented geometry make up the various *test implants* which are exposed to the test milieu as well as to *biomechanical influences* (with and without loading). Both short- and long-term tests should be conducted, and the animal implantations should be done in various species. At the conclusion of the animal tests, the tissues in proximity to the implant are examined both macroscopically and microscopically, and the cellular and tissue constituents are identified with respect to their location and time of appearance.

For example, the time of appearance and the persistence of granulocytes, lymphocytes, plasma cells, histiocytes, foreign-body giant cells, connective tissue cells, fibers and vessels are important as parameters for the incorporation of the test implants and the occurrence of foreign-body reactions.

The tissue should also be examined analytically for the presence of any substances that may have passed from the implant into the tissue. Finally, the test implant is removed, and the material itself is examined for surface changes, structural integrity, and other physical and chemical changes.

Trial implantations in human patients should commence only after animal studies have been completed. At that point the *clinical testing* should be monitored in a prospective study.

The testing procedure outlined above is a very costly one. Yet the more carefully the individual tests are performed, the greater the likelihood of recognizing potential hazards and avoiding later failures and unexpected problems. It must be understood, however, that both the *in vitro* and *in vivo* investigations are basically nothing more than screening tests, and extreme care must be taken when applying their results to human implantation – for mechanical and biological tests provide only a crude approximation of the conditions and stresses to which an implant is subjected during service in the human body [42].

Consequently, the decision as to whether a material is suitable for a particular implant usually is made only after the material has proved its value in clinical usage, either as a short-term implant (plates, screws, pins, etc.) or long-term prosthesis (e.g., joint replacement arthroplasty). In this respect, variations in the design features of implants often are of decisive importance, even when the same materials are used!

In the past, we have found repeatedly that materials entering clinical trials after very successful preliminary testing (and often amid much enthusiasm) proved highly disappointing when implanted in human patients. Examples are Teflon [7], polyester [34] and, more recently, certain endoprostheses constructed of Al_2O_3 ceramic, including those combined with metal stems [10, 11, 12, 23–25, 29]. All the blame cannot be placed on the implant material, of course; certain design flaws were partly responsible for the failures (Figs. 1 and 2).

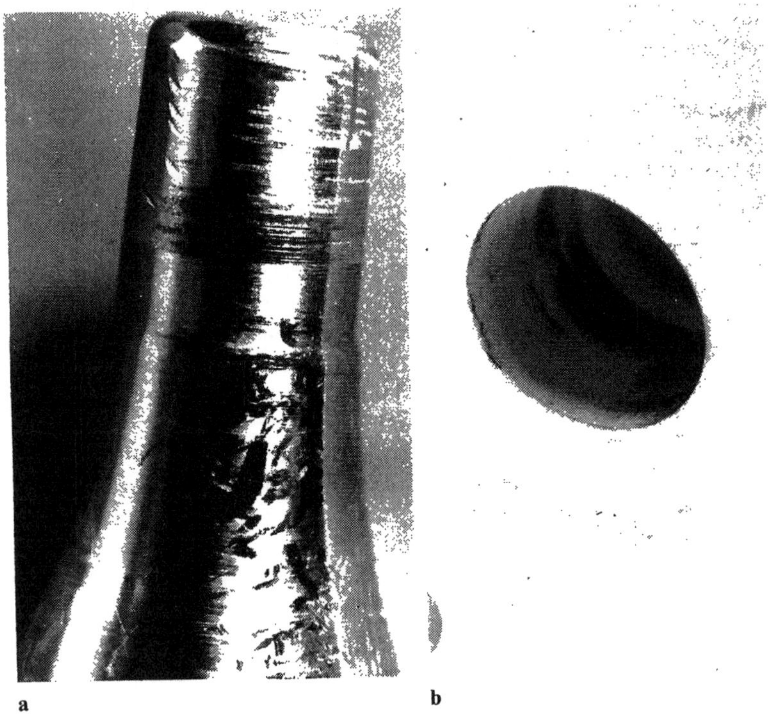

a b

Fig. 1. A press-fit conical connector that deviates from the original design of Sulzer-Feldmuhle, resulting in a loose fit of the ceramic head. **a** Deep wear grooves are visible in the cone (in addition to processing artifacts and damage incurred at reoperation), and **b** there is a corresponding discoloration of the ceramic

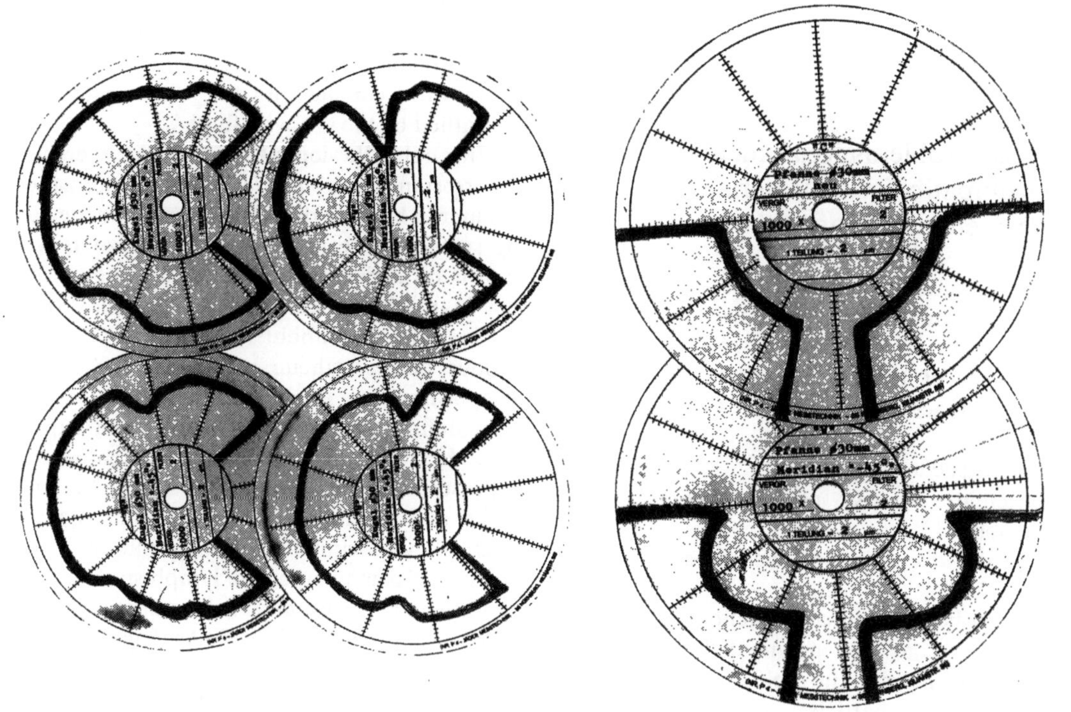

b

Fig. 2a, b. Manufacturing flaws such as incongruities, unwanted play and faulty grain size lead to excessive wear when components made of Al_2O_3 are paired in prosthetic systems. The Figure shows diagrams of a roundness test of an Al_2O_3 head and matching Al_2O_3 socket. **a** A perfect sphere would be represented by a circular line in the diagram. The wear-induced deviations appear as deep indentations on the spherical surface. **b** The diagram of a new acetabular socket is compared with that of a worn socket. The wear observed in this system is attributed to a slight, unwanted play between the head and socket. (We thank J. Hinterberger of the Biomechanics Laboratory of the Orthopedic Clinic of Munich for conducting these studies and communicating the results)

Implant Materials for Use Without Cement

A number of *implant materials* are used in the production of endoprosthetic components designed for cementless fixation:

Metallic materials: CoCrMo alloys
CoNiCrMo alloys
TiAlV alloys
pure metals (Ti, Ta, Nb)
Polymers: polyethylene
polyacetal
polytetrafluorethylene
silicone rubber
Ceramic materials: Al_2O_3 ceramic
glass ceramic
Carbons

With regard to biocompatibility, more or less extensive studies have been published on this subject for all implant materials that are in current use.

For some materials, such as stainless steel AISI 316L, CoCr-base alloys, Ti alloys, silicone rubber, polyacetal and polyethylene, years of clinical experience already are available for various types of short- and long-term implants and for endoprostheses that have been implanted without cement.

For other materials, not enough has been learned about their performance as uncemented implants to make a definitive evaluation. In these cases we must rely on experience with the cemented fixation of these materials.

For additional material-specific details, the reader is referred to the pertinent literature [3, 5, 8, 9, 17, 36, 38, 46–48]. Of particular interest is the multi-volume *CRC Series in Biocompati-*

bility recently published by D. Williams, in which authorities on material science report on their respective fields of expertise.

Special Problems Relating to the Biocompatibility of Materials for Uncemented Endoprostheses

Efforts to eliminate the use of bone cement in joint replacement arthroplasty are motivated by a desire to avoid the *side-effects and disadvantages* of the *in situ* polymerizing polymethylmethacrylate. These undesired effects include:

- local tissue toxicity;
- systemic toxicity of methylmethacrylate monomer;
- possible disruption of the low-strength cement bed;
- foreign-body giant-cell reaction of the implant bed to the polymethylmethacrylate, either in the implant itself or in the form of fragments and particles; and
- possible hypersensitivity reactions.

All these effects can contribute to loosening of the implant, thereby jeopardizing the long-term success of the joint replacement.

However, the elimination of bone cement also sacrifices some important *advantages* of cement fixation:

- encasement of the anchoring components of the endoprosthesis;
- correction of incongruities between the implant and its bed,
- option of orienting the prosthetic components independently of the shape of the bone bed, and
- immediate stable fixation of the components.

When an artificial joint is attached without cement, *two areas of contact* are recognized between the implant material and the tissue:

1. The contact area between the artificial *joint components* and the surrounding joint capsule, and
2. the contact area between the *anchoring components* and the implant bed.

1. Contact between Joint Components and Capsule

In joint replacements, the problems associated with the cementless implantation of endoprostheses are essentially the same as those of cemented prostheses: In the immediate vicinity of the articulating surfaces, the *implant materials* are in direct contact with the joint capsule and are bathed by the synovial fluid.

Through adhesion, abrasion, fatigue, erosion or corrosion, small *particles* of the endoprosthetic material become dislodged from the articulating surfaces. The phenomenon of *wear* is well known in engineering and is a common problem in machine bearings, for example. Much has been learned about the wear properties of various endoprosthetic materials used in arthroplasties and the associated effects on the surrounding tissues, though most such experience has been gained with cemented endoprostheses: The wear particles enter the joint cavity and are absorbed by the joint capsule, where they precipitate a foreign-body reaction. The particles may enter the lymph spaces of the periarticular tissue and subsequently be removed from the area (Fig. 3). As long as the volume of wear debris does not overtax the ability of the tissue to remove it, an equilibrium can be established between material wear and tissue reaction. Apparently this can enable the artificial joint to function normally for a long period of time [39, 43].

In *endoprostheses attached with bone cement,* we have observed that this equilibrium is upset when the volume of wear debris increases to the point that a massive granulomatous foreign-body reaction is precipitated in the periarticular tissue, causing phagocytosis and debris removal to become decompensated. Even tissues elsewhere in the implant environment can become involved in this decompensation process – most notably the reticuloendothelial system in the bone marrow and the connective tissue at the bone-cement interface. Here a foreign-body granulation tissue develops that is capable of resorbing the bone and thus creating looseness in the implant bed. We have demonstrated the involvement of the bone bed in the granulomatous foreign-body reaction to wear debris for the materials Teflon, Fluorosint, polyester, polyethylene, CoCr-base metal alloys, silicone rubber and polymethylmethacrylate. The tissue reaction in terms of cell content, fiber formation, granulomatous response, etc. varies depending on the type of material that is accumulated. However, it is our experience that the nature, extent and severity of the tissue reaction depend

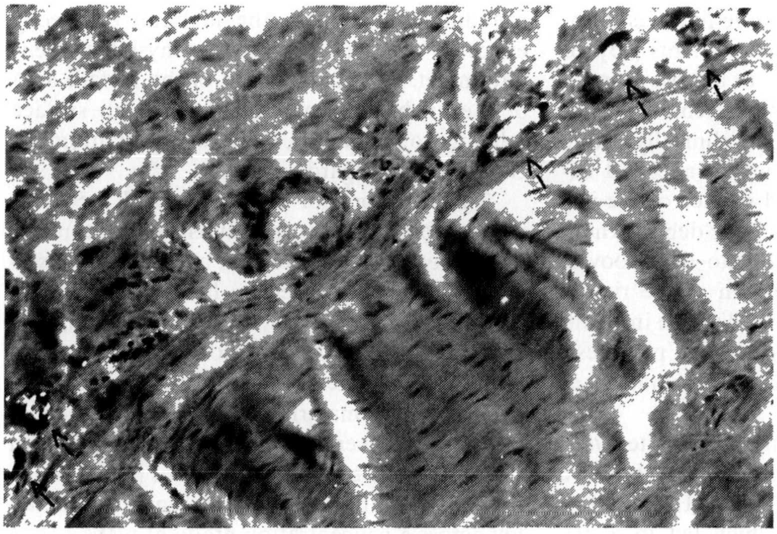

Fig. 3. Removal of minute wear particles in periarticular lymph spaces (*arrows* indicate bright polyethylene particles). Capsule tissue, polarized light, ×145

more on the volume and size of the particles than on the chemical composition of the material.

This problem adds yet another dimension to the question of biostability and biocompatibility: Materials which in solid form are highly biostable and biocompatible exert effects in particulate form that can lead to failure of the prosthesis.

The connection between material wear, bone resorption and implant loosening also demonstrates the fallacy of the notion that the problem of endoprosthetic wear can be solved simply by periodic replacement of the prostheses. Whenever excessive material wear becomes evident radiologically or clinically, the bone surrounding the implant generally shows such heavy resorption that a complete revision of the anchorage becomes necessary (assuming there is sufficient bone stock to permit it). As a rule, an artificial joint fails not because its moving parts become worn, but because the surrounding tissue becomes deficient and the anchorage loosens.

Because *uncemented endoprosthetic components* for artificial joints are made from essentially the same materials as conventional cemented prostheses, it would be reasonable to assume that the problem of material wear is similar for both fixation modalities. Nevertheless, the elimination of bone cement precludes extreme forms of wear produced by the abrading action of methylmethacrylate and x-ray contrast media in cases where, for example, traces of cement are inadvertently left between the articulating surfaces at operation, or acrylate particles from a disrupted cement sheath migrate into the joint cavity and come between the articular surfaces.

But even in *cementless implantations,* wear particles from the articulating surfaces can migrate into the surrounding bone and evoke reactions that weaken the integrity of the anchorage, as Plenk et al. [20, 21; Plenk H. Jr., 1982, personal communication] have demonstrated in animal experiments and human implantations for *steel and Al_2O_3 ceramic* as well as for *tantalum* and *polyethylene.* When a *ceramic implant and steel screw* combination was used in experimental animals, loosening of the implant gave rise to wear debris which (4 months postoperatively) was found both around the screw and in the wide connective tissue layer around the ceramic socket. The massive accumulation of wear debris at these sites prevented appositional bone growth around the implant, even though new bone formation was demonstrable by fluorescent microscopy [20]. Electron beam microanalysis showed the debris to consist of aluminum and stainless steel constituents.

In proximity to *Al_2O_3 ceramic femoral cups* that had undergone massive wear (due to fracture of the socket), Plenk et al. [20] also found ceramic particles deposited in the connective tissue between the bone and the still firmly-seated ceramic implant.

These authors made the same findings in total hip replacements in human patients [25]. In one revisional operation due to a loose stem, a more or less thick fibrous tissue membrane was removed from the vicinity of a clinically stable Al_2O_3 ceramic socket. This membrane had become molded to the grooved surface of the implant and contained ceramic wear debris. There had been no bony ingrowth into the grooves, but apparently bony overgrowth at the rim of the socket was sufficient to stabilize the implant. Thus, wear debris in this uncemented prosthesis had interfered with the desired formation of new bone.

Animal experiments with uncemented *tantalum femoral endoprostheses* revealed massive wear of the tantalum head (Plenk H. Jr., 1982, personal communication), which led to a discoloration of the capsule (metallosis) after only 6 weeks. After 7 months the debris-containing granulation tissue still hindered appositional bone growth, especially in the proximal portion of the implant. In other animal experiments Plenk et al. [21] found massive amounts of polyethylene wear debris in the fibrous tissue surrounding polyethylene screw-in sockets (Endler type) – yet another case of foreign-body granulation tissue interfering with new bone formation around an uncemented implant.

These results of Plenk et al. show that when material wear is excessive, essentially the same processes can occur in the abscence of bone cement as when a cement mantle is present.

It remains to be seen what long-term significance the presence of wear debris at the articulating surfaces of endoprostheses will have with respect to cementless fixation. However, it is clear that efforts must be made to obtain tissue samples from the interfacial area of uncemented endoprostheses for careful morphological and analytical evaluation whenever the opportunity arises (revisions, autopsies). The surfaces of the retrieved implants also should be carefully examined using advanced material science techniques.

2. Contact between Anchoring Components and Implant Bed

The *anchoring components* of an uncemented implant are sites where the material is in direct contact with the tissue of the implant bed. Because there is no protective cement sheath surrounding the implant, the material is directly exposed to the (corrosive) physiologic environment. The enlargement of the surface area of the anchoring components through surface relief, porous coatings, etc. has important implications in this regard.

The formation of chemically and mechanically stable "passivating films" gives conventional *metal alloys* protection against the physiologic milieu. The protective film, which consists mainly of oxides of the alloying elements, prevents or delays material decomposition through electrochemical reactions. As the corrosion resistance of the material increases, the effects of even highly adverse ambient conditions (oxygen lack, Cl^- ions) become less serious [30]. The belief that the diffusion of metal ions from the alloy across a concentration gradient plays only a minor role in this process [8] is called into question by more recent investigations [17] (Fig. 4). The passivating film can become damaged by friction between the articulating members of the joint or between the anchoring components and the implant bed (except for PMMA bone cement or contact tissue) [31, 32].

The mechanical strength and adherence of a passivating film on an implant determine the nature of the products formed by abrasion of the protective layer. These products are visible both macro- and microscopically [16]. Biochemical reactions with organic compounds and enzymatic reactions have been demonstrated *in vitro,* and intracellular collections of wear debris have been detected in tissue from the vicinity of removed implants [46–48]. The Co and Ti alloys are most apt to spontaneously form a new passivating film subsequent to surface damage [30, 45]. This process of "limited corrosion" releases alloy constituents that do not contribute to formation of the oxide film. Thus, corrosion products as well as wear products can be demonstrated in body tissues by microanalytical methods [39].

The selective excretion of certain metal salts by virtue of their special solubilities (in urine, stool, hair and nails) leads to an accumulation of metal ions that are bound in oxides, salts or organic tissue constituents. This is especially marked for the elements Co and Cr in CoCrNi alloys, which show a reversal of metal ion concentrations in favor of Cr [39].

Polymeric materials are of course immune to the electrochemical decomposition that affects

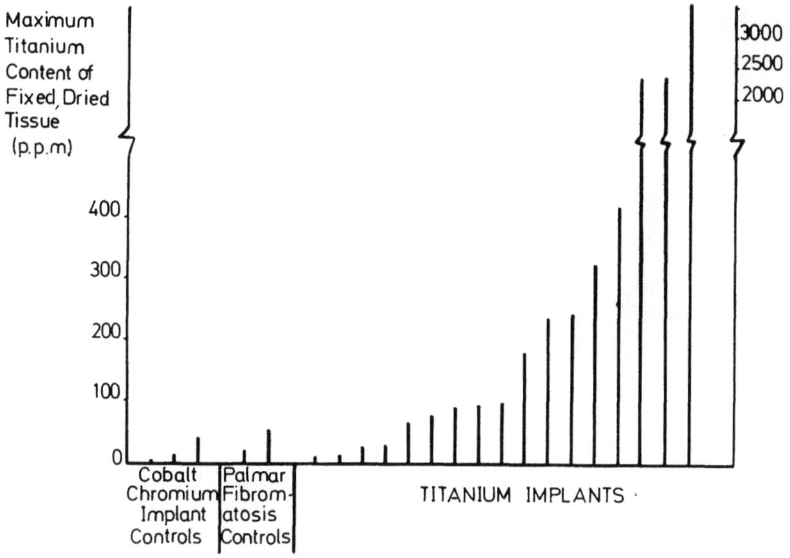

Fig. 4. The quantity of metallic compounds in the tissue surrounding the implant varies considerably among the different titanium implants investigated by Meachin [13]

metals, but they are subject to composition changes due to the uptake of body fluids (oxidation, hydrolysis, imbibition, dilution, etc.) [2, 13]. Besides discoloration – a sign that an extraneous substance has invaded the material (often seen in polyester and Silastic) – attention must be given to the possibility of mechanical strength losses through degradation of the polymer [1, 26, 27, 35]. So far the changes have been investigated only in connection with the wear behavior of articulating surfaces. When polymeric materials are used for anchoring components, however, precautionary design measures are indicated to counteract the gradual fatigue to which polymers are subject, both on a microscopic and macroscopic scale (Fig. 5).

Primary *mechanical rest* at the tissue-implant interface can be achieved only by a solid primary fixation of the endoprosthetic components [49]. If this condition is satisfied, the implant can become stably incorporated into bone [6, 14, 15, 28, 33].

If motion is allowed between the implant and bone, a fibrous tissue membrane of varying thickness will form in the interfacial zone [12, 18, 37].

Movements of the implant can also lead to wear phenomena on the anchoring surfaces, allowing foreign substances to enter the tissue and precipitate an undesired reaction. Hence, the uncemented implant must have anchoring components that are highly abrasion-resistant.

The changes that can result from a loose-fitting implant are illustrated by the Silastic endoprostheses used for the replacement of interphalangeal and metacarpophalangeal joints. They are anchored by means of uncemented stems impacted into the medullary cavity of the bones. In some cases this allows constant motion between the bone, soft tissues and implant,

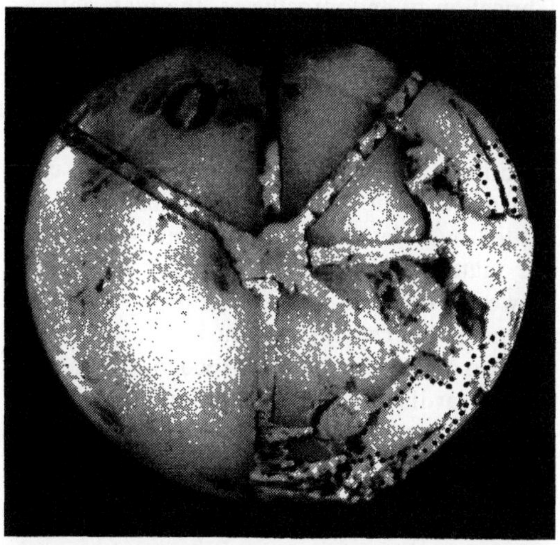

Fig. 5. A view of the outer surface of a polyethylene socket shows considerable deformation and an almost uniform, faint discoloration (dots outline areas not discolored). Bone cement fills the fixation grooves and covers a portion of the implant surface. Areas that are roughened or recessed are filled with dark blood residue

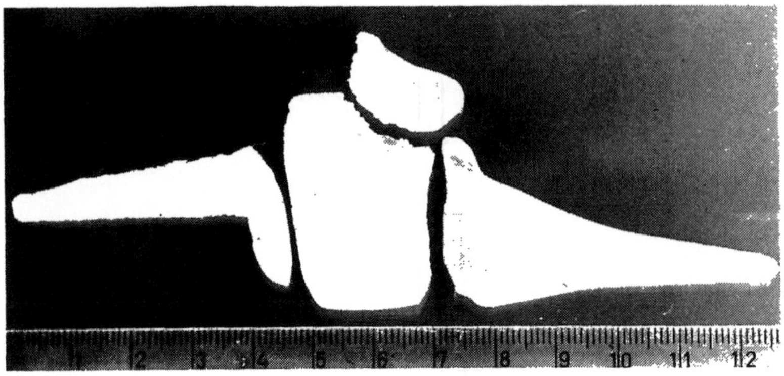

Fig. 6. Fractured Silastic elbow-joint implant with abraded anchoring stem

which Swanson describes as a "piston effect" (Fig. 6). Despite the fact that an isolating fibrous tissue capsule forms around the Silastic implant, particles of silicone rubber become abraded from the prosthesis and accumulate in this tissue, where they provoke a granulomatous foreign-body reaction. Extensive resorption of the implant bed results from the fibrous tissue proliferation.

Summary

A material may be designated as a biomaterial if it remains biostable and biocompatible for the life of the implantation. When used for the fabrication of endoprostheses, the material also must meet rigorous mechanical and in some cases tribological criteria. These properties must be demonstrated in both mechanical and biological tests.

Efforts to anchor endoprosthetic components without PMMA bone cement are motivated by a desire to eliminate side-effects and the material-related disadvantages of cement. However, this also means sacrificing important advantages of cement fixation.

Two areas of contact are recognized in uncemented artificial joints: 1) the articulating surfaces and surrounding capsular tissue and 2) the anchoring components and bone bed (bone-implant interface).

The entry of wear debris into the joint capsule stimulates a foreign-body reaction and impairs the function of the capsular tissue in varying degrees, depending on the volume of foreign material.

If wear is excessive, the particles also enter the bone marrow and bone-implant interface, where bone resorption by granulation tissue can weaken the bony anchorage of the implant.

Direct contact between the anchoring components and the implant bed raises the possibility of direct interactions between the implant and tissue (e.g., corrosion of metals or degradation of polymers), especially when the surface area of these components is increased by surface irregularities or porous coatings.

Besides biocompatibility, "mechanical rest" at the bone-implant interface is an essential prerequisite for permanent implant fixation.

References

1. Anderson JM, Barenberg S, Hiltner A (1981) Prosthetic valve wear products-embolization and systemic presentation. In: Weinstein A, Gibbons D, Brown S, Ruff W (eds) Implant retrieval: Material and biological analysis. NBS, Special publication 601, U.S. Department of Commerce, pp 283–298
2. Autian J (1964) Toxicity, untoward reactions and related considerations in the medical use of plastics. J Pharm Sci 53/11: 1289–1301
3. Black J (1981) Biological performance of materials, fundamentals of biocompatibility. Dekker, New York Basel
4. Brown S (1979) Developing biocompatibility test methods ASTM committee F-4. Medical device and diagnostic industry, vol 1, No. 5, pp 25–32
5. Bruck SD (1980) Properties of biomaterials in the physiological environment. CRC Press, Boca Raton
6. Cameron HU, Pilliar R, Macnab I (1973) The effect of movement on the bonding of porous metal to bone. J Biomed Mater Res 7: 301–311
7. Charnley J (1963) Tissue reactions to polytetrafluorethylene. Lancet II: 1379
8. Conzen H, Straumann F, Paschke E (1967) Grundlagen der Alloplastik mit Metallen und Kunststoffen. Thieme, Stuttgart
9. Dumbleton JH (1981) Tribology of natural and artificial joints. Elsevier, Amsterdam Oxford New York

10. Geduldig D, Dörre E, Happel M, Lade R, Prüssner P, Willert HG, Zichner L (1975) Welche Aussicht hat die Biokeramik als Implantatmaterial in der Orthopädie? Med Orthop Technik 6: 138–143
11. Hinterberger J, Ungethüm M (1978) Untersuchungen zur Tribologie und Festigkeit von Aluminiumoxydkeramik-Hüftendoprothesen. Z Orthop 116/3:294–303
12. Knahr K, Salzer M, Plenk H Jr, Grundschober F, Ramach W (1981) Experience with bioceramic implants in orthopaedic surgery. Biomaterials 2/4:98–104
13. Leininger RI (1972) Polymers as surgical implants. CRC Press, Boca Raton, pp 333–381
14. Linder L, Lundskog J (1975) Incorporation of stainless steel, titanium and vitallium in bone. Br J Accident Surg 6/4:277–285
15. Lundskog J (1972) Heat and bone tissue – An experimental investigation of the thermal properties of bone tissue and threshold levels for thermal injury. Elanders, Göteborg
16. Meachim G (1976) Histological interpretation of tissue changes adjacent to orthopaedic implants. In: Williams D (ed) Biocompatibility of implant materials. Sector, London, pp 120–127
17. Mears DC (1979) Materials and orthopaedic surgery. Williams & Wilkins, Baltimore
18. Muhr G, Stockhusen H, Müller O (1976) Die Hüftarthroplastik mit isoelastischen Totalendoprothesen im Tierexperiment. Arch Orthop Unfallchir 86: 115–128
19. Pflüger N, Böhler F, Grundschober H, Plenk H Jr, Schider S (1980) Die Verankerung von porös beschichteten bzw. Oberflächenstrukturierten Tantal-Totalendoprothesen im Tierexperiment. In: Jäger M, Hackenbroch MH, Refior HJ (Hrsg) Grenzschichtprobleme der Verankerung von Implantaten unter besonderer Berücksichtigung von Endoprothesen. Thieme, Stuttgart New York, S 166–172
20. Plenk H Jr, Locke H, Punzet G, Salzer M, Zweymüller K (1980) Tissue reactions to debris from bioceramic endoprostheses. In: Winter GD, Leray JL, de Groot K (eds) Evaluation of biomaterials. Wiley & Sons, Chichester New York Brisbane Toronto, pp 431–439
21. Plenk H Jr, Endler M, Gritler D, Grundschober F, Schnabl A (1981) Tissue reaction to a cement-free screw type HDPE socket endoprosthesis for the hip joint. Secon European Conference on biomaterials, Gothenburg, pp 71–72
22. Plenk H Jr (1982) Persönliche Mitteilung
23. Plitz W, Griss P (1981) Clinical, histo-morphological and material related observations on removed alumina-ceramic hip joint components. In: Weinstein A, Gibbons D, Brown S, Ruff W (eds) Implant retrieval: Material and biological analysis. NBS, Special publication 601, U.S. Department of Commerce, pp 131–156
24. Salzer M, Knahr K, Locke H, Stärk N (1978) Cement-free bioceramic double-cup endoprosthesis of the hip-joint. Clin Orthop 134:81–86
25. Salzer M, Knahr K, Plenk H Jr (1981) Long-term clinical and histological evaluation of bioceramic total hip endoprosthesis. Intern Orthopedics 4/11:1231–1240
26. Scales JT (1972) Some aspects of Stanmore total hip prostheses and their development. In: Chapchal G (ed) Arthroplasty of the hip. Thieme, Stuttgart, S. 113–120
27. Schoen FJ, Titus JL, Lawrie GM (1981) Materials degeneration causing late failure of mechanical heart valve prostheses: problems and promise. In: Weinstein A, Gibbons D, Brown S, Ruff W (eds) Implant retrieval: Material and biological analysis. NBS, Special publication 601, U.S. Department of Commerce, pp 269–282
28. Schroeder A, Pohler O, Sutter F (1976) Gewebsreaktion auf ein Titan-Hohlzylinderimplantat mit Titan-Spritzschichtoberfläche. SMfZ/RMSO 86/7:713–727
29. Stock D, Gottstein J, Harms P, Kuhlmann GP (1982) Gewährleisten die zur Verfügung stehenden Aluminiumoxyd-Keramik-Hüftendoprothesenmodelle beim derzeitigen Stand der Entwicklung eine ausreichende Zuverlässigkeit? Med Orthop Techn 1:14–17
30. Süry P, Semlitsch M (1978) Corrosion behaviour of cast and forged cobalt based alloys for double – alloy joint endoprostheses. J Biomed Mater Res 12/5:723–741
31. Thull R (1978) Implantatwerkstoffe für die Endoprothetik. Schiele & Schön, Berlin
32. Thull R, Schaldach M (1980) Mechanisch induzierte Korrosion an Gleit- und Fixierungselementen hoch belasteter Endoprothesen. In: Jäger M, Hackenbroch MH, Refior HJ (Hrsg) Grenzschichtprobleme der Verankerung von Implantaten unter besonderer Berücksichtigung von Endoprothesen. Thieme, Stuttgart, S. 161–165
33. Uhthoff HK (1973) Mechanical factors influencing the holding power of screws in compact bone. J Bone Joint Surg [Br] 55/3:633–639
34. Weber BG, Stühmer G, Semlitsch M (1974) Erfahrungen mit dem Kunststoff Polyester als Komponente der Rotationstotalprothese des Hüftgelenkes. Z Orthop 112/5:1106–1112
35. Weightman B, Paul JL, Rose R, Simon S, Radin EL (1973) A comparative study of total hip replacement prostheses. J Biomech 6:299–311
36. Weinstein A, Gibbons D, Brown S, Ruff W (1981) Implant retrieval: Material and biological analysis. NBS, Special publication 601, U.S. Department of Commerce
37. Willert HG, Schreiber A (1969) Unterschiedliche Reaktionen von Knochen- und Weichteillager auf autopolymerisierende Kunststoffimplantate. Z Orthop 106/2:231–252
38. Willert HG, Semlitsch M (1980) Biomaterialien und orthopädische Implantate. In: Witt AN, Rettig H, Schlegel KF, Hackenbroch M, Hupfauer W (Hrsg) Orthopädie in Praxis und Klinik, Bd II: Allgemeine Orthopädie. Thieme, Stuttgart
39. Willert HG, Semlitsch M, Buchhorn G, Kriete U (1978) Materialverschleiß und Gewebereaktion bei künstlichen Gelenken. Orthopäde 7:62–83
40. Willert HG, Buchhorn G, Ungethüm M (1980) Proposed guideline for the biological testing of

orthopaedic implant materials and implants. Biomaterials 1/10: 179–182
41. Willert HG, Buchhorn G, Semlitsch M (1980) Die Reaktion des Gewebes auf Verschleißprodukte von Gelenk-Endoprothesen der oberen Extremitäten. Orthopäde 9: 94–107
42. Willert HG, Buchhorn U, Prüssner P (1981) Aussagewert biologischer Tests im Rahmen der Überprüfung von Biomaterial. In: Rettig H, Weber U (Hrsg) Symposium über Biomaterialien. Gentner, Stuttgart
43. Willert HG, Buchhorn G, Buchhorn U, Semlitsch M (1981) Tissue response to wear debris in artificial joints. In: Weinstein A, Gibbons D, Brown S, Ruff W (eds) Implant retrieval: Material and biological analysis. NBS, Special publication 601, U.S. Department of Commerce, pp 239–267
44. Willert HG, Buchhorn G, Semlitsch M (1981) Recognition and identification of wear products in the surrounding tissues of artificial joint prostheses. In: Dumbleton JH (ed) Tribology of natural and artificial joints. Elsevier, Amsterdam Oxford New York, pp 381–419
45. Williams DF (1977) Titanium as a metal for implantation, part 1: Physical properties. J Med Eng Technol 1/4: 195–198, 202
46. Williams DF (1981) Systemic aspects of biocompatibility, vol 1, 2. CRC series in biocompatibility. CRC Press, Boca Raton
47. Williams DF (1981) Biocompatibility of clinical implant materials, vol 1, 2. CRC series in biocompatibility. CRC Press, Boca Raton
48. Williams DF (1982) Biocompatibility of orthopaedic implants, vol 1, 2. CRC series in biocompatibility. CRC Press, Boca Raton
49. Zweymüller K, Semlitsch M (1982) Concept and material properties of a cementless hip prosthesis system with Al_2O_3 ceramic ball heads and wrought Ti-6Al-4V stems. Arch Orthop Trauma Surg 229–236

The Induction of Bone Resorption by Prosthetic Loosening

S. M. Perren

Prosthetic loosening represents a major complication of joint replacement arthroplasty. In our studies of the undesired loosening of implants for the internal fixation of fractures (Perren et al., 1975), we have observed that micromovements in the contact zone between plate screws and the bone lead to superficial bone resorption and secondary instability. Similarly, the loosening of endoprostheses is based upon a change in the geometry of the contact zones between the bone, cement and implant. This may occur as a result of excessive mechanical loading or a biological resorption of the surrounding bone. In the present article we shall show how discoveries from internal fixation experiments with mechanically induced bone resorption can be applied to the problem of prosthetic loosening.

Motion-Induced Bone Resorption

Weight-bearing bones undergo a cyclic deformation during walking. If a plate is attached to the bone with screws at one end but is left unattached at the other, then relative movement will occur between the free end of the plate and the bone (Fig. 1). If the free end is attached to the bone with a loose-fitting screw, this screw will wobble as weight is alternately placed upon the limb and removed. Viewed more closely, this wobbling motion of the screw takes place about an axis that is located in the far cortex (Fig. 2). On both sides of this axis, the contact zone alternately becomes compressed and unloaded by the movement of the screw. Should the contact surface become loaded in the opposite direction, creating an alternation between compression and tension, then the contact zone will open. Though the relative movements between the bone and metal may have an amplitude of only a few micrometers, they are sufficient to cause bone resorption and implant loosening, provided there is a significant transverse motion component across the contact zone.

The superficial bone resorption caused by micromovements and the replacement of the bone by connective tissue and cartilage are shown schematically in Fig. 3. Through bone resorption, the primary mechanical microinsta-

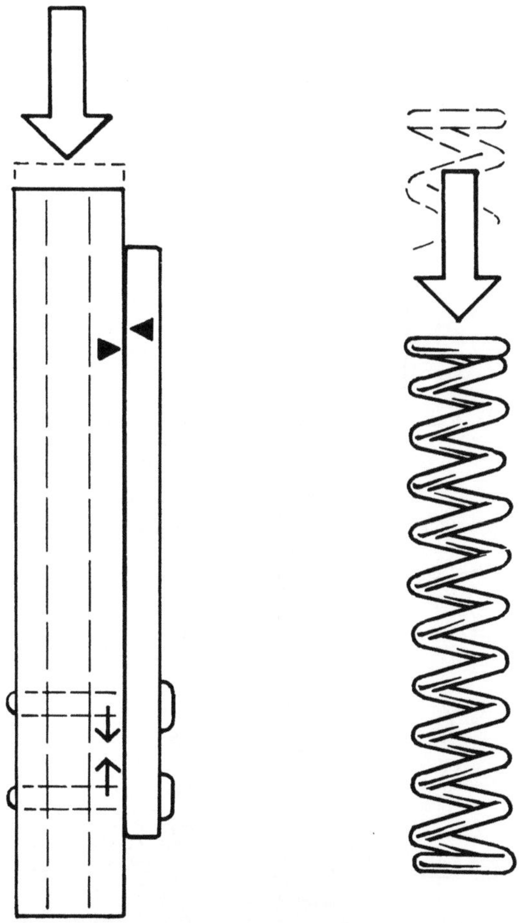

Fig. 1. Production of micromovements in vivo. If a plate is attached to a long bone at one end only, loading of the bonde during weight-bearing will cause the bone to move a short distance relative to the end of the plate

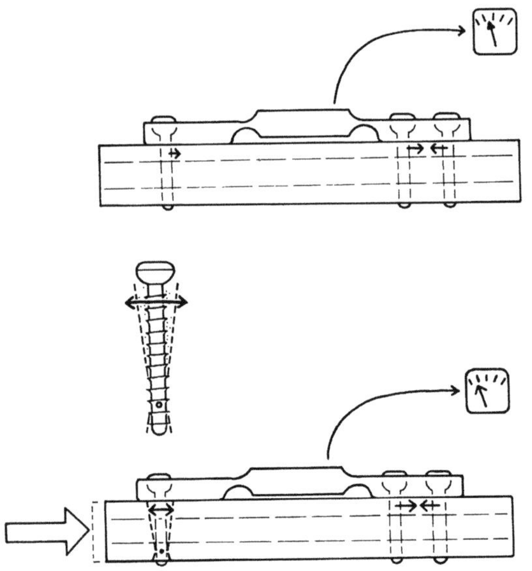

Fig. 2. Movement of a plate screw in vivo. If the free end of the plate in Fig. 1 is loosely attached to the bone with a screw, axial wobbling of the screw will occur with each stride. This movement takes place about an axis located in the far cortex

bility has led to a marked loosening of the implant that is apparent on gross inspection. In experiments in which the contact zones were prestressed when the plates were applied, thereby prohibiting movement at the screw-bone interface, no resorption took place. The behavior of the bone in the zones near the axis of the wobbling movements is interesting: Despite a tangential displacement of the contact zones, no bone resorption occurs (Fig. 5).

It is appropriate to compare the two different types of bone reaction with the behavior of the bone surrounding a prosthesis. It is known that the collar of a femoral endoprosthesis cannot reliably prevent subsidence of the prosthesis in the face of bone resorption and, owing to its effect as an asymmetric bearing, promotes movement of the prosthesis within the bony canal (Schneider, 1982), analogous to the wobbling movements of the screw described above. The clinically interesting behavior of the "collarless" straight-stem prosthesis (Mueller, 1979) can be explained mechanically by second-

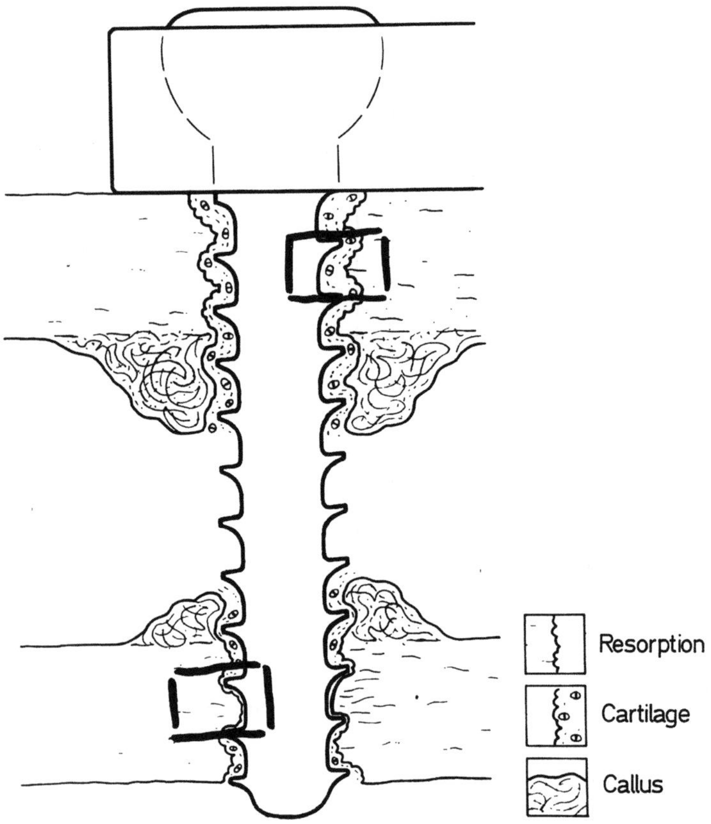

Fig. 3. Survey of bone reaction. The movement of the loose screw leads to a resorption of the bone surrounding the screw. The rectangles indicate the areas depicted in the micrographs in Figs. 4 and 5

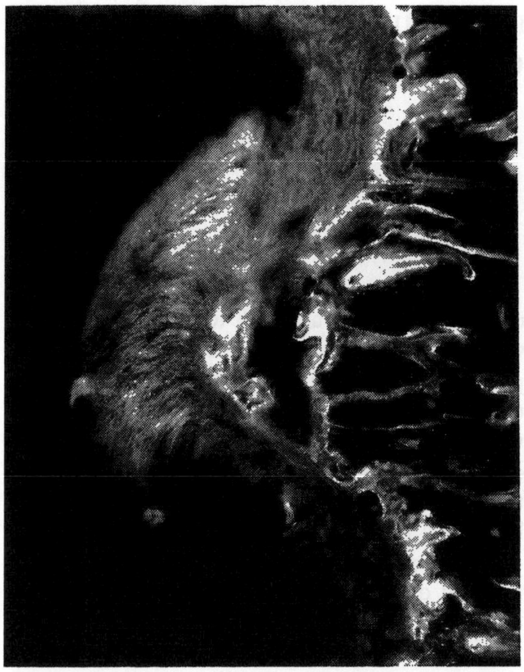

Fig. 4. Biological reaction of bone to micromovement of an implant. The thin section from the threaded zone in the near cortex shows superficial bone resorption and replacement by connective tissue and cartilage. Secondary loosening of the screw has occurred. We compare this type of motion with the intermittent engagement of a prosthetic collar against the bone

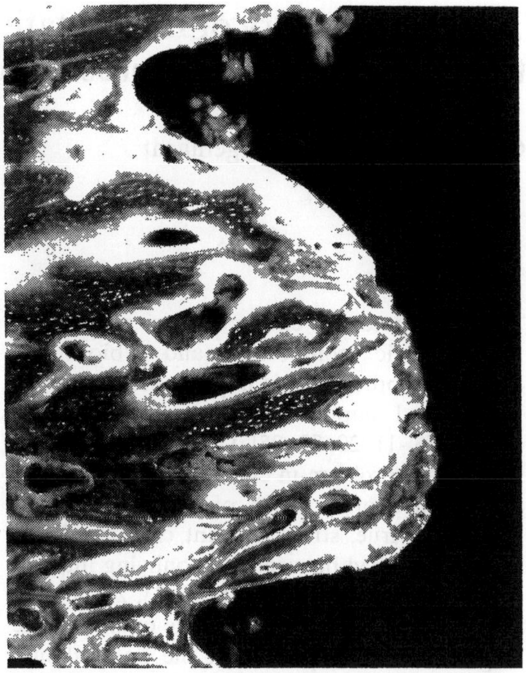

Fig. 5. Near the axis of rotation of the wobbling movement no resorption is apparent. Here the motion of the implant surface is essentially tangential. This movement is analogous to that of the stem of a collarless, straight-stem prosthesis within a bony canal

ary impaction into the femoral canal, but it may also be explained in terms of differences in the biologic behavior of the bone under two different modes of relative movement. The relative importance of quantitative differences alone and/or qualitative difference between tangential movement and movement with a normal component remains unclear.

Summary

Superficial resorption has been induced in the cortical bone of a sheep by micromovements across the contact zone. The finding that no resorption occurred in the zones of tangential motion is extrapolated to the contact zone between a prosthetic stem and the femur, and differences in the behavior of hip prostheses of different designs are discussed.

References

Müller ME, Elmiger B (1979) Coxarthrose. 10-Jahres-Ergebnisse der sog. Setzholz-Totalprothese. Orthopäde 8:73

Perren SM, Ganz R, Rüter A (1975) Oberflächliche Knochenresorption um Implantate. Med Orthop Techn 95:6–10

Schneider R (1982) Die Totalprothese der Hüfte. Huber, Bern Stuttgart Wien

The Biochemistry of Implantation: Bonding of Living Bone to Stress-Bearing Endoprosthetic Components – A Survey

G. P. Zoephel and A. Engelhardt

The development of endoprostheses made from metal-ceramic composites and "bioactive" glasses has brought new hope to the search for uncemented implant systems with long-term stability [6–11, 20, 22, 25]. Despite all advances, the greatest problem in endoprosthetics remains the absence of a mode of fixation that establishes a true, stress-resistant chemical bond to be established between the nonliving implant and the living bone [1, 2, 4, 5, 15, 23, 24, 26–28]. Such a bond should approach the quality of the original tissue. In particular, the bond should be free of microtoxicity and capable of transferring combined tensile, shear and compressive stresses. During the implantation, there should be minimal interference with the pattern of biochemical and biophysical impulses within the living tissue. In the present paper we shall discuss biochemical principles which we believe have an important bearing on the problem of cementless implant fixation.

In our estimation, no implant system has yet been devised in which a true chemical bond is established between a load-bearing endoprosthesis and the living bone. It is understandable, therefore, that a bewildering variety of terms has evolved to characterize the concept of a "bond" forming between the implant and bone [10, 13, 14, 16, 18, 19, 21, 25]. Terms such as "close apposition of bone and implant," "interlocking," "*true* bonding," "polar interactive forces," "adhesion," "dispersion forces" and "interdiffusion of charged groups" reflect the inaccessibility of chemical bonding with purely morphologic instrumentation. Moreover, such terms are used with little if any regard for the question of what *atoms* or *groups of atoms* of what structural elements are to be bonded together.

It is known that chemical bonding cannot be demonstrated directly, even with electron microscopy. Surface spectroscopy provides a means of indirect demonstration, but this technique cannot be applied to *in vivo* bonding without modification. Thus, it appears that implant-tissue bonding can be confirmed only through the use of biochemical techniques. We venture to state that such tests would quickly demonstrate the inadequacy of fixation methods that are claimed to establish a "bone-implant bond."

Concepts of endoprosthetic fixation can be roughly divided into those based upon the geometry of the implant and those based upon its material. The demonstration of fixation on a material basis is possible only on a molecular level. We believe that many of the "bonds" reported to date are more a product of preparation technique than chemical bonding forces. The preparation technique was shown to be a decisive factor in the metallic and nonmetallic implant materials investigated by Harms and Mäusle [16]. In all cases, electron microscopy of the unstressed test implants showed a layer of macrophages between the tissue and implant. It is clear that cellular elements do not permit the establishment of a stress-resistant material bond. Only since the development of bioactive glasses has the possibility of achieving a chemical bond between bone and implant been seriously discussed [6, 9–11, 13, 14, 16, 18–22, 25]. However, the arguments and experimental results presented to date are not convincing from a biochemical standpoint.

1. The alleged "close bonding" or preferential adhesion of bioactive glasses to bone is dependent on the solubility (leaching) of the glasses.
   Too little is known as yet about the influence of the leached ions on osteogenic cells.
   The low total concentration of liberated material does not necessarily imply freedom from significant toxicity.
   Most toxicologic test procedures for biomaterials are simplified short-term tests that give

little information on the long-term behavior of foreign materials in the body [17, 29].
Too few dynamic, biochemical measurements have been made of the special synthetic activities of more highly differentiated cells.

2. The leached, active boundary layer of the implant has a porosity that reduces its mechanical stability.
3. The binding elements between the bone and the ceramic or glass are unknown. Speculations on this point are presented below.
4. If the solubility of the glasses and ceramics is reduced, then a "good bond" is no longer formed between the supporting tissue and implant material, and these materials lose much of their advantage over conventional implant materials.
5. The existence of the aforementioned "good bond" has not been proved under conditions of physiologic loading [12, 16].

Based on these considerations, we are doubtful that the alleged bond is anything more than a close mechanical "interlock" between the biomaterial and bone, made possible by the solubility of the material surface. Nevertheless, in the light of our own clinical results and from a biochemical perspective, glasses and glass ceramics combined with metallic prosthetic cores are clearly the most favorable materials that have been developed to date for the fabrication of endoprostheses having long-term stability in the human skeleton. In materials that contain silicon oxide, the silanol groups in the surface of the implant are practically the only components that could enter into a direct chemical and bond with the tissue, although the metal hydroxides or metal complex clusters in the silicon oxide ceramic surface might possibly contribute to some degree. However, all surface groups must first be converted to a reactive form through suitable hydrolytic processes. The hydrolysis of these bonds would require energy conditions that are not easily attained *in vivo*.

On the tissue side, the organic constituents of the bone matrix, type 1 collagen with small amounts of glucosaminoglycanes and noncollageneous proteins, and the crystalline phase of the bone mineral, an apatite of varying composition, are available for bonding. Attempts have been made to establish a structural continuity between the implant and living tissue via the mineral phase of the supporting tissue [13, 18, 20, 21]. But parts cannot simply be taken away from a composite material if the properties of the composite are to remain intact. Such concepts are based on a misunderstanding of the biochemical processes involved in the development and regeneration of supporting tissue. Another error is to equate calcium phosphates with the same gross chemical formulas or with identical physical parameters in *one respect* as being structurally and thus functionally equivalent. Because unphysiologically high concentrations of bone mineral generally lead to resorption, leaving behind the substrate of synthetic apatite, we need not answer the question of how a soluble crystal lattice could bring about a stable chemical bond between bone and implant in an aqueous milieu.

Thus, it appears that the fixation of endoprostheses to living tissue must rely upon the true structural elements of the supporting and connective tissue, the collagen matrices. Chemical groups on the protein side include:

- the amino group $-NH_2$, basic amino acid radical in side chains
- the alcohol group –OH, also occurring in side chains
- the thiol group –SH, present in sulfur-containing amino acid radicals or bound in disulfide bridges (–S–S–)
- the carboxyl group –COOH, acidic amino acid radical,

and several reductive or oxidative forms of the foregoing groups. In the body, these groups and *only* these group, together with their hydrate and salt envelope, accompanying polymers and protective groups, must be brought into such close proximity with the silanol (or metal hydroxide) groups of the glass or ceramic surface that a hydrolytically stable Si–O–C–(Si–C) bond is able to form there.

It is important to recall that virtually all forces acting within and between molecules are electrical in nature. However, these forces or potential fields vary greatly in magnitude and thus in their range of influence. In nature, permanent structures that are subject to large mechanical stresses derive their stability almost exclusively from homopolar (covalent) bonds (intermolecular cross-links in collagen, fibrin, elastin and other biopolymers). All other forms of physicochemical bonding are inherently inferior in strength to the covalent bond and, significantly, are found in structures that require only transitory fixation or flexibility and derive protection through other means (tertiary and quarternary structures of proteins and enzymes, DNA and RNA spatial structures, etc.). Besides ion-ion interactions in salt-containing crystals and metallic bonding, the interaction between permanent dipoles in the form of hydrogen bonding is undoubtedly a relatively stable bond type. However, its domain is the temporary and secondary stabilization of *conformations,* or specific spatial arrangements, in many biopolymers that function under shielded or low-stress conditions. This bond type does not possess a true hydrolytic stability. Its lability in an aqueous milieu is, however, an essential property that renders it suitable for biological applications. In contrast to electrostatic Coulombian interactions, whole potential energy is inversely proportional to distance, and the ion-dipole interaction with a potential proportional to r^{-4}, the "van der Walls" forces (dipole-dipole interaction, dipole-induced dipole interaction, London's dispersion forces and overlap energies) act between molecules only over extremely short distances. Their potential energy is inversely proportional to the sixth power of the intervening distance.

The basic problem with such forces is nicely summed up by Buonocore: "The key to lasting adhesion lies not only in bringing surfaces into molecular proximity but also in keeping them there" [3]. No one has yet shown convincingly how this can be done under the biochemical conditions of implantation, with a contaminated wound bed, relative interfacial movements and organic biomolecules. The problem on the mechanical side, i.e. an improved surface geometry to optimize contact between implant and tissue; is based mainly on the changeability of the living implant bed on the one hand, and the deficient transfer of tensile and shear stresses on the other. We believe that the absence of a physiologic stimulus pattern in the interfacial zone underlies the high incidence of bone resorption and endoprosthetic subsidence. An altered stimulus pattern inevitably causes an alteration of metabolic processes at the interface, perhaps leading to the synthesis of insufficient matrix.

Another problem that remains to be solved pertains to the biochemical toxicity of implant materials. The key questions are 1) What is the fate of wear debris and of ions and molecules leached from wear debris and the implant? and 2) *What modes of administration* of substances act upon *what cell compartments* in the *long term* and in *what manner?*

Only a careful analysis of the biosynthesis of the supporting tissue can point the way toward endoprosthetic designs with long-term stability that can form a biologically stable chemical bond with the living tissue. In a complex series of delicate steps, collagen aggregates that are largely "prefabricated" at the cellular level are joined extracellularly to form the fiber bundles of osteoid. Presumably the adhesion of growing fibers to the cell surface and basement membrane is a necessary step in this process. Mineralization of the formed matrix is the final step that ensures structural stability.

If a way can be found to anchor the growing fibers chemically with the nonbiologic prosthetic material, then the problem of the *in vivo* fixation of implants will come a step closer to being solved. Bone is the ideal composite material for load-bearing supporting elements of the human body. An endoprosthesis that disregards and makes no attempt to imitate the process of its synthesis will be unable to solve the problem of long-term stability in the interfacial zone.

References

1. Asshof H (1980) Beitrag zur Vermeidung der Hüftprothesenlockerung. Z Orthop 118:134–136
2. Bryan WJ, McCaskill BL, Tullos HS (1981) Hip endoprosthesis stabilization with a porous low modulus stem coating. Clin Orthop 157:125–132
3. Buonocore MG (1981) Retrospection on bonding. Dent Clin North Am 25:241–255
4. Carlsson AS (1981) 351 total hip replacement according to Charnley. Acta Orthop Scand 52:339–344
5. Chandler HP (1981) Total hip replacement in patients younger than thirty years old. J Bone Joint Surg [Am] 63:1426–1434
6. Ebert R, Baurschmidt P, Schaldach M (1980) Keramische Werkstoffe in der Ersatzteilchirurgie. Biomed Tech (Berlin) 25:74–80
7. Engelhardt A (1982) Endlich eine ausgereifte Total-Endoprothese? Ärztl Prax 8:226–233
8. Engelhardt A, Sencar M, Scharbach H, Grell H, Andreef J (1981) Erfahrungen mit zementlos verankerten Implantaten. Z Orthop 119:789–791
9. Fuchs GA (1982) Biologische und biomechanische Eigenschaften glaskeramikbeschichteter Metallimplantate als einfaches Modell belasteter zementloser Hüft-Endoprothesen. Biomed Tech (Berlin) 27:24–29
10. Fuchs GA, Deubcher K (1981) Glass-ceramic coated implant. Arch Orthop Trauma Surg 98:121–126

11. Griss P, Heimke G (1981) Five years experience with ceramic-metal composite hip endoprostheses. Arch Orthop Trauma Surg 98:157–171
12. Griss P: Die Aussagefähigkeit histologischer Befunde zur Beurteilung von Knochenersatzwerkstoffen.
13. Gross UM, Strunz V (1980) The anchoring of glass ceramic of different solubility in the femur of the rat. J Biomed Mater Res 14:607–618
14. Gross UM (1981) The ultrastructure of the interface between glass ceramic and bone. J Biomed Mater Res 15:291
15. Gschwend N, Debrunner MU (Hrsg) (1976) Total hip prosthesis. Huber, Bern
16. Harms J, Mäusle E (1980) Biokompatibilität von Implantaten in der Orthopädie. Springer, Berlin Heidelberg New York
17. Hench LL (1981) Guest editorial. J Biomed Mater Res 15:3–7
18. Hench LL, Ogino M (1980) Formation of calcium phosphate films on silicate glasses. J Non-Crystalline Solids 38, 39:673–678
19. Hench LL (1971) Bonding mechanisms at the interface of ceramic prosthetic materials. J Biomed Mater Res 2:117–141
20. Hench LL (1977) Analysis of bioglass fixation of hip prostheses. J Biomed Mater Res 11:267–282
21. Hench LL (1980) Compositional dependance of the formation of calcium phosphate films on bioglass. J Biomed Mater Res 14:55–64
22. Hench LL (1981) Toxicology and biocompatibility of bioglasses. J Biomed Mater Res 15:805–817
23. Holz U, Weller S, Lohfert H (1980) Erfahrungen mit dem alloplastischen Gelenkflächenersatz am Hüftgelenk. Z Orthop 118:681–690
24. Jolley MN, Salvati EA, Brown GC (1982) Early results and complications of surface replacement of the hip. J Bone Joint Surg [Am] 64:366–377
25. Köhler S, Retemeyer K, Berger G (1981) Untersuchung zur Haftvermittlung von Bio-Vitrokeramik und Titan im tierischen Knochen. Z Exp Chir 14:139–143
26. Ring PA (1981) Uncemented total hip replacement. J R Soc Med 74:719–724
27. Salvati EA (1981) A ten-year follow-up study of our first one hundred consecutive Charnley total hip replacements. J Bone Joint Surg [Am] 63:753–767
28. Stock D (1982) Gewährleisten die zur Verfügung stehenden Aluminiumoxyd-Keramik-Hüftendoprothesen beim derzeitigen Stand der Entwicklung eine ausreichende Zuverlässigkeit? Med Orthop Techn 102:14–17
29. Williams D (1976) Biocompatibility of implant materials. Pitman Turnbridge Wells

Possibilities and Limitations of the Cementless Fixation of Endoprosthetic Components *

K. Draenert and Y. Draenert

The evolution of technology differs from the phylogenesis of biological systems in that it is mediated by the human intellect. Biological development follows inevitably from the laws that relate form with function and is a continuous process. As technology progresses, on the other hand, it is easy to lose sight of the problems that the technology was originally intended to solve. The fixation of a femoral head prosthesis with polymethylmethacrylates by Charnley (1960) was the culmination of many attempts to replace natural joints or joint components with artificial parts. The early attempts of Groves (1890), the Judet prosthesis (1956), and the "mould arthroplasty" of Smith-Petersen (1939, 1948) all failed due to problems of attachment to the bone. The introduction of Charnley's bone cements was celebrated as a "therapeutic breakthrough" (Schlegel, 1975). The impressive results of cement fixation were attributed to the large surface area made available for the transfer of loads: "Mechanical tests have shown an improvement of 200 times in the load-bearing capacity of the prosthesis compared to the condition without cement" (Charnley, 1970).

Subsequent experimental and pathohistologic studies of prosthetic implants yielded highly diverse results. However, it was generally agreed that polymethylmethacrylates became encapsulated by a fibrous tissue membrane when implanted in the body (Feith, 1975; Charnley, 1965). On the other hand, there have been reports in recent years of "bioactive materials" that form strong bonds with the bone through the establishment of collagen fiber insertions on the implant surface (Hench, 1970).

In a number of experiments on rabbits, dogs and monkeys, and based on pathohistologic studies of tissue samples obtained at revision or autopsy, two fundamental discoveries have been made:

1. Endogenous tissue can never become anchored in an artificial implant. Fiber insertions on a ceramic surface should be interpreted not as true molecular bonds, but rather as a mortise- and-tenon effect at the bone-implant interface that cannot withstand large tensile forces.
2. All implants have a weight that is subject to gravitational forces. In addition, cemented implants acquire an aggregate weight as the cement shrinks onto the implant and away from the bone bed during polymerization, forming a cement-implant complex.

The bony anchorage of an implant depends less on its bioactive properties than on the stresses acting at the bone-implant interface and the directions of force transmission. In model experiments in which animal femurs were filled with bone cement, a direct bone-cement contact could be clearly demonstrated (Draenert, 1981). The bony anchorage of the implant depends both upon relative interfacial movement and upon the transfer of stresses across the interfacial zone. Relative movements lead to demineralization, resorption and remodeling of the surrounding bone, to the replacement of the original, stable lamellar bone by a rapidly-formed bony mesh, and finally to the replacement of the bone bed by connective tissue. A rigid layer of fibrous connective tissue or even fibrocartilage may form, depending on specific load conditions.

The forces that act on an implant are partially absorbed by the implant and partially transmitted to the implant bed, in accordance with the properties of the implant material. In a system of this type, where bonding at a molecular level is not achieved, only compressive forces can be optimally transmitted. As soon as tension is exerted on an artificial interface, contact between the tissue and implant is lost, and a gap is

* Study supported by the Deutsche Forschungsgemeinschaft, project DR 121/1

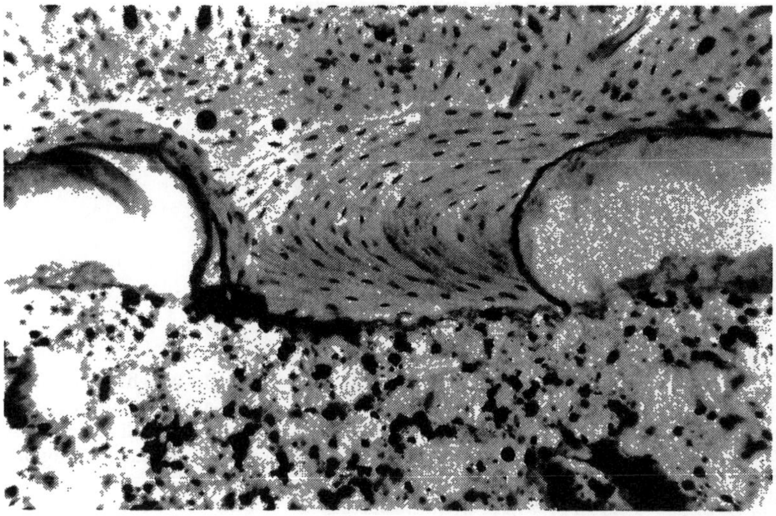

Fig. 1. The morphologic correlate of the "bony anchorage" of an implant is the perpendicular orientation of the trabeculae with respect to the implant surface, with no intervening fibrous tissue. The micrograph is a detail of a section taken from the posterior circumference of a rabbit femur and photographed in polarized light. The medullary cavity had been filled with bone cement (1 year)

created. This gap will close only when compressive forces are applied perpendicular to the implant surface.

All implants with bony anchorage show trabeculae that are oriented at right angles to the implant surface (Fig. 1). The lines of force that govern stress transfer from the bone to the implant and from the implant to the surrounding bone are determined by the forces resulting from muscular exertion and body weight. Taking an artificial joint as an example, we may conclude from this that stress transfer can be optimum only along lines of compression. Tensile stresses can be compensated only indirectly by one of two methods:

1. Creating a mechanical interlock by enclosing the bony trabeculae in plastic cement so that tension on the cement will exert compression on the trabeculae (Fig. 2). This has the net effect of converting tension to compression.
2. "Prestressing" as used by the ASIF to obtain stable interfragmental compression of bone fractures. This technique creates a high primary compression that is not nullified by tension.

Prestressing is effective in all cases where bone viscoelasticity and remodeling produce only a very slow decay of the primary compression (Perren et al., 1969). Prestressing is not an ideal means of anchoring a prosthesis in the area of the proximal femur, first because the femoral bone structure is designed for a radial dispersion of forces, and second because long-term implants such as joint prostheses cannot escape the effects of viscoelasticity and remodeling.

The viscoelastic behavior of the bone leads very rapidly to a relaxation of the primary compression, and remodeling carries this process further until forces in the compact bone are essentially transmitted passively along the pressure-bearing surfaces. In the region of the cancellous bone, the primary compression decays immediately owing to the elasticity of the trabeculae. Thus, it appears that prestressing of-

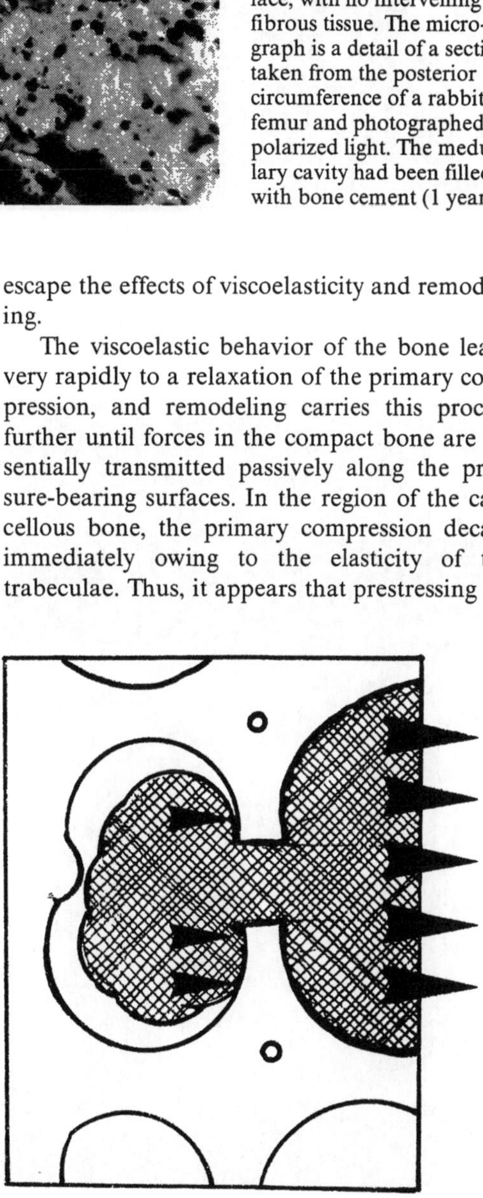

Fig. 2. Mechanical locking of the bone cement about the trabeculae provides a limited degree of tension resistance, in effect by converting tension to compression

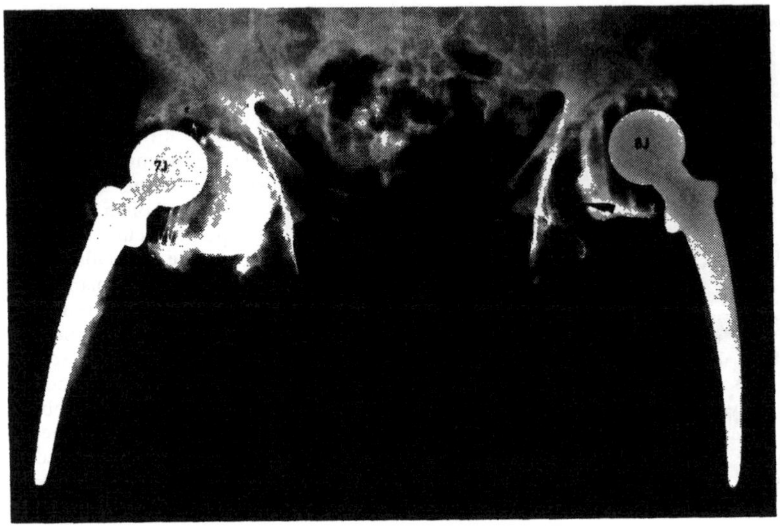

Fig. 3. Weight distributions that are asymmetric to the resultant of all forces cause excessive head loading of the implant with consequent loosening

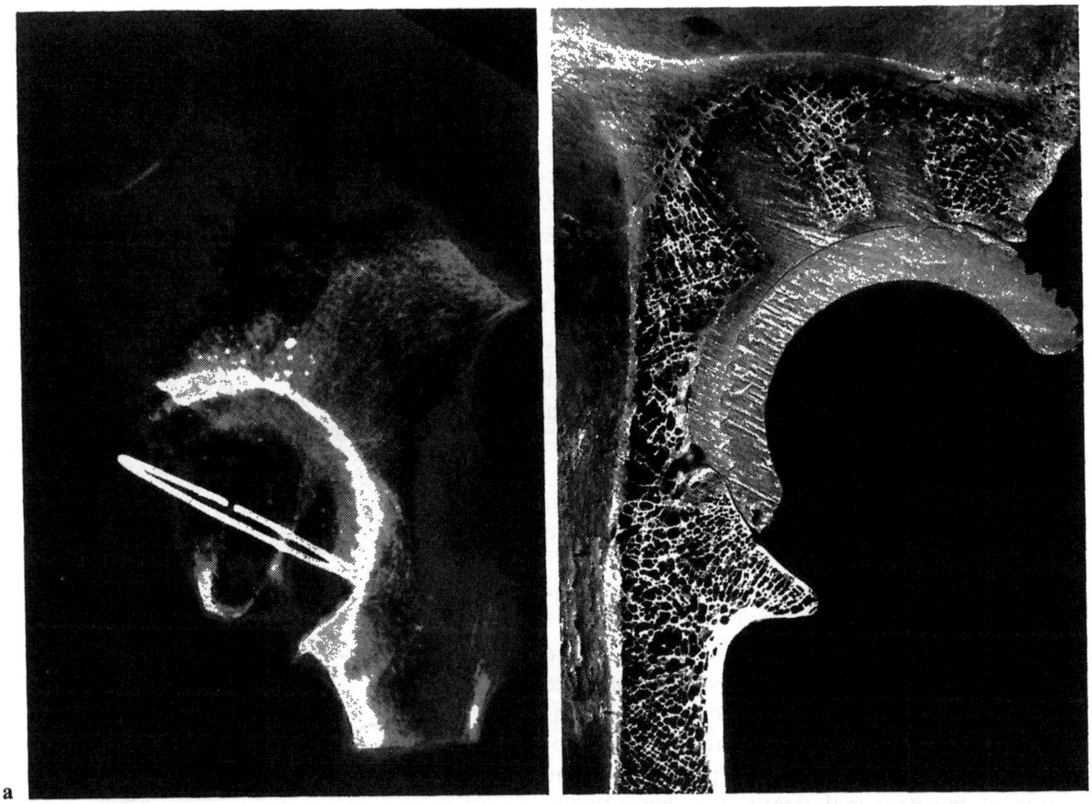

a b

Fig. 4a. The acetabular component should be positioned such that the weight of the cement-implant system is distributed symmetrically with respect to the resultant force R (Agfa contour photo of an anatomic specimen). **b** Anchoring the acetabular component with bone cement is prudent only in the roof of the acetabulum, where pure compressive stresses can be transferred to the bone fers no definitive solution to the problem of permanent prosthetic anchorage.

Histomorphologic analysis confirms these findings. Along compression lines are found sites of bony contact at which a mature, lamellar bone is formed. At sites acted upon by tensile forces, on the other hand, relative movements between the implant and bone lead to a resorption of bone substance, which ultimately is replaced by a bed of rigid fibrous tissue.

The forces transmitted from the implant to the bone and the dynamic deformation of the bone determine the stresses that develop at the interfaces. The magnitude of these stresses is determined by the moment arms and material properties of the implant as well as by the surface area available for its anchorage.

The conclusions to be drawn from these considerations with respect to the anchoring of prostheses are different for the acetabular component of a total hip replacement than for a femoral cup or femoral endoprosthesis.

In the past, little attention has been given to the weight of an implant and the consequent gravitational forces to which it is subjected; yet these factors represent the major cause of acetabular socket loosenings. The large pressure-bearing surface that the acetabulum provides can serve as an anchoring surface for a prosthetic socket. However, weight distributions that are asymmetric to the resultant force R cause excessive head stresses to be exerted on the implant from the moment weight is borne on the system, causing the socket to loosen (Fig. 3). The aggregate weight of the socket-cement complex must be taken into account when cemented prostheses are used.

Only a weight distribution that is symmetric to the resultant force R creates conditions that are optimum for bony anchorage. This cannot, of course, eliminate the interfacial stresses that result from the frictional moments of the articulating components. Given the fact that only compressive forces can be transmitted across the interface, the only correct position for an acetabular prosthesis is that in which its weight is distributed symmetrically with respect to the resultant of all forces (Fig. 4a, b). A cement-free anchorage is conceivable.

In the case of the femoral component, pure compression is possible only in the area of its posteromedial circumference, i.e., in the calcar area. In a stem prosthesis, an enlargement of

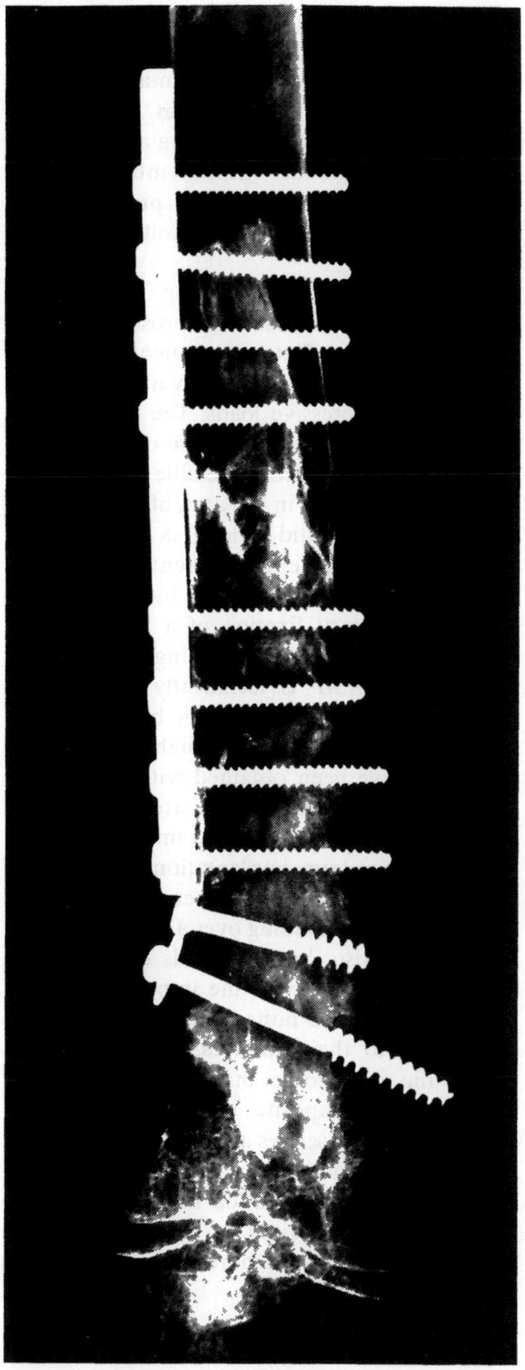

Fig. 5. Composite internal fixation 19 years after operation. The bone cement can only withstand compressive loading on a long-term basis. But if this condition is satisfied, experience has shown that the cement can provide a stable, reaction-free anchorage for many years. The cement filling the medullary cavity is buttressed for its entire length by strong bony trabeculae oriented at right angles to its surface

this pressure-bearing surface can be achieved only by anchoring the implant transversely in the bone with the aid of plastic material, in effect creating cross-members that provide additional surface area for receiving and transferring compressive loads. These members can also reduce relative movements that promote bone resorption and hinder appositional bone growth.

Another way of eliminating these movements would be to attach the prosthesis to the bone with screws. But with cement fixation, a much larger surface area is available for the transfer of compressive loads. The concept that highly porous surfaces like those offered by ceramic implants or porous metallic coatings promote bony ingrowth in the area of the proximal femur cannot be valid as long as disruptive interfacial shear prevents differentiation of the pluripotent mesenchymal tissue into bone.

The temporary fixation of a femoral stem prosthesis with screws according to the principles of the ASIF is technically difficult and very costly. Fixation with plastic bone cement is simple by comparison. The highly diverse results that have been obtained with cement fixation in total hip replacements are an indication that the technique is of crucial importance for a successful long-term implantation. Owing to its material properties, bone cement can withstand only compressive loading over a prolonged period of time. Also, because loads can be transferred from the body to the implant and from the implant to the bone only along lines perpendicular to their surfaces, compression remains the only force that can be optimally transmitted. Composite internal fixations, in which plates and screws are used in conjunction with bone cement to secure the internal fixation, provide the best illustration that cemented implants subjected mainly to compressive loads can remain stably anchored for many years (Fig. 5).

Conclusions

Morphologic findings at the bone-cement interface confirm the biomechanical theory of Perren (1982) that relative motion between the implant and bone leads to bone resorption.

A load can be optimally transmitted by an implant only when applied at right angles to its surface. This offers direct evidence that physiologic implantation angles in the acetabular region should not be imitated. Similar discoveries in the femoral region have already led to the adoption of a larger neck-stem angle for the femoral component.

The magnitude of interfacial stresses is inversely proportional to the surface area that is available for load transfer. This area is far greater in cemented implants than in uncemented protheses.

The roof of the acetabulum offers a possible site for the cement-free attachment of a prosthesis. However, its spherical geometry requires interlocking or screw fixation of the implant within the acetabular roof.

Mindful of the weight of the implant-cement system and the associated gravitational forces, the acetabular component should not be implanted at an upright angle or with a large medial cement mass, as this would tend to increase head stresses on the implant.

In the region of the proximal femur, a cemented stem prosthesis still offers the only means of creating a surface area sufficient for the transfer of pure compressive loads. The material properties of an implant determine load transfer at the interface. Isoelastic materials have favorable properties in terms of interfacial movement but should not create the impression that anything other than compressive stresses can be transferred across the interface, despite the behavior of the material.

In summary, it is clear that the original law postulated by Julius Wolff (1892), stating that strong compression leads to bone resorption, is incorrect (Matzen, 1952; Mueller and Perren, 1972).

Bone resorption results from relative movement between the fragments of a bone fracture (Mueller and Perren, 1972) or between an implant and its bed (Perren, in press). Morphologic evidence restricts implant-to-bone stress transfer to those forces acting at right angles to the implant surface.

References

Charnley J (1960) Anchorage of femoral head prosthesis to the shaft of the femur. J Bone Joint Surg [Br] 42:28–30

Charnley J (1965) A biochemical analysis of the use of cement to anchor the femoral prosthesis. J Bone Joint Surg [Br] 47:354–363

Charnley J (1970) Acrylic cement in orthopaedic surgery. Livingstone, Edinburgh London

Draenert K (1981) Histomorphology of the bone-to-cement interface: remodelling of the cortex and revascularization of the medullary canal in animal experiments. In: Salvati EA (ed) The Hip. Proceedings of the ninth open scientific meeting of the Hip Society. Mosby, St. Louis Toronto London

Feith R (1975) Side effects of acrylic cement implanted into bone. Doctoral dissertation. Brakkenstein Nijmegen

Hench LL, et al. (1970) Investigations of bonding mechanism at the interface of prosthetic material. Report XO, 1–6. U.S. Army Med Res Dev Command Contract No 17–70 0001/75

Judet J, Judet R (1956) The use of an artificial femoral head for arthroplasty of the hip joint. J Bone Joint Surg [Br] 32:166

Matzen PF (1952) Vom Einfluß mechanischer Einwirkungen auf die Kallusbildung. Brun's Beitr Klin Chir 184:147–179

Müller ME, Perren SM (1972) Callus und primäre Knochenheilung. Monatsschr Unfallheilkd 75:442–454

Oest O, Müller K, Hupfauer W (1975) Die Knochenzemente. Enke, Stuttgart, S 53

Perren SM (1983) Reaktion des Knochengewebes auf Implantate. In: Morscher E (Hrsg) Die zementlose Fixation von Hüftendoprothesen. Springer, Berlin Heidelberg New York Tokyo

Perren SM, Straumann F, Müller ME, Allgöwer M (1969) A method of measuring the change in compression applied to living cortical bone. Acta Orthop Scand [Suppl] 125:7–16

Schlegel KF (1975) Geleitwort. In: Oest O, Müller K, Hupfauer W (Hrsg) Die Knochenzemente. Enke, Stuttgart

Smith-Petersen MN (1939) Arthroplasty of the hip. A new method. J Bone Joint Surg [Br] 21:269

Smith-Petersen MN (1948) Evolution of mould arthroplasty of the hip joint. J Bone Joint Surg [Br] 30:59

Wolff J (1892) Das Gesetz der Transformation der Knochen. Hirschwald, Berlin

Histologic Studies on the Incorporation of Uncemented Implants *

R. K. Schenk and W. Herrmann

Introduction

To study the bony incorporation of prostheses, it is necessary that the implant-tissue interface be made accessible to microscopic examination. Uncemented implants generally are better suited for such examination than cemented ones, for bone cement is easily lost during histologic processing. Prostheses made of insoluble plastic materials (polyethylene, polyacetal) provide specimens that can be sawed, ground and even sectioned to some degree using ordinary embedding techniques developed for undecalcified bone. With newer processing methods, even metal-tissue interfaces can be examined by light microscopy with a high degree of resolution. This enables us to obtain general insights into the tissue reactions occurring at prosthetic interfaces by examining specimens obtained from laboratory animals or taken from human patients during revisional surgery or autopsy.

In the present paper our object is not to make a comparative evaluation of different types of prosthesis and prosthetic materials, but rather to explore the basic patterns of tissue reaction to selected implants while demonstrating the possibilities offered by an improved technique of microscopic examination.

Methods

The specimens are fixed and embedded using proven techniques for the processing of undecalcified bone. The fresh specimen is placed in 40% alcohol that has been precooled to 4–7 °C and is stored in a refrigerator until completely infiltrated (1–5 days). Then it is dehydrated in graded alcohols, placed in 2–3 changes of xylene, and transferred to methylmethacrylate, to which 25% Plastoid N has been added as a softening agent. Two to three weeks are allowed for complete infiltration, whereupon the specimen is placed in the embedding medium, to which 2% benzoyl peroxide has been added as a catalyst. No effort is made to remove the stabilizer in the methacrylate. With larger specimens, time is allowed for spontaneous polymerization at room temperature, as this significantly reduces the danger of bubble formation due to overheating. In contrast to an earlier work (Schenk, 1965), we no longer stain the specimen with basic fuchsin during dehydration; given the unavoidably large section thicknesses above 100 μm, transillumination would lead to a heavy superimposition of superficial and deep structures if this were done. The blocks are cut into sections 0.5–0.7 mm thick with a circular saw or diamond blade (e.g., Buehler Isomet). A microfraise (Jung Co., Nussloch bei Heidelberg) is then used for facing the surface to be examined, that surface is stained, and the lower surface that is not to be examined is cut away with the fraise. With a suitable microscopic and microphotographic technique, the surface staining method makes it possible to examine cells and tissue structures with a resolution that ordinarily is achieved only in semithin sections. The principle of surface staining was described previously by Gross and Strunz (1977), and the improvements and modifications made possible with the introduction of the microfraise are reported elsewhere (Schenk et al., in preparation).

Findings

Isoelastic Femoral Head Prostheses

Initial histologic observations on the tissue reaction to a femoral head prosthesis implanted in

* Supported by the Education and Research Fund of the Association for the Study of Internal Fixation

an 86-year-old woman who died 6 weeks postoperatively already indicate intensive bony callus formation around the prosthetic stem, accompanied by trabecular filling of the surrounding medullary cavity (Morscher et al., 1981). In direct contact with the polyacetal resin was a layer of connective tissue, 30–120 μm wide, with relatively strong collagen fibers and a moderate cell density. Isolated foreign-body giant cells were observed, either in contact with the implant surface or suspended in the surrounding bone marrow. Rigid connective tissue or fibrocartilage, which would have been evidence of microinstability, was not observed. Analogous findings were made in the femur of a 76-year-old woman who died 7½ weeks postoperatively, and in whom the situation had been complicated by an intraoperative fracture of the severely osteoporotic cortex. Bony callus formation was evident both in the fracture area and in the medullary cavity surrounding the prosthetic stem, and a portion of the fracture site had already been bridged by bone. The primary stability achieved at operation and the splinting action of the prosthetic stem apparently were sufficient to enable a primary ossification to occur. In both cases, however, the morphologic basis for this primary stability remained unclear.

Therefore, in a third patient – a 95-year-old man who died from cardiac failure 4 weeks postoperatively – we cut cross-sectional specimens from the entire length of the prosthetic stem in an effort to obtain a ramdom sampling (Fig. 1a–g). We found that a primary press-fit had been achieved in the distal third of the stem at the time of implantation. Cross-sections from this region show that the implant almost completely fills the cylindrically-reamed medullary cavity, and they reveal good circumferential contact between the implant surface and the compact bone (Fig. 1b–d). Some reciprocal deformation of the implant and bone occurred during insertion of the prosthesis, this is especially marked on the implant side. In addition, because some destruction of medullary vessels occurred when the cavity was prepared and the implant was inserted, the cortical bone is avascular over a considerable area and shows little vital reaction after 4 weeks. On the other hand, the gaps between the implant and bone have become invaded by new medullary vessels. They are consistently surrounded by loose, relatively cell-rich connective tissue, and a lively, reactive ossification is evident on the inner surface of the cortex and along the surface of the cancellous trabeculae. This ossification marks the first step toward filling the gaps between the implant and cortex and is particularly evident in the recesses on the implant surface (Fig. 1e–g). However, nowhere has new bone been laid down directly on the polyacetal resin. The interfacial zone consists of a delicate network of fine connective-tissue filaments that contain isolated giant cells. Bone formation occurs in an "implantopetal" direction, i.e., starts in the bone bed and proceeds in the direction of the foreign body. Direct bone-implant contact, where present, is mediated by preexisting bone with which the implant has come in contact during primary press-fitting or postoperative weight-bearing.

Findings on the Incorporation of Implants with a Titanium Spray Coating

Studies on the incorporation of titanium plasma-coated hollow cylindrical implants in the mandible have shown that a very solid bony attachment is achieved within a short time (Schroeder et al., 1976, 1978). Apparently this is attributable not only to the inert metal, but also to the rough surface finish created by the coating. The success of this experiment prompted us to conduct similar experiments on femoral head prostheses. We used a specially-developed cylindrical shell prosthesis that was fitted into the femoral neck of dogs with the aid of a special instrument set (Sutter et al., 1982). To date we have made histologic evaluations of 6 prostheses that had been implanted for 8 weeks (Fig. 2a–g). We have found the tissue compatibility to be extremely good, and have observed intensive new bone formation in the vicinity of the prosthesis and in contact with the metal surface. The round, 3-mm perforations in the hollow cylinder have already been largely filled with new cancellous bone (Fig. 2c, d). Particularly noteworthy is the solid contact of the newly-formed trabeculae with the metal surface. Examination of stained sections reveals no tissue interposed between the bone and metal, and mineralized bone matrix containing osteocytes is in direct apposition to the titanium plasma (Fig. 2e, f). It could be shown by means of sequential fluorescent labeling that the bone is

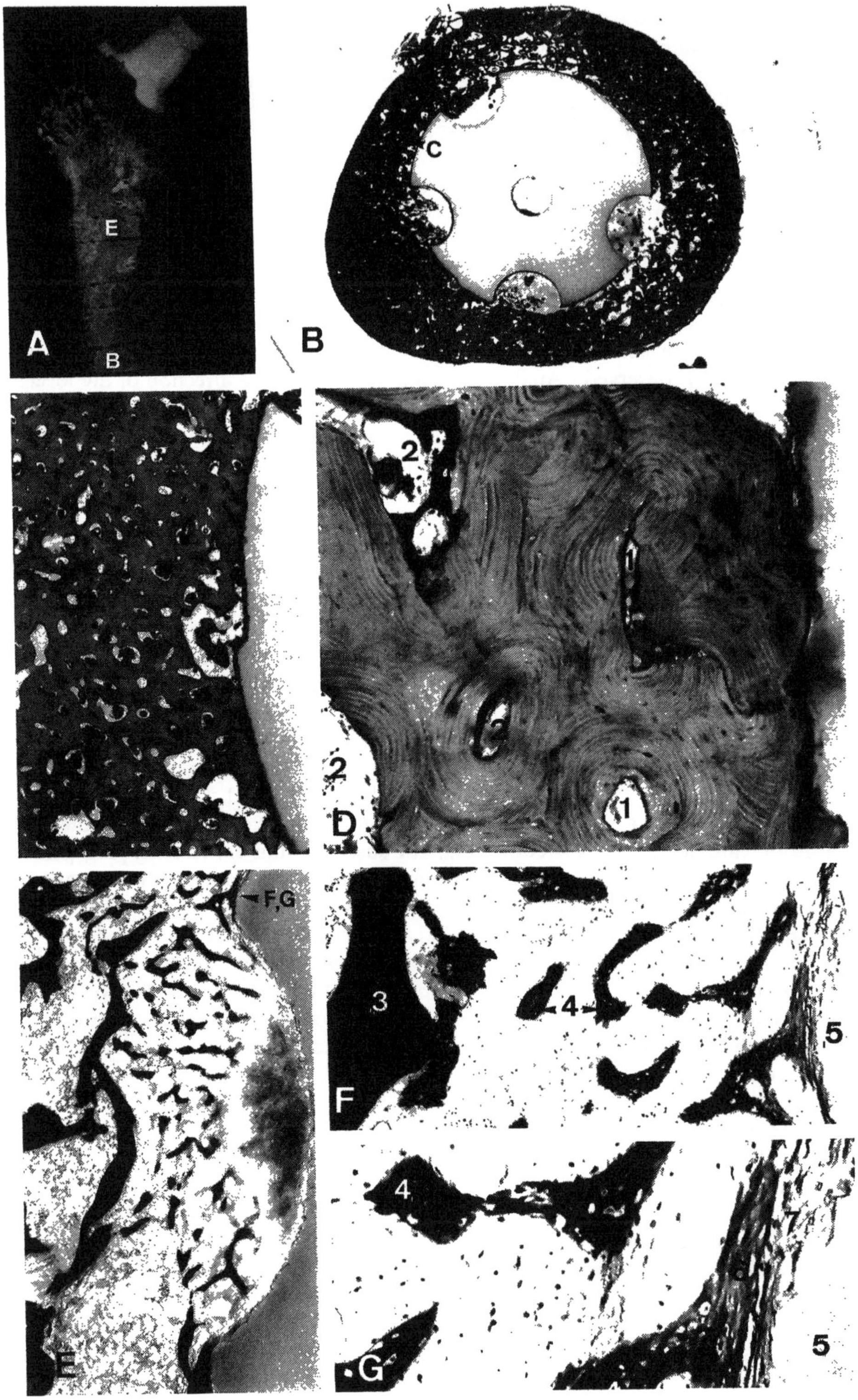
A
B
E
B
C
2
2
1
D
F,G
E
3
4
5
F
4
5
G

laid down directly on the metal and from there proceeds in an "implantofugal" direction to establish a connection with the bone bed. The direct contact between the implant and bone enables weight-bearing loads to be transferred directly to the surrounding bony framework, thus leading early to a true integration of the implant into the cancellous bone.

Discussion

The processes of differentiation that occur along the tissue-implant interface raise the fundamental question of whether and to what extent these processes are caused by material properties or by mechanical influences associated with relative movement. In discussing this question, we may draw on concepts and hypotheses concerning tissue differentiation during fracture healing. The classic concepts of Roux, Pauwels, Krompecher and others concerning the effect of mechanical factors on tissue differentiation have proved valid to the extent that bone formation is confined to "mechanically neutral" zones, i.e., is contingent upon rest and stability. If micromovements [or relative movements after Schneider (1982)] occur, the bone tissue reacts with resorption (Perren et al., 1975), and connective tissue and fibrocartilage form from the granulation tissue. However, recent findings have cast doubt on the notion that the direction of the forces acting on the bone (tension, compression, shear) has a critical bearing on the formation of connective tissue or cartilage. Today it is thought that the magnitude of local tissue deformations is the decisive factor in this regard (Perren and Cordey, 1977). The occurrence of fibrous and cartilaginous tissue during the course of spontaneous or delayed fracture healing is always intermediary, i.e., it is replaced by bone tissue at the edge of the fracture site or bony callus during the process of desmal or chondral ossification. In the case of fibrocartilage, this replacement is initiated by mineralization process, whose failure is a significant factor in the etiology of pseudarthrosis (Mueller et al., 1968; Schenk et al., 1968).

A knowledge of this reaction pattern is helpful in differentiating it from fibrous-tissue encapsulation caused by the properties of the material. The class of biocompatible materials include compounds that release substances which may well precipitate a foreign-body reaction when present in sufficient concentration, but which are not damaging to the tissues (Rahn, personal communication). The tissue reaction to such substances is characterized by the formation of a fibrous connective tissue, accompanied by the appearance of macrophages and possibly giant cells. It is not characterized by an infiltration of round- or polymorphonuclear cells or even necrosis like that seen in incompatibility or inflammatory reactions. Foreign body reactions of this type are seen with certain bone cements (residual monomer?) as well as with the polyacetal prostheses discussed in the present articles (formaldehyde residues?). Only such reactions can explain the fact that gaps between the implant and bone are bridged exclusively in an "implantopetal" direction, while the prosthetic surface remains separated from new bone by a fibrous tissue layer – this despite good primary stability and the proximity of stable contact zones. This interpretation is also supported by the absence of fibrocartilage, which invariably appears after several weeks of instability. The formation of intermediary supportive tissue is governed by the same principles that apply to the "gap healing" of fractures. Schneider (1982) has shown that the processes initiated by relative movements along a bone-cement interface may be either compensated or decompensated, and that even after years, direct bony contact can be achieved through gap healing.

◄

Fig. 1 A–G. Isoelastic femoral prosthesis in a 95-year-old man who died 4 weeks postoperatively (from the clinic of Prof. R. Bombelli). **A** Autopsy specimen prepared for removal of cross-sections (cross-sections B and E are labeled). **B** Distal cross-section with press-fit, 2.5 : 1. **C** Detail showing large contact area between implant and cortex, 15 : 1. **D** The press-fit leads to slight deformation of the implant through the configuration of the inner cortical surface, 80 : 1. *1* – Avascular, devitalized osteons; *2* – Channels with vital contents and reactive bone formation (newly synthesized bone is stained dark). **E** Detail of a proximal shaft cross-section with reactive bone formation in the area of a groove on the prosthetic stem, 15 : 1. **F** "Implantopetal" bone formation, 60 : 1. *3* – Original cancellous bone; *4* – Reactive fiber bone; *5* – Implant **G** Tissue-implant interface, 160 : 1. *6* – Osteoid; *7* – Connective tissue

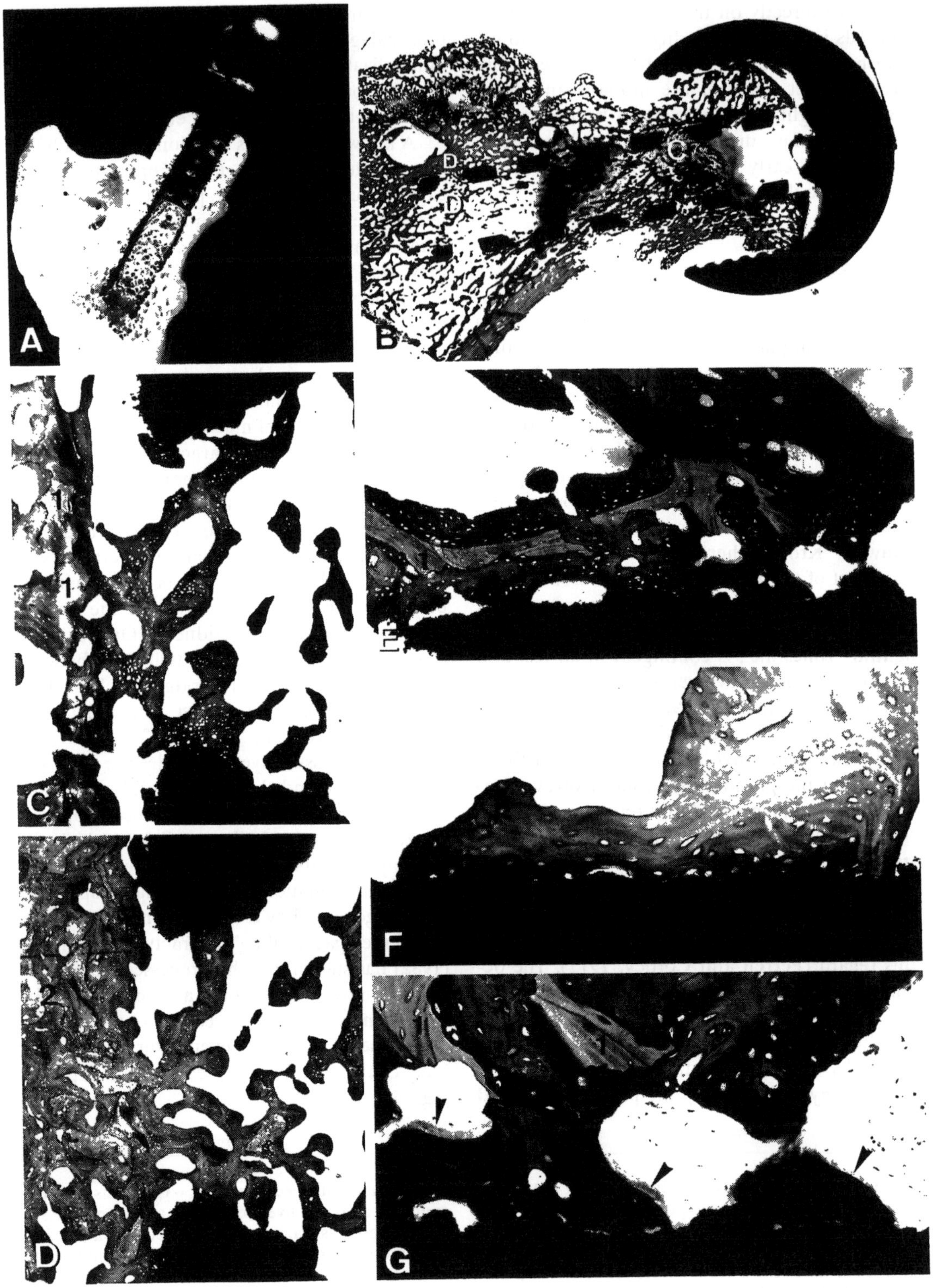
A
B
C
D
E
F
G

Of course a postoperative observation time of 8 weeks provides little basis for predicting the long-term integration of polyacetal prostheses. However, extensive experiments with isoelastic total hip prostheses have been done in sheep in which histologic studies were performed up to 51 weeks after implantation (Muhr et al., 1976). These experiments showed frequent loosening of the femoral component as a result of design factors, while the acetabular components remained clinically stable. In all cases, however, the prosthesis remained isolated from the bone by a rigid connective tissue layer. In the acetabula the fiber architecture of the connective tissue capsule showed a definite alignment with prevailing load lines and was interpreted as a "buffer zone," especially since round cells and giant cells were absent. Cartilage formation was also observed on the unstable femoral prostheses, "particularly at the edges, where the implant and host tissue were in close proximity." Further long-term studies are needed before the chances of producing bony contact can be accurately evaluated.

An opposite pattern of integration is illustrated by the hollow cylindrical implants with a titanium plasma coating. Titanium has proved to be bioinert both experimentally and clinically, although it occasionally leads to a dark discoloration of the tissue and, in small particles, is ingested and removed by macrophages. The titanium plasma coating provides the implant surface with a microstructure which promotes appositional bone growth and substantially enlarges the anchoring surface. In all previous experiments, a direct metal-to-bone contact within the bony implant bed was the rule, and the presence of intervening connective or cartilaginous tissue was a rare exception observed only when instability was grossly apparent. The improved adhesion between the bone and metal has been confirmed by measuring the forces required to loosen cortical bone screws (Hutzschenreuter et al., 1976). It is unclear whether this adhesion is a purely mechanical phenomenon derived from the enlarged interfacial area, or is the result of interactions at a material level.

It has already been mentioned that direct contact between bone and implant enables a direct stress transfer to the bone. This must be taken into account in the design of the prosthesis and during the healing period if damage to the growing bone from excessive stresses is to be avoided. In experiments with mandibular implants, a stress-free postoperative period can be maintained without difficulty. On the other hand, the dogs used in the femoral prosthesis experiments placed full weight on the operated limb only a few days after surgery. Nevertheless, the prosthesis broke loose in only 1 out of 6 cases, and this was due at least in part to an extensive avascular zone in the femoral neck resulting from an intraoperative vascular injury. Thus, the absence of a connective-tissue buffer zone did not prove to be a disadvantage, and direct bony contact indeed appears to promote functional adaptation of the cancellous bed to the forces transferred by the prosthesis, to the extent that a true "osseointegration" (Brånemark et al., 1977) may be said to exist, analogous to that occurring in mandibular implants.

Summary

Advances in histologic preparation techniques, especially the use of the microfraise and surface staining, have made differentiation processes at the tissue-implant boundary even more accessible to microscopic examination. Using specimens of isoelastic femoral prostheses recovered at autopsy, the development of a bony mantle and fibrous tissue capsule during the first 8 weeks is demonstrated and discussed in the light of hypotheses relating to tissue differentiation during fracture healing.

Fig. 2A–G. Experimental cylindrical shell prosthesis with titanium plasma-coated surface. Implantation time = 8 weeks. **A** Demonstration specimen with predrilled prosthesis channel and prosthesis partially inserted. **B** Overview of an operated dog femur, 2.5 : 1. C. D – Location of perforations. **C** Proximal perforation filled with newly-formed trabeculae and supported by old cancellous bone (1), 30 : 1. **D** Distal perforation permeated with new cancellous bone and supported by compact bone (2), 30 : 1. **E** Direct bony apposition has established contact between the implant and old cancellous trabeculae (1), 80 : 1. **F** Bone-metal interface. The white spaces represent osteocyte lacunae and contain vital cells, 160 : 1. **G** "Implantofugal" bone formation, 160 : 1. Note osteoid seams at sites of advanced bone apposition (*arrows*)

The bony integration of femoral head prostheses that are constructed of titanium alloy and coated with titanium plasma was investigated experimentally in dogs. A direct deposition of bone on the titanium plasma layer could be observed, leading to early contact between the implant and adjacent cancellous or cortical bone and resulting in a firm bony anchorage that transfers loads directly to the bone without the formation of a buffer zone.

References

Brånemark PI, Hansson BO, Adell R, Breine U, Lindström J, Hallén O, Oehman A (1977) Osseointegrated implants in the treatment of the edentulous jaw. Scand J Plast Reconstr Surg [Suppl] 11:16

Gross UM, Strunz V (1977) Surface staining of sawed sections of undecalcified bone containing alloplastic implants. Stain Technol 52:217

Hutzschenreuter P, Claes L, Pohler O (1976) Lösemomente bei Corticaliszugschrauben mit unterschiedlicher Oberfläche und ihre histologischen Korrelate. Helv Chir Acta 43:765

Morscher E, Bombelli R, Schenk R, Mathys R (1981) The treatment of femoral neck fractures with an isoelastic endoprosthesis implanted without bone cement. Arch Orthop Traum Surg 98:93

Muhr G, Stockhusen H, Müller O (1976) Die Hüftarthroplastik mit isoelastischen Totalprothesen im Tierexperiment. Arch Orthop Unfallchir 86:115

Müller J, Schenk R, Willenegger H (1968) Experimentelle Untersuchungen über die Entstehung reaktiver Pseudarthrosen am Hunderadius. Helv Chir Acta 35:301

Perren SM, Cordey J (1977) Die Gewebsdifferenzierung in der Frakturheilung. Unfallheilkunde 80:161

Perren SM, Ganz R, Rueter A (1975) Oberflächliche Knochenresorption um Implantate. Med Orthop Tech 75:6

Schenk R (1965) Zur histologischen Verarbeitung von unentkalkten Knochen. Acta Anat (Basel) 60:3

Schenk R, Müller J, Willenegger H (1968) Experimentell-histologischer Beitrag zur Entstehung und Behandlung von Pseudarthrosen.Hefte Unfallheilkd 94:15

Schneider R (1982) Die Totalprothese der Hüfte. Ein biomechanisches Konzept und seine Konsequenzen. Aktuel Probl Chir Orthop 24

Schroeder A, Pohler O, Sutter F (1976) Gewebereaktion auf ein Titan-Hohlzylinderimplantat mit Titan-Spritzschichtoberfläche. SSO Schweiz Monatsschr Zahnheilkd 86:713

Schroeder A, Stich H, Straumann F, Sutter F (1978) Über die Anlagerung von Osteozement an einen belasteten Implantatkörper. SSO Schweiz Monatsschr Zahnheilkd 88:1051

Sutter F, Schenk R, Butler H, Schürch H, Straumann F (1982) Entwicklung einer Hohlzylinder-Schalenprothese als Femurkopfersatz. Med Orthop Tech 82:103

Metallic Implant Materials for Hip Joint Endoprostheses Designed for Cemented and Cementless Fixation

M. Semlitsch

Introduction

Since the 1940s metallic implant materials have been predominantly used for the manufacture of artificial hip joints. In the 1960s artificial acetabular sockets were also manufactured from polymers, and femoral components made from these materials were tested in the 1970s. Aluminium oxide ceramic, which was also introduced in 1970s, has since found acceptance as an implant material for the femoral and acetabular components of various total hip systems. In the last few years carbon has also been tested as a material for total hip prostheses (Willert – Semlitsch, 1981).

Choice of Metallic Implant Materials

The choice of implant materials (Semlitsch – Willert, 1981) used for the manufacture of artificial hip joints is relatively large today (Table 1). At first the choice was limited mainly to cast CoCrMo alloy ISO 5832-4 and stainless steel ISO 5832-1B, as well as to wrought TiAlV alloy ISO 5832-3 for a very small number of hip prosthesis models.

In the early 1970s the range of these three cobalt-, iron- and titanium-base alloys was extended by the addition of wrought CoNiCrMo alloy ISO 5832-6. For many years now this high-strength and extremely corrosion-resistant implant material has been used for the manufacture of femoral stems. Clinical experience gained over ten years with more than 450,000 series-produced hip prostheses has demonstrated the high fracture resistance of anchoring stems made of this implant material.

The next implant material introduced in the late 1970s was a CoCrMo alloy produced by powder metallurgy (P/M) and forging. The chemical composition of this high-strength alloy is practically identical to that of the cast CoCrMo alloy ISO 5832-4.

A further addition to these three cobalt-base implant materials was the cast and wrought CoCrNiMo alloy ISO 5832-7, which is used mainly in France.

The early 1980s saw the introduction of a stainless steel variant alloyed with nitrogen (ISO 5832-1C), accepted within the scope of ISO Standard 5832-1. In addition to this, there has been an ISO proposal for an FeCrNiMnMoNbN stainless steel of enhanced strength and corrosion resistance (Smethurst, 1981).

In recent years researchers have conducted a number of experimental animal studies with the NiTi memory alloy (Bensmann, 1979) and have also been investigating the pure metals tantalum and niobium produced by powder metallurgy processes (Schider, 1982).

Tabelle 1. Metallic materials for total hip prostheses

Standard	Condition	Composition
ISO 5832-1B -1C	WF CW WF	Fe-18Cr-14Ni-3Mo Fe-18Cr-14Ni-3Mo-N
ISO Proposal	CW WF	Fe-21Cr-9Ni-4Mn-3Mo-Nb-N
ISO 5832-3 -	WF C	Ti-6Al-4V
- - -	C WF WF	Ti-5Al-2,5Fe Ti-
ISO 5832-4 ASTM Proposal	C PM WF	Co-28Cr-6Mo
ISO 5832-6 ASTM 562-78	WF CW	Co-35Ni-20Cr-10Mo
ISO 5832-7 ISO Proposal	WF C	Co-20Cr-17Ni-7Mo
-	WF	Ni-45Ti
ASTM F 560-78 -	PM PM	Ta 100 Nb 100

C.....cast CW....cold worked
WF....wrought + forged PM....powder metallurgy

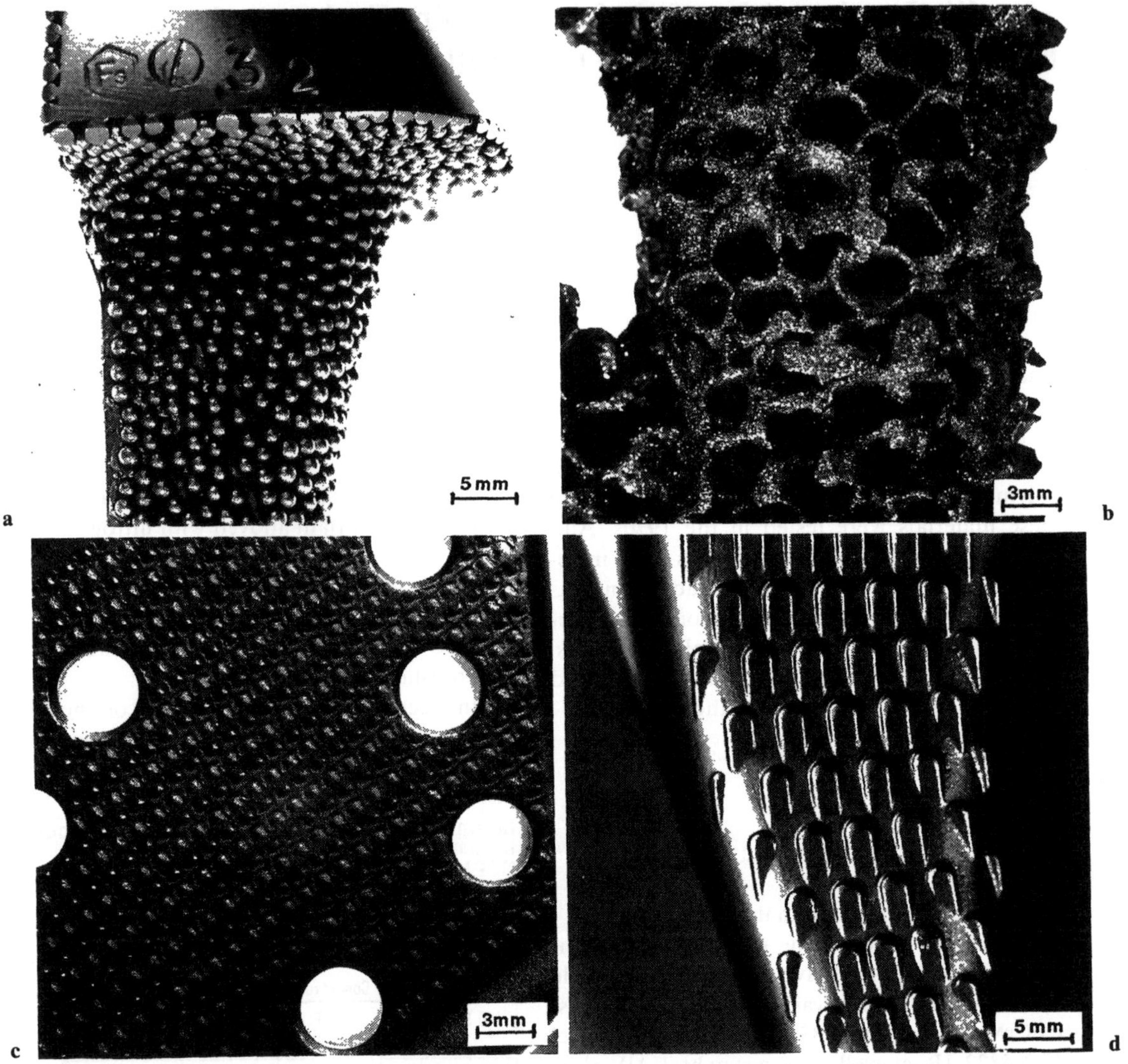

Fig. 1a–d. Surface microstructures of metallic femoral prostheses designed for cement-free implantation. **a** Cast-on CoCrMo globules (Lord prosthesis). **b** Cast-on CoCrNiMo craterlets (Judet prosthesis). **c** Machined surface relief on TiAlV (Zweymüller prosthesis) **d** Tear-shaped surface projections on TiAlV (Parhofer prosthesis)

As an addition to the TiAlV implant alloy, which has proved itself in clinical application since the 1950s (Laing, 1981), further titanium-base alloys, e.g. TiAlFe in cast and forged condition, are also being considered as candidates for the manufacture of hip prostheses (Zwicker, 1980).

In the case of ten total hip prostheses implanted without cement, where there is direct contact between the bone and the metallic femoral stem (Fig. 1) and to some extent the metallic acetabular socket, both implant components are manufactured from the two cast CoCrMo and CoCrNiMo alloys, as well as from TiAlV alloy in forged and cast condition (Table 2).

Wear Properties

An implanted total hip prosthesis is subjected to severe corrosive and mechanical stresses within the body (Fig. 2). The latter result from the millionfold motion of the head in the socket, eventually leading to wear of the articulating

Author	used since	Stem		Ball head		Hip socket			
		Metal		Metal	Ceramic	Polymer	Metal		Ceramic
		C	WF	C			C		
SIVASH	1965		TiAlV	CoCrMo		(PE)	CoCrMo	TiAlV	
RING	1967	CoCrMo		CoCrMo			CoCrMo		
URIST-MOORE	1969	CoCrMo		CoCrMo			CoCrMo		
SBARBARO-MOORE	1970	CoCrMo		CoCrMo			CoCrMo		
JUDET	1971	CoCrNiMo		CoCrNiMo		PE	CoCrNiMo		
LORD	1973	CoCrMo		CoCrMo	(Al_2O_3)	PE	CoCrMo		
MITTELMEIER	1974	CoCrMo			Al_2O_3				Al_2O_3
BOUTIN	1975		TiAlV		Al_2O_3				Al_2O_3
ZWEYMULLER	1979		TiAlV		Al_2O_3	PE			
PARHOFER (PM)	1980		TiAlV		Al_2O_3	PE		TiAlV	

Metal: C .... Cast alloys Ti-6Al-4V, Co-28Cr-6Mo, Co-20Cr-17Ni-7Mo
WF........ Wrought alloy Ti-6Al-4V
Ceramic: Al_2O_3..... Sintered ceramic
Polymer: PE........ Ultra-high molecular weight polyethylene
( ).....alternative

Tabelle 2. Total hip prostheses with direct contact between the bone and metal stem, as well as between the bone and acetabular socket made of metal, ceramic or polyethylene

surfaces (Willert – Semlitsch, 1978). Since the inception of hip joint replacement, various material combinations have proved effective in clinical use (Table 3).

The metal/metal combination (cast CoCrMo alloy ISO 5832-4) in the original Mueller hip prosthesis with an optimal clearance of about 0.2 mm shows only minimal wear even after 10 years implantation. Nevertheless, the metal-on-metal concept came under fire in the late 1960s because of a "microfit" between the head and socket of another hip prosthesis (McKee, 1982) in which the thinwalled acetabular component showed a tendency to distortion that caused seizing of the metal head. This resulted in severe abrasion of metal particles from the articulating surfaces of the components, and these eventually caused severe foreign-body reactions in the tissue. Moreover, the socket and stem tended to loosen because of the increased frictional forces

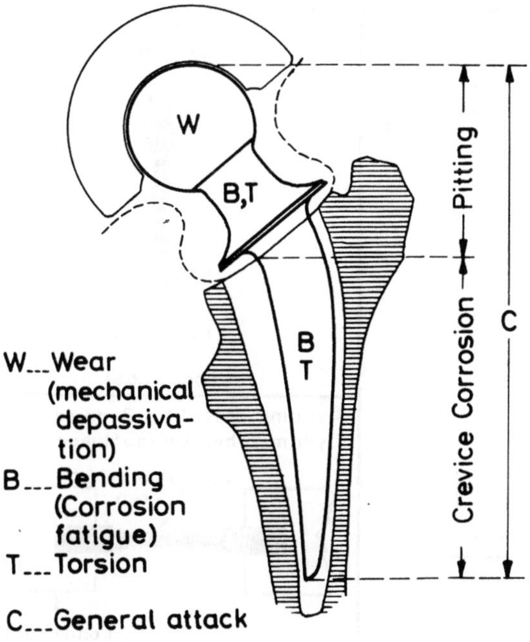

Fig. 2. Mechanical and chemical effects on a total hip prosthesis implanted in the body

Table 3. Material combinations for the socket and head of total hip prostheses

Hip socket	Ball head
Co Cr Mo – C	Co Cr Mo – C
UHMW-Polyethylene	Fe Cr Ni Mo – WF Fe Cr Ni Mn Mo – WF
	Co Cr Mo – C Co Cr Ni Mo – C
	Hard chromium on Co Ni Cr Mo – WF
	Ti Al V – WF
	Al_2O_3-ceramic
Al_2O_3-ceramic	Al_2O_3-ceramic
Carbon, isotropic	Carbon, SiC-infiltrated

C .... Cast alloy
WF.......... Wrought+forged alloy

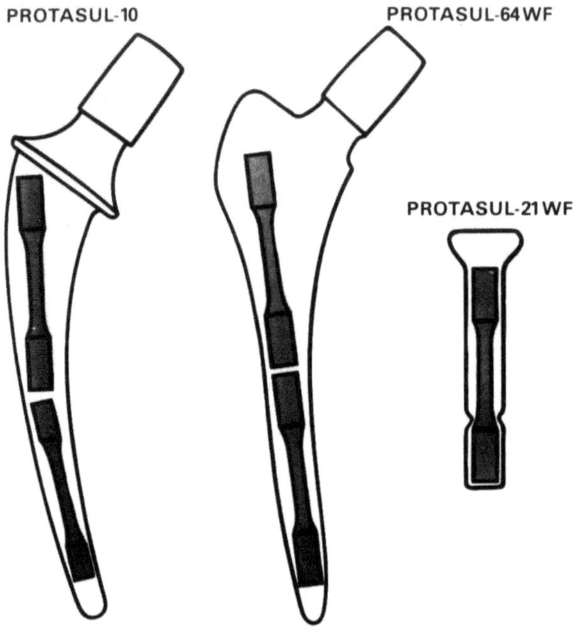

Fig. 3. Sources of cylindrical test specimens in forged femoral components.

transmitted to the anchoring zone between the acrylic cement and the bone.

Most of the total hip replacements in current use feature a metal/polyethylene combination for the head and socket. Past experience has shown that an annual wear rate of 0.05 –0.25 mm in the polyethylene socket is a reasonable estimate. A femoral ball made of extremely high-purity and high-strength Al_2O_3 ceramic (e.g. Biolox quality) in combination with a polyethylene socket (Semlitsch, 1976), which has been in clinical use since the mid-1970s, shows good promise of a lower long-term wear rate for the polyethylene socket (Niederer, 1978, Weber, 1981).

As an alternative to these material combinations, clinicians can also make use of ceramic/ceramic and carbon/carbon combinations.

Corrosion Resistance

Since a total hip prosthesis implanted in the body is subject to corrosive attack as illustrated in Fig. 2, utmost attention should be paid to the selection of the material for long-term implants. It is generally known that cobalt- and titanium-base alloys possess a higher corrosion resistance than high-alloy iron-base implant materials. With cobalt- and iron-base alloys, this can be expressed by the corrosion resistance index (Table 4). An unsuitable combination of metallic materials in a total hip prosthesis may give rise to galvanic corrosive processes (e.g. iron-

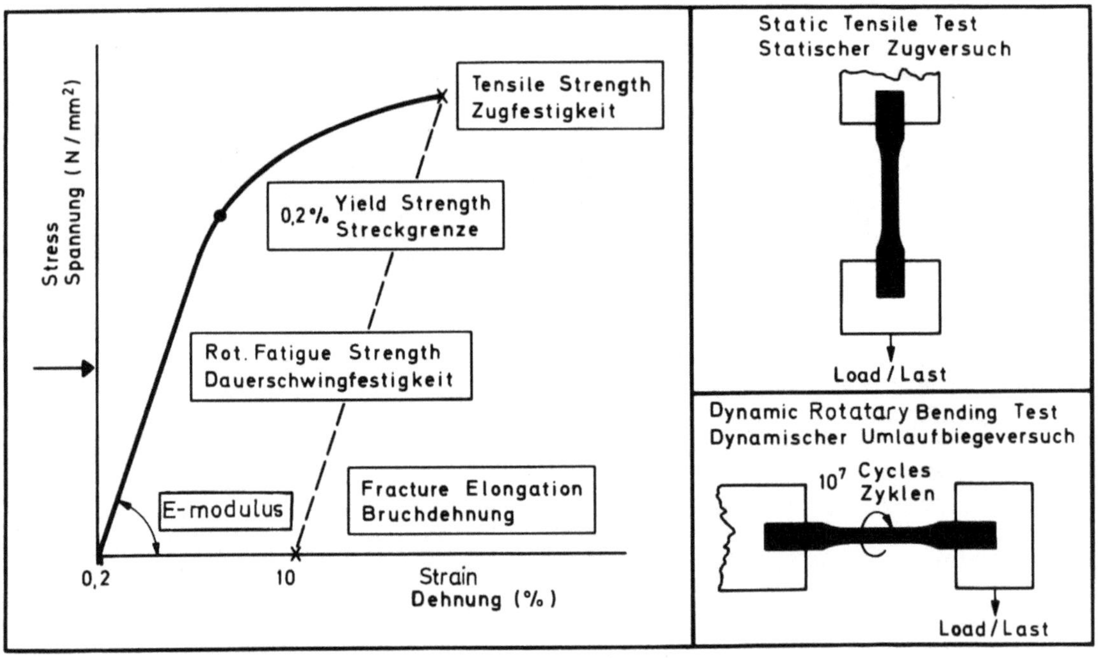

Fig. 4. Mechanical properties of metallic materials, determined in tensile tests and rotary bending tests

Table 4. Corrosion resistance of implant alloys

Implant Alloys	Structure	Elements in Weight %: C	Cr	Mo	N	Corrosion Resistance: Index Cr + 3.3 Mo + 16 N	Level (1 L, 2 M, 3 H)
Fe Cr Ni Mo AISI - 316 L	Austenite	0,03	18	3	-	28	
Fe Cr Ni Mo Mn Nb N St. St. ORTRON - 90	Austenite	0,05	21	3	0,4	37	
Co Cr Mo PROTASUL - 2 PROTASUL - 21 WF	Austenite plus Carbides	0.25	28	6	-	45	
Co Ni Cr Mo PROTASUL - 10	Austenite	0,025	20	10	-	53	

3... High 2... Medium 1... Low Corrosion Resistance Level

Table 5. Modulus of elasticity E of implant ceramic, metals, carbons and polymers compared with Young's modulus of bone

Materials	0 – 100 – 200 – 300 – 400 x 10^3 N/mm²
Ceramic	
Al_2O_3	380000
Metals	
Co Ni Cr Mo	230000
Co Cr Mo	220000
Fe Cr Ni Mo	200000
Ta	190000
Nb	115000
Ti Al V	110000
Carbons	
CFRC	140000
SiC/C	100000
ISC	25000
Polymers	
Polyacrylat	2500 - 4000
Polyacetal	2800 - 3200
Polyester	2800 - 3100
Polypropylene	1000 - 1600
Polyethylene	500 - 1000
Polysilicon	10
Bone	
Corticalis	8000 - 24000
Spongiosa	700 - 4000

base alloys like ISO 5832-1 with cobalt- or titanium-base alloys). On the other hand, the currently used cobalt- and titanium-base surgical implant alloys can be safely combined with each other because they show outstanding corrosion resistance in the physiologic environment.

Mechanical Properties

An accurate knowledge of the mechanical properties of the implant material is an essential prerequisite for the design of fracture-resistant femoral prosthetic stems. The mechanical strength values are determined in static tensile tests and dynamic rotary bending tests (Fig. 4), preferably on cylindrical test specimens taken from the femoral components themselves (Fig. 3). The following significance is attributed to the relevant mechanical properties of surgical implant materials:

- *Modulus of elasticity E* as the measure of the elasticity and stiffness of the implant,
- *0.2% yield strength $R_{p0.2}$* as the measure of resistance to permanent deformation of the implant,
- *ultimate tensile strength R_m* as the measure of resistance to fracture of the implant under loading,
- *fracture elongation A_5* as the measure of the toughness of the implant,
- *Rotary bending fatigue strength σ_{bW}* as the measure of the fracture resistance of an implant subjected to many million loading cycles.

In total hip prostheses that are implanted without cement, and particularly in the case of anchoring stems, the elastic modulus of the implant material is a matter of crucial importance (Table 5). It is always compared with the elastic modulus of the adjacent bone (Fig. 5). Strictly

Alloy	ISO-No	N/mm²
▶ Fe Cr Ni Mo	5832 - 1	
annealed		290 - 370
cold - worked		800
hot - forged		1000 - 1070
▶ Fe Cr Ni Mo Mn Nb N	—	
ORTRON^{R} - 90 cold - worked		810 - 950
▶ Ti Al V	5832 - 3	
PROTASUL^{R} - 64WF hot-forged, annealed		900 - 1080
▶ Co Cr Mo	5832 - 4	
cast		450 - 600
▶ Co Cr Mo	—	
hot - forged		
PROTASUL^{R} - 21 WF		900 - 1200
VITALLIUM^{R} - FHS		860 - 930
ENDOCAST^{R} - SL		1000
powder metallurgy		
ZIMALOY - Micro Grain		820 - 920
▶ Co Ni Cr Mo	5832 - 6	
PROTASUL^{R} - 10 hot-forged, hard		1000 - 1600
BIOPHASE^{R} cold - worked		1585

Table 6. 0.2% yield strength of implant alloys for total hip prostheses

speaking, we should consider the elasticity and/or stiffness of an implant cross-section in relation to the surrounding bone cross-section in order to be able to estimate the magnitude of relative movements between the implant and bone.

On the basis of their mechanical properties (Tables 6–9) the implant alloys currently in clinical use may be divided into three strength categories: low, medium and high (Table 10). For economic reasons some manufacturers are still using low-strength implant alloys for highly-stressed endoprosthetic stems. In this connection particular attention should be given to larger stem cross-sections as a means of reducing stresses along the lateral surface of the stem under physiologic loading conditions. High-strength implant alloys allow much greater latitude in design with a greater safety margin against fracture of the implant.

Fatigue Strength of Femoral Prostheses

On the basis of 10 years' experience with over 450,000 series-produced fracture-proof femoral prostheses made from high-strength wrought Protasul alloys, it is advisable to subject every stem of new design to static and dynamic strength testing. For these tests, the femoral prosthesis is placed in neutral position into the standard femur proposed by Ungethuem (Fig. 6). The stem is embedded at levels up to 50 mm below the collar of the prosthesis. This allows extreme loosening of the stem to be simulated. Clinical experience has shown that the possibility of stem loosening of any femoral endoprosthesis cannot be eliminated entirely. In the event of loosening, the fracture always starts on the heavily-loaded lateral side of the stem. Hence, the stresses that develop there under a static load F (1000–11,000 N) are of particular

Table 7. Ultimate tensile strength values of implant alloys for total hip prostheses

Alloy	ISO-No	0 … 800 1000 … 1800 N/mm²
▶ FeCrNiMo	5832-1	
annealed		480-600
cold-worked		860
hot-forged		1100-1170
▶ FeCrNiMoMnNbN	—	
ORTRON® - 90 cold-worked		1030-1150
▶ TiAlV	5832-3	
PROTASUL® - 64WF hot-forged, annealed		1000-1120
▶ CoCrMo	5832-4	
cast		665-1000
▶ CoCrMo	—	
hot-forged		
PROTASUL® - 21WF		1400-1600
VITALLIUM® - FHS		1200-1280
ENDOCAST® - SL		1250-1400
powder metallurgy		
ZIMALOY - Micro Grain		1200-1300
▶ CoNiCrMo	5832-6	
PROTASUL® - 10 hot-forged, hard		1200-1700
BIOPHASE® cold-worked		1790

Alloy	ISO-No	Elongation (0–50 %)
FeCrNiMo	5832-1	
annealed		40
cold-worked		12
hot-forged		10-14
FeCrNiMoMnNbN	—	
ORTRON®-90 cold-worked		15
TiAlV	5832-3	
PROTASUL®-64WF hot-forged, annealed		10-15
CoCrMo	5832-4	
cast		8-25
CoCrMo	—	
hot-forged		
PROTASUL®-21WF		8-20
VITALLIUM®-FHS		15
ENDOCAST®-SL		15
powder metallurgy		
ZIMALOY-Micro Grain		15
CoNiCrMo	5832-6	
PROTASUL®-10 hot-forged, hard		10-15
BIOPHASE® cold-worked		8

Table 8. Elongation values of implant alloys for total hip prostheses

interest. The distribution of stresses along the lateral aspect of the stem are determined by means of strain gauges attached to the stem surface (Fig. 7). With increasing load F, the maximum bending stresses always arise at the junction (gauge position 3) of the embedded and unembedded portions of the stem. It is here that the crack would be initiated in a loosened endoprosthetic stem.

The smallest stems of the Zweymüller prosthesis (Figs. 7a and b) can be subjected to a multiple load of 3000 N (about three times the body weight of 100 kg) without permanent deformation. Moreover, the higher the 0.2% yield strength of the material used for the stem (900–1080 N/mm^2 for the wrought Ti–6Al–4V alloy Protasul-64 WF), the higher the elastic load capacity of the stem (8000 and 11,000 N corresponding to 760 and 720 N/mm^2, respectively, along the lateral side of the stem).

In order to determine the safety margin against fracture of the stem, the structural strength of the simulated loose stem should also be tested under dynamic loading conditions (Semlitsch – Panic, 1981).

These tests are performed in an air-fluxed physiologic saline solution at a temperature of 37 °C with pulsating loads of up to 5–10 million cycles applied at a frequency of 5–10 Hz (Fig. 8, right). The test results obtained with twenty Zweymüller femoral prostheses of two different models are plotted in a Woehler diagram (Fig. 8, left). This reveals that the smallest model 10 of the 7-stem modular system can be subjected to pulsating fatigue loads of 5500–6000 N (about six times the body weight of 90–100 kg) without breaking even under these extremely harsh test conditions.

In the case of the larger prosthesis model 12.5 S, the pulsating load can be as high as

Table 9. Rotary bending fatigue strength of implant alloys for total hip prostheses

Alloy	ISO-No	N/mm²
▶ Fe Cr Ni Mo	5832 - 1	
annealed		250
cold - worked		350
hot - forged		340-380
▶ Fe Cr Ni Mo Mn Nb N	—	
ORTRON[R] - 90 cold - worked		580
▶ Ti Al V	5832 - 3	
PROTASUL[R] - 64 WF hot-forged, annealed		500-660
▶ Co Cr Mo	5832 - 4	
cast		190-400
▶ Co Cr Mo	——	
hot - forged		
PROTASUL[R] - 21 WF		600-870
VITALLIUM[R] - FHS		500-750
ENDOCAST[R] - SL		550-625
powder metallurgy		
ZIMALOY - Micro Grain		620-790
▶ Co Ni Cr Mo	5832 - 6	
PROTASUL[R] - 10 hot-forged, hard		500-800
BIOPHASE[R] cold - worked		540-600

Table 10. Mechanical properties of metallic materials, determined in static tensile tests and dynamic rotary bending tests

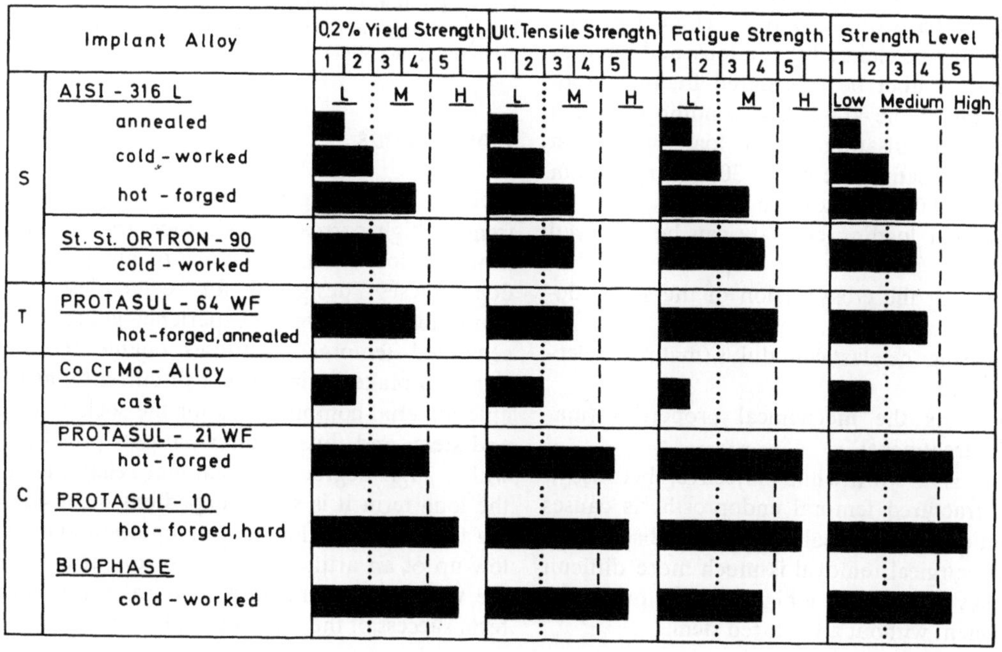

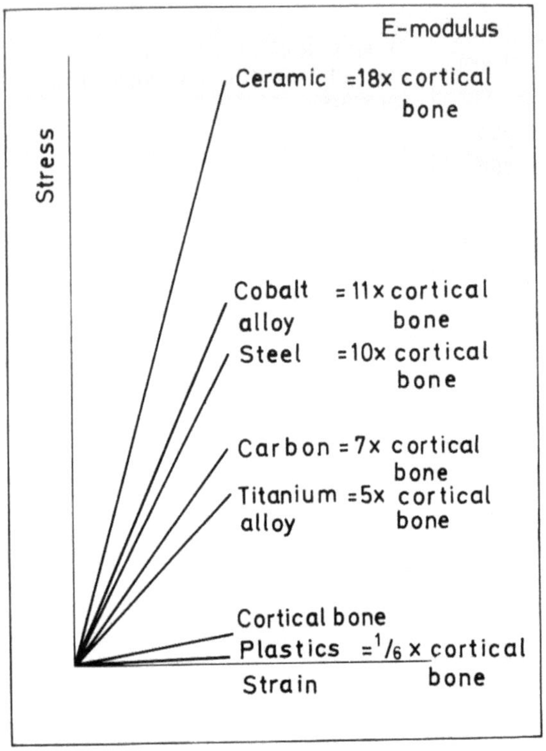

Fig. 5. Elasticity of various implant materials, expressed as a multiple of the elasticity of cortical bone

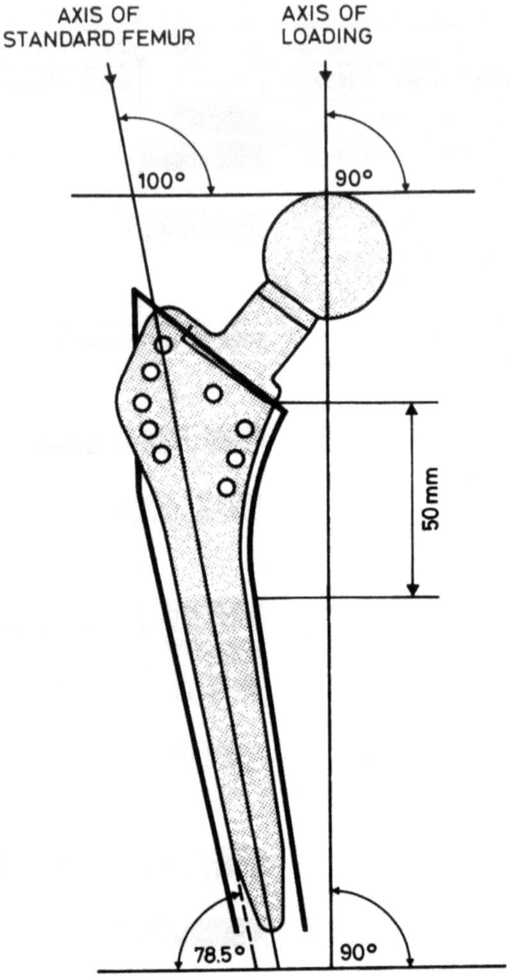

Fig. 6. Position of simulated loose Zweymüller femoral prosthesis in the standard femur (stem fixed 50 mm below collar)

9000–9500 N. These values signify a high safety margin against fracture that can scarcely be attained with some femoral prostheses designed for implantation without cement.

On the basis of many years' clinical experience, it may be claimed that a loosened femoral prosthesis cannot be considered fracture-proof unless, under the above test conditions, it can withstand a pulsating fatigue load of at least 2800 N (pulsating between 300 N = minimum load and 3100 N = maximum load).

A higher loading capacity can be achieved by:

- increasing the cross-section of the stem (design),
- increasing the elastic modulus (material selection) and
- improving the mechanical properties (material treatment).

This is a worthwhile objective, because a loose, fractured femoral endoprosthesis causes the patient a great deal of pain and discomfort, and its surgical removal is much more difficult and risky than that of a high-strength prosthetic component without a fractured stem.

Conclusions

Several high-strength implant alloys of extremely high corrosion resistance are currently available for the manufacture of hip joint endoprostheses designed for cementless implantation. Many years' experience gained with cemented femoral prostheses enable the designer to make optimum use of currently available material combinations for the socket, head and stem, and thus to offer patients prostheses with a high degree of functional reliability. In the long term it is surely expedient – considering the high costs for the implantation and follow-up of an artificial hip – not to cut costs in the wrong areas and thus jeopardize the long-term success of the total hip replacement.

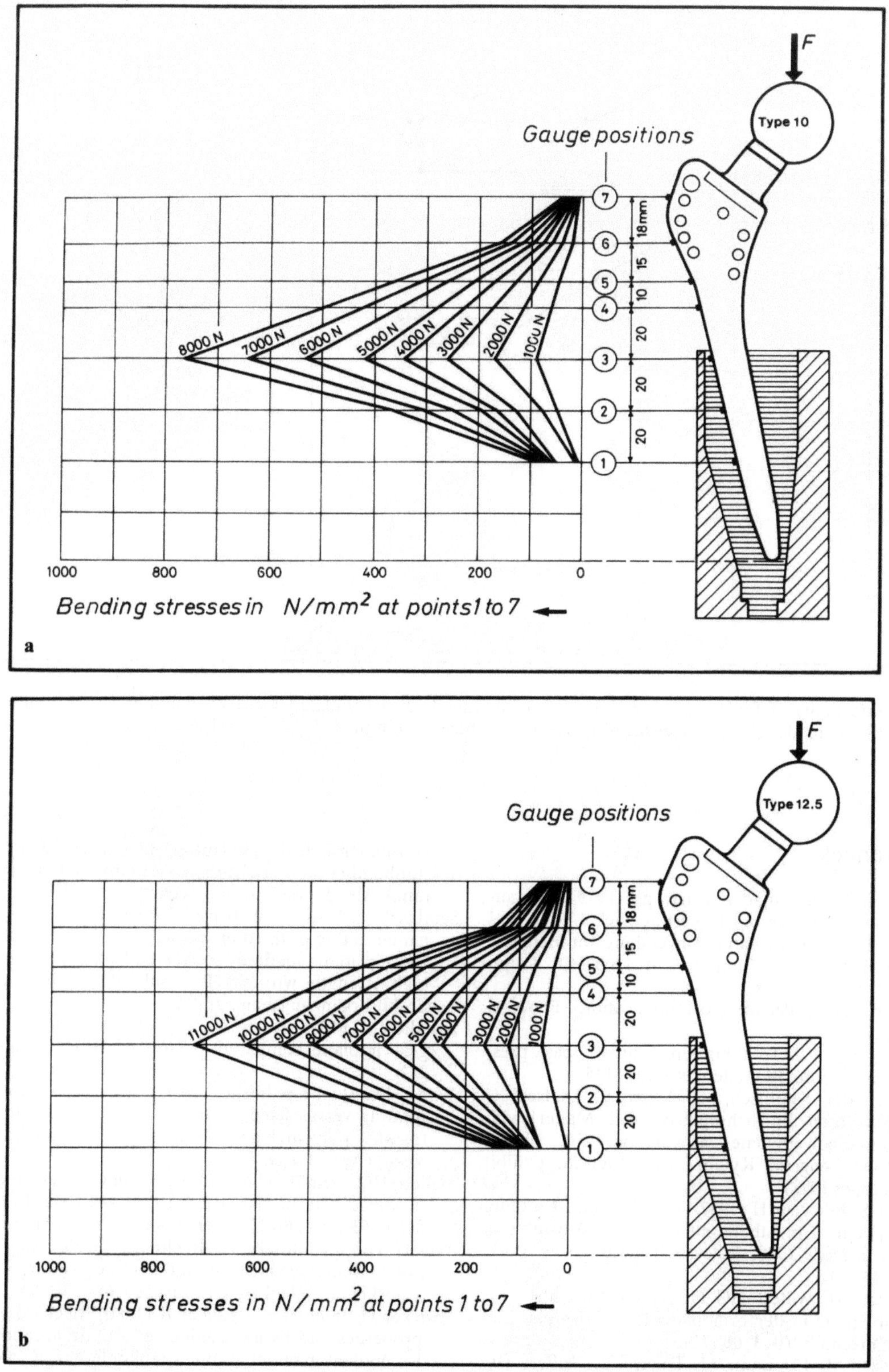

Fig. 7. Distribution of bending stresses along the lateral surface of a simulated loose Zweymüller femoral stem, model 10 (a) and model 12.5 S (b), under static loads of 1000–11,000 N

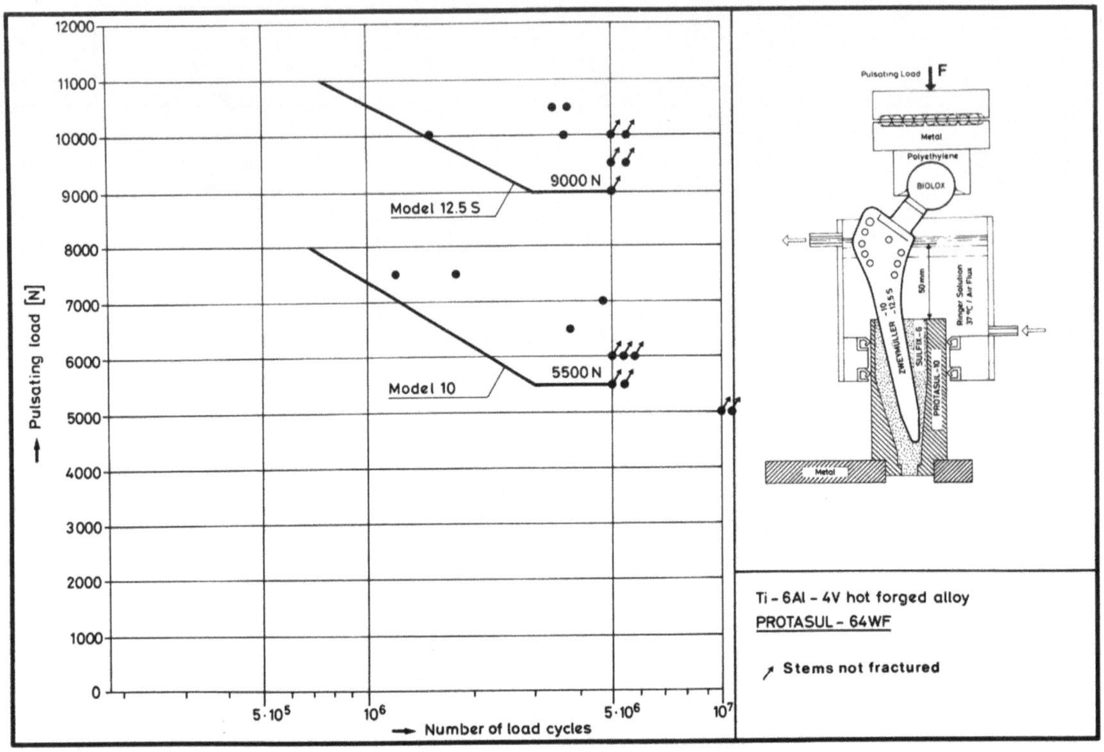

Fig. 8. Safe limits of functional corrosion fatigue loading F of a simulated loose Zweymüller femoral stem (model 10 and model 12.5 S) under the test conditions indicated at right

References

Bensmann G, Baumgart F, Hartwig J (1979) Untersuchungen der Memory-Legierung Nickel-Titan und Überlegungen zu ihrer Anwendung im Bereiche der Medizin. Forschungsbericht. Tech Mitt Krupp 37/1:21–34

Laing P (1981) Personal communication (Phoenix, USA)

McKee GK (1982) Total hip replacement – past, present and future. Biomaterials 3:130–135

Niederer PG, Semlitsch M, Doerre E, Dietschi C (1978) Total hip arthroplasty (M.E. Müller) with ceramic-polyethylene articulation. 14. World SICOT Congress, Kyoto/Japan, Scientific Exhibit (Oktober 1978)

Schider S, Bildstein H (1982) Tantalum and Niobium as potential prosthetic materials. In: Advances in biomaterials 1980. Wiley, Chichester New York, pp 13–20

Semlitsch M, Willert HG (1981) Biomaterialien für Implantate in der orthopädischen Chirurgie. Medizintechnik 101:3, 66–72

Semlitsch M, Lehmann M, Doerre E, Willert HG (1976) Neue Perspektiven zu verlängerter Funktionsdauer künstlicher Hüftgelenke durch Werkstoffkombination Polyäthylen-Aluminiumoxidkeramik-Metall. Med Orthop Techn. 96:152–160

Semlitsch M, Panic B, Weber H, Schoen R (1981) Dynamic testing of the dimensional stability of artificial hip joints made of cobalt- and titanium-base high strength wrought Protasul alloys. Biomed Techn Ergänzungsband 26:94

Smethurst E (1981) A new stainless steel alloy for surgical implants compared to 316 S 12. Biomaterials 2:2

Weber BG (to be published) Total hip replacement, rotating versus fixed, metal versus ceramic heads (against polyethylene). Orthop. Res. Society Las Vegas (April 1981)

Willert HG, Semlitsch M (1981) Biomaterialien und orthopädische Implantate. In: Orthopädie in Praxis und Klinik, Bd II. Thieme, Stuttgart New York

Willert HG, Semlitsch M, Buchhorn G, Kriete U (1978) Materialverschleiß und Gewebereaktion bei künstlichen Gelenken. Orthopäde 7:62–83

Zwicker U, Buehler K, Mueller R (1980) Mechanical properties and tissue reactions of a titanium alloy for implant material. 4. Int. Titankonferenz, Kyoto (Mai 1980)

The Use of Polymers for Endoprosthetic Components

R. Mathys and R. Mathys, Jr.

Introduction

The outstanding chemical stability and tribologic properties of polymers have favored their introduction as implant materials. In 1946 the Judet Bros. [5] introduced polymethylmethacrylate as a material for femoral endoprostheses. In 1958 Charnley used polytetrafluoroethylene (Teflon) for an acetabular prosthesis which was cemented into place with cold-curing polymethylmethacrylate. When the Teflon showed an unacceptable degree of wear, Charnley [2, 3] introduced high-density polyethylene as an alternative material for acetabular prostheses.

Structure of the Polymers

Polymers can be divided into two main groups: duroplastics and thermoplastics.

The duroplastics form a three-dimensional cross-linked macromolecule during polymerization (Fig. 1). Once the polymer has formed, it cannot be remolded even by heating. Because of this, molding is usually done concurrently with polymerization.

The thermoplastics form linear macromolecules on polymerization (Fig. 1). These chain-like molecules may form an irregular, tangled mass (amorphous state) or may be in close contact with one another, forming crystalline zones (semi-crystalline state). All thermoplastics have a characteristic melting point which is determined by the covalent bonding energy of their atoms.

In thin sections of semi-crystalline polymers, the crystalline zones can be visualized by polarized light. These zones are called spherolites.

The molecular structures of the polymers currently used as implant materials range from

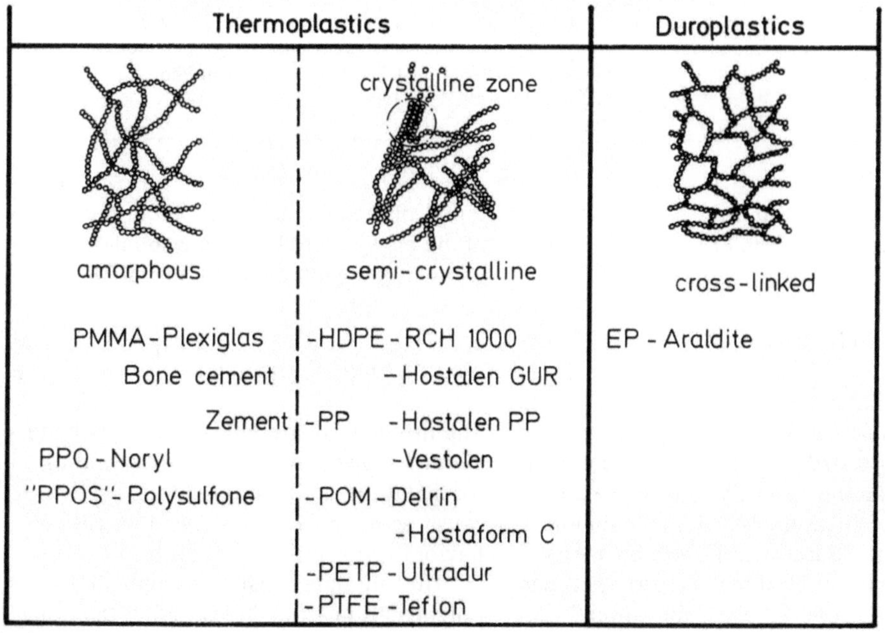

Fig. 1

Table 1. Chemical Structure of Polymers

Name of polymer	Structural formula	Density g/cm³	Crystallinity (in %)	Molecular weight
Polyethylene (PE, HDPE)	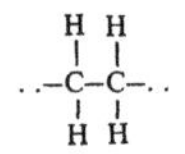	0.915 0.935 0.965	55 70 95	$3.5 \cdot 10^6$ $4 \cdot 10^6$
Polypropylene (PP)	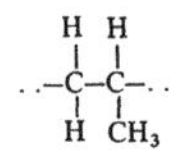	0.900 0.907	60 70	$4 \cdot 10^5$ $8 \cdot 10^5$
Polytetrafluoroethylene (PTFE, Teflon)	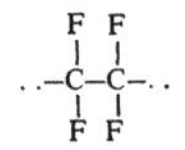	2.0 2.3	55 62	$4 \cdot 10^5$ $8 \cdot 10^5$
Polyacetal (POM) Homopolymer	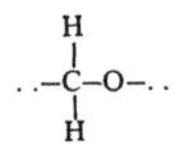	1.41 1.42	70 80	$4 \cdot 10^4$ $9 \cdot 10^4$
Copolymer	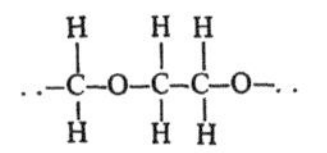	1.41	70 75	$4 \cdot 10^4$ $9 \cdot 10^4$
Polyethylene glycol terephthalate (PETP)	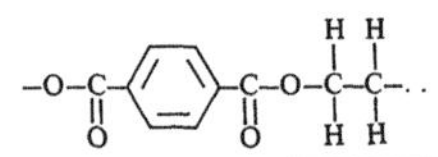	1.38	30 40	$3 \cdot 10^4$ $4 \cdot 10^4$
Polymethylmethacrylate (PMMA)	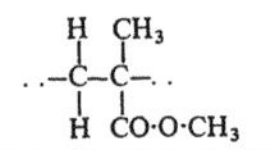	1.18	amorphous	$1 \cdot 10^6$ $1.5 \cdot 10^6$
Polyphenylene oxide (PPO)	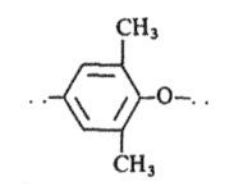	1.06	amorphous	
Polysulfone (PPOS)	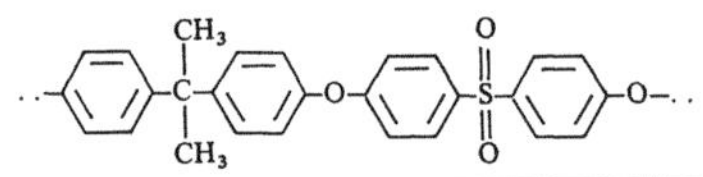	1.24	amorphous	
Epoxy resin (EP)	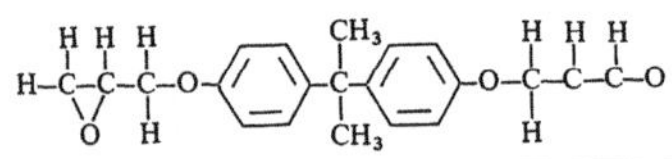	1.2	cross-linked	

the simple, linear high-density polyethylene to the cross-linked epoxy resin (Table 1).

Tissue Compatibility

As a rule, the initial testing of a new biomaterial is conducted *in vitro,* i.e., in cell cultures. Then the material is tested *in vivo* for tissue compatibility by implanting specially shaped specimens into experimental animals. At the Laboratory for Experimental Surgery in Davos, Switzerland [4], for example, a dumbbell-shaped specimen measuring 4×7 mm is used for animal implantations. Based on the types of cells that are found on histologic examination, the suitability of the new material can be evaluated in relation to other, known biomaterials (Fig. 2).

Mechanical Properties

The mechanical strength values of polymers are about 10 times lower than corresponding values for metals. It is difficult to give exact figures, because some polymers show a viscoelastic behavior during testing.

The ultimate tensile strength of the "soft" polymers is near the lower end of the range that is reported for bone [1] (10–150 N/mm²). The

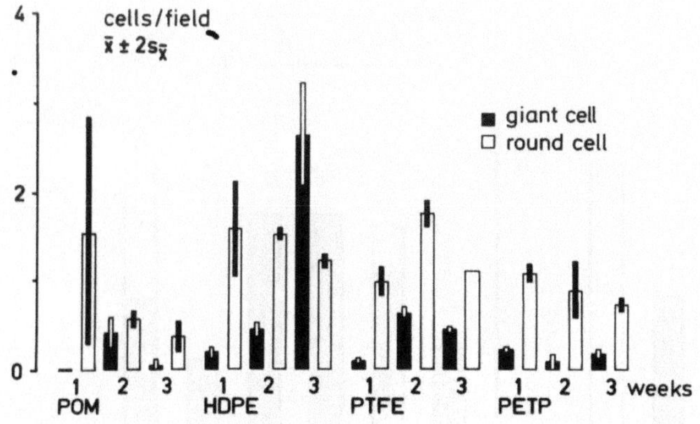

Fig. 2. Types of cells found on examination of histologic sections from animal implantations

typical high-strength polymers fall near the middle of this range. Similar relationships apply with regard to elastic modulus. The strength and E modulus of polymers can be increased dramatically by fiber reinforcement (Fig. 3). The maximum tensile strength that can be achieved for cold-curing methylmethacrylate is about 60 N/mm². If fluid inclusions enter the cement at the time of implantations, its strength will be greatly reduced.

In addition to biocompatibility, the selection of a polymer for prosthetic components is based upon the stress that may be applied for a given time before the material exceeds a given deformation (creep stress, Fig. 4a) and upon its fatigue strength (Fig. 4b). Assuming that a mere 3.7 N/mm² of pressure is exerted on the projected surface of a femoral ball 32 mm in diameter with a load of 3000 N at the hip, we find that Teflon, polyethylene and polypropylene will undergo a slight degree of deformation after 1000 hours.

The fatigue testing of polymers is quite difficult, and the values measured at a test frequency of f = 10 Hz are not easily applied to conditions of clinical use, for the materials will have little opportunity to undergo plastic deformation when 10^7 load cycles are applied within a mere 300 hours. This particularly applies to polyethylene and polypropylene. We

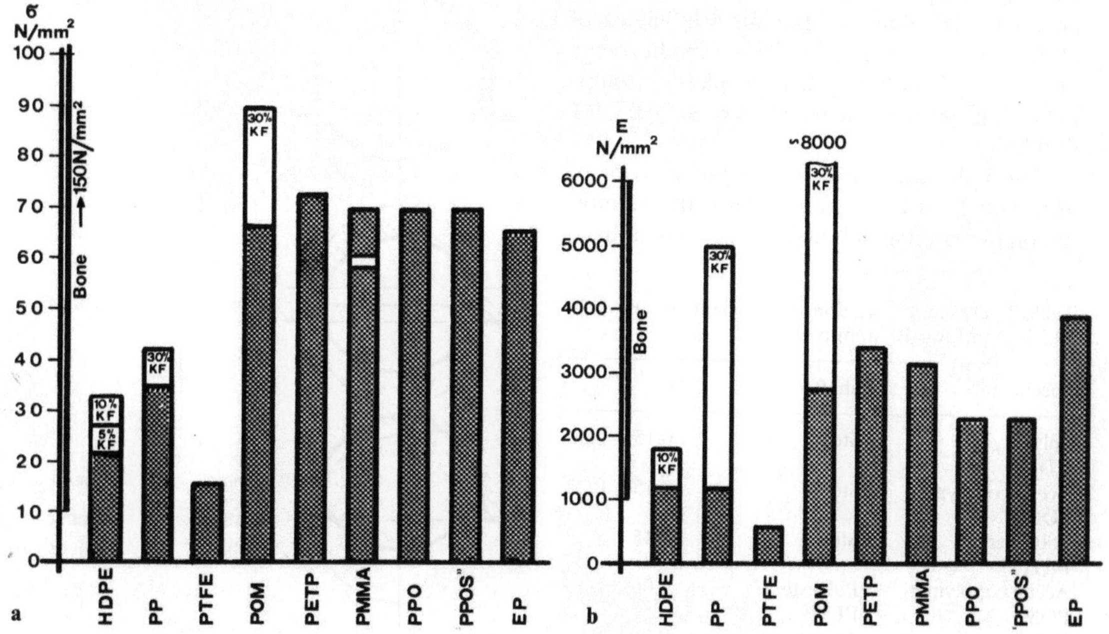

Fig. 3a, b. Mechanical properties. **a** Yield stress (tensile strength at RT) of bone σ = 10–150 N/mm². **b** Elastic modulus of bone = 1000–6000 N/mm²

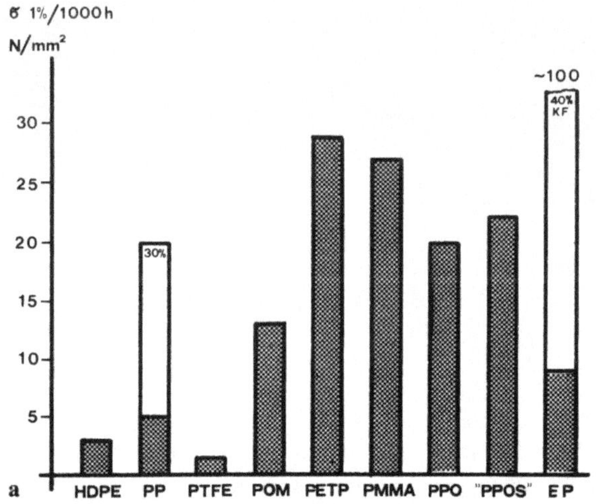

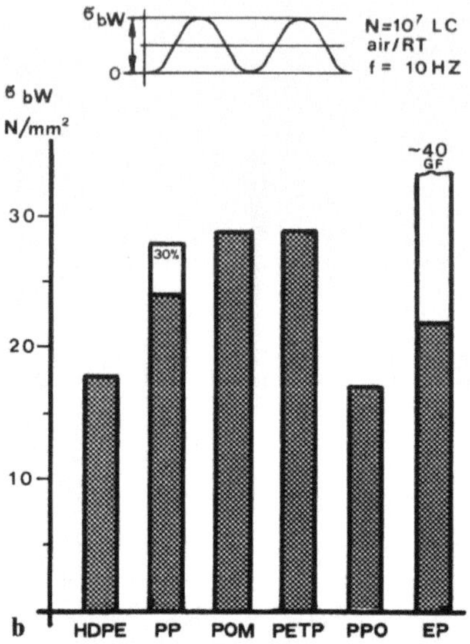

Fig. 4a, b. Mechanical properties. **a** Creep stress: stress that causes 1% deformation after 1000 hrs. **b** Alternating bending strength: 10^7 cycles (LC) in air, test frequency f= 10 Hz

believe that the permissible creep stress is also an important criterion for dynamically-loaded components of prosthetic joints.

Friction and Wear

One of the outstanding features of polymers is their low friction when in contact with other materials. The dynamic friction coefficients of plastic-on-metal combinations are in the range of 0.1–0.2 [7], while plastic-on-plastic combinations have coefficients as low as 0.05–0.1 (Table 2).

Fig. 5 illustrates how the wear behavior of articulating surfaces varies with the combination of materials selected. When a metal head is combined with a plastic socket, for example, we find that wear is limited almost entirely to the plastic component, and the metal ball sinks into the socket. The geometry of the articulation remains essentially intact, however, and only the range of joint motion is reduced. Converse-

Table 2. Dynamic Eriction Coefficient μ. p=2.5–22.5 Kp/cm², v = 10 m/min

Specimen	Shaft	μ
Polyethylene HDPE	Steel	0.15 ÷ 0.20
Acetal copolymer POM	Steel	0.15 ÷ 0.20
Polyester PETP	Steel	0.15
Acetal copolymer POM	Polyester PETP	0.05 ÷ 0.10
Polyester PETP	Acetal copolymer POM	0.05 ÷ 0.08

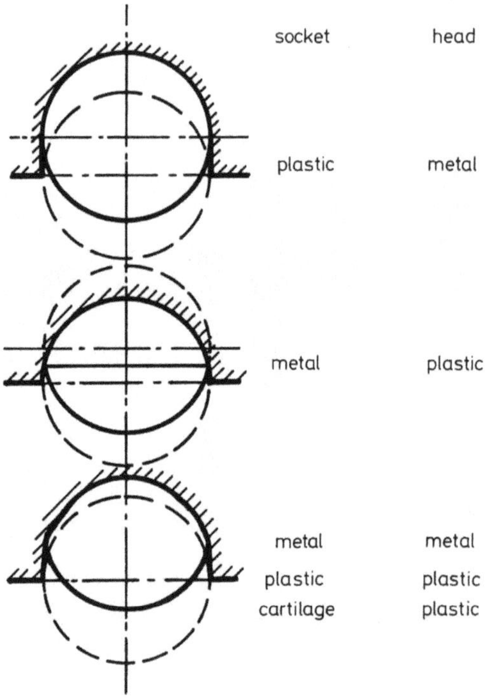

Fig. 5. Typical modes of wear of endoprosthetic components

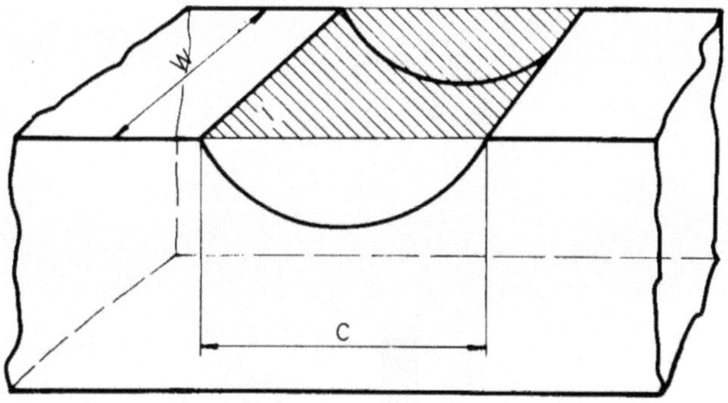

Fig. 6. Wear test specimen. Wear is measured by the chord length S. *W* = width; *C* = chord; *I* = interface

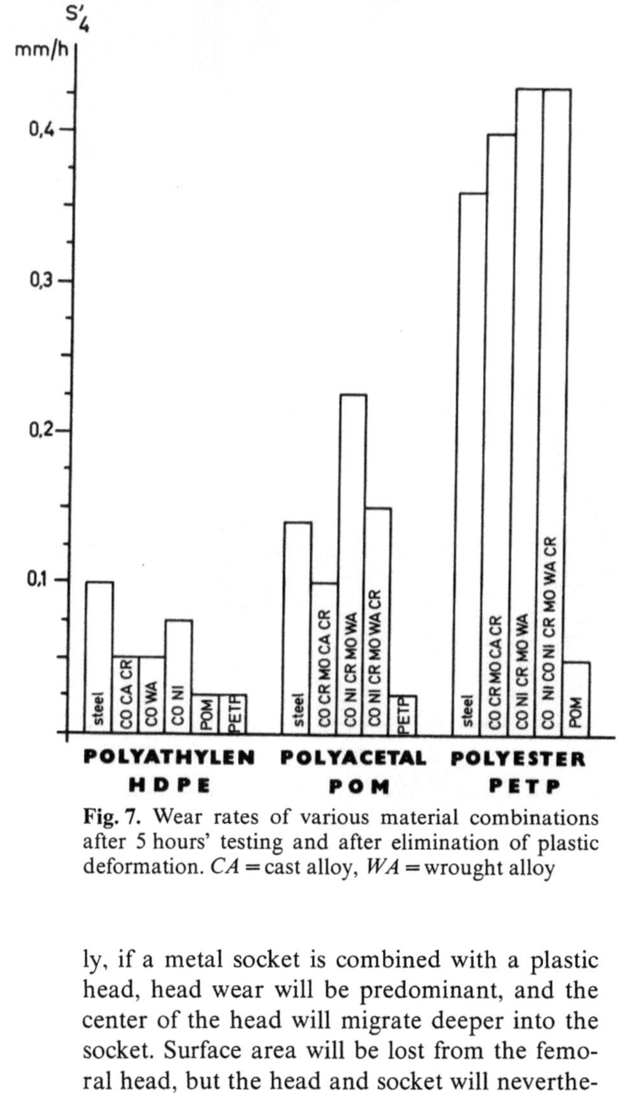

Fig. 7. Wear rates of various material combinations after 5 hours' testing and after elimination of plastic deformation. *CA* = cast alloy, *WA* = wrought alloy

ly, if a metal socket is combined with a plastic head, head wear will be predominant, and the center of the head will migrate deeper into the socket. Surface area will be lost from the femoral head, but the head and socket will nevertheless remain congruent.

If the head and socket are made of the same material, then both components will experience an equal amount of wear. In the process, the articulating surfaces will decrease in area and lose their congruity. This can also occur when an Al_2O_3-on-Al_2O_3 system is used.

Experience with Teflon has shown that a low coefficient of friction does not necessarily imply low wear. Exhaustive tests are needed to evaluate the suitability of materials for sliding joint surfaces.

We have devised a simple, reproducible test to screen for suitable material combinations [7]: A shaft is rotated back and forth in a medium of Ringer's solution, and the test specimen is pressed against the shaft under a constant load of 100 N. Wear is measured by the chord length S of the circular impression made in the specimen (Fig. 6). This produces an increase of interfacial area, which is equivalent to reducing the contact pressure.

A graphic representation of the wear rate as determined after five hours' testing and after eliminating plastic deformation (Fig. 7) indicates that polyethylene, combined with metals or other polymers, has the most favorable wear properties. Clinical experience has confirmed these findings. Charnley [3] reports wear rates of 0.09–0.3 mm/year for polyethylene on steel, and 2.4–3.6 mm/year for Teflon on steel. For sockets made of acetyl resin, we found wear rates between 0.5 and 1.4 mm/year. The frequent discrepancies between experimental findings and clinical results again demonstrate the danger of applying experimental results to practice.

Resistance to Degradation

The generally high resistance of polymers to chemical attack is well known. However, this resistance is limited in some polymers or is highly polymer-specific. Owing to the widespread use

	strong acids	oxidizing	strong organic	weak alkalis acids	strong alkalis	fatty oils
HDPE	⊕	−	+	+	+	+
PP	−	−	+	+	+	⊕
PTFE	+	+	+	+	+	+
POM	−	−	+	+	+	+
PETP	+	−	+	+	−	+
PMMA	○	⊖	−	+	○	+
PPO	⊕	+	+	+	⊕	
"PPOS"	+	−	⊕	+	+	+
EP	−	−	⊖	+	○	+

+ resistant ⊕ generally resistant
○ moderately resistant ⊖ weakly resistant
- not resistant

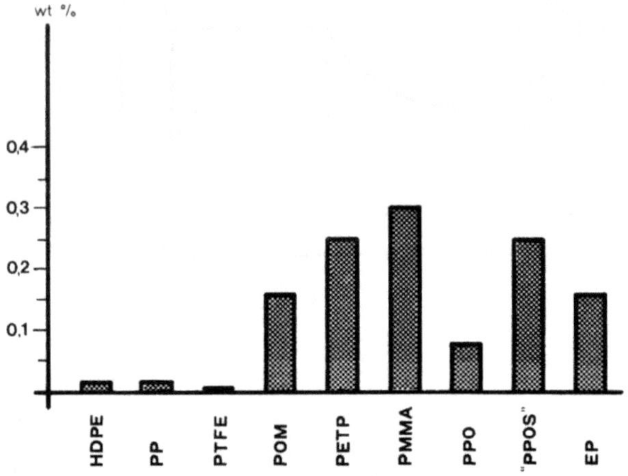

Fig. 8. Chemical resistance of selected polymers. **a** Resistance to various media. **b** Moisture uptake at 50% rel. hum. and 23 °C

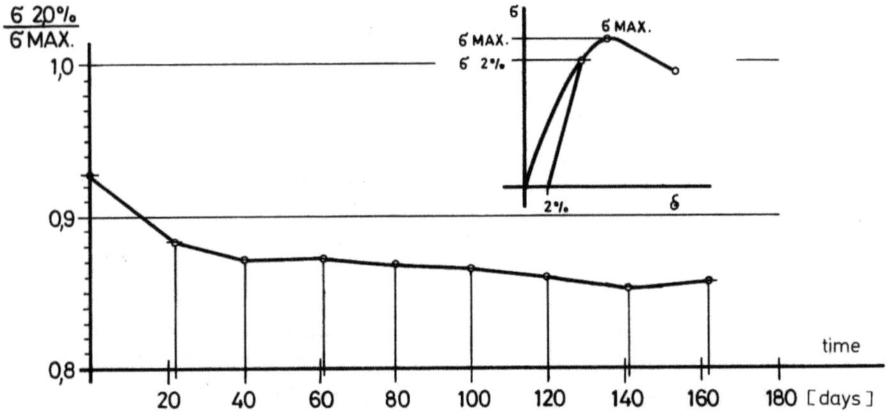

Fig. 9. Aging resistance of Polyoxymethylene. The graph shows tensile strength, expressed as the ratio σ 2% / σ max., as a function of boiling time in Ringer's solution (~100 °C, darkness, 0–162 days)

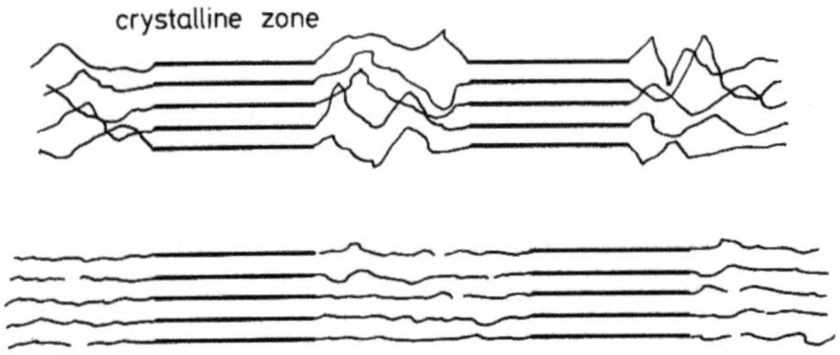

Fig. 10. Mechanical degradation of polymers (semi-crystalline). The mechanically weaker, noncrystalline zones form sites of predilection for rupture

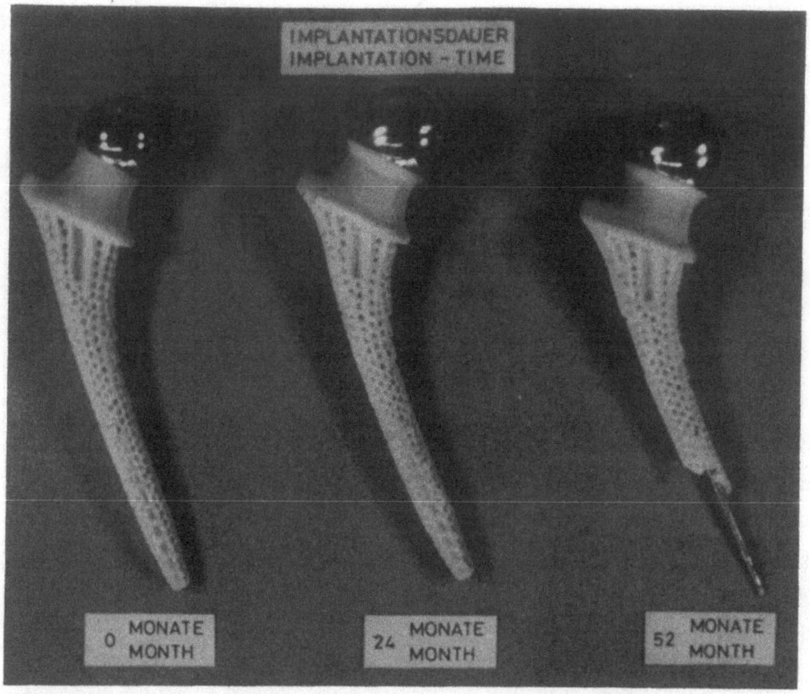

Fig. 11. Implantation of plastic prostheses. No gross changes are apparent after implantation times of 24 and 52 months. At revision, the 52-month specimen had to be fractured because distal bone ingrowth prevented removal of the prostheses

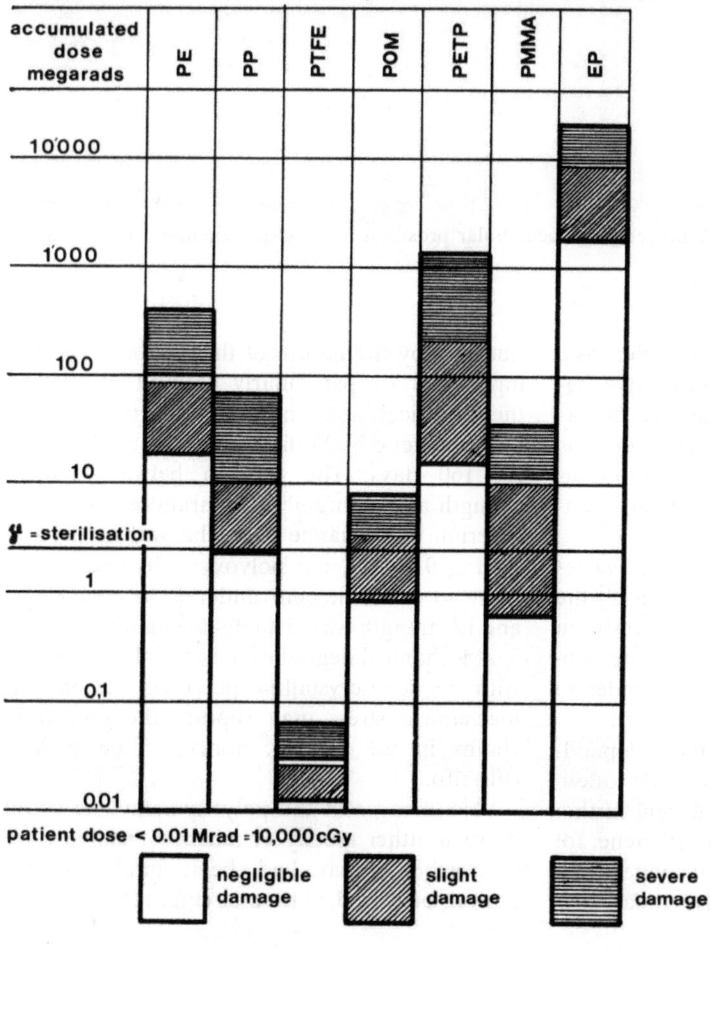

Fig. 12. Resistance to γ-irradiation. γ-ray sterilization (2.5 Mrad) is destructive to polypropylene, polytetrafluoroethylene, polyoxymethylene and polymethylmethacrylate

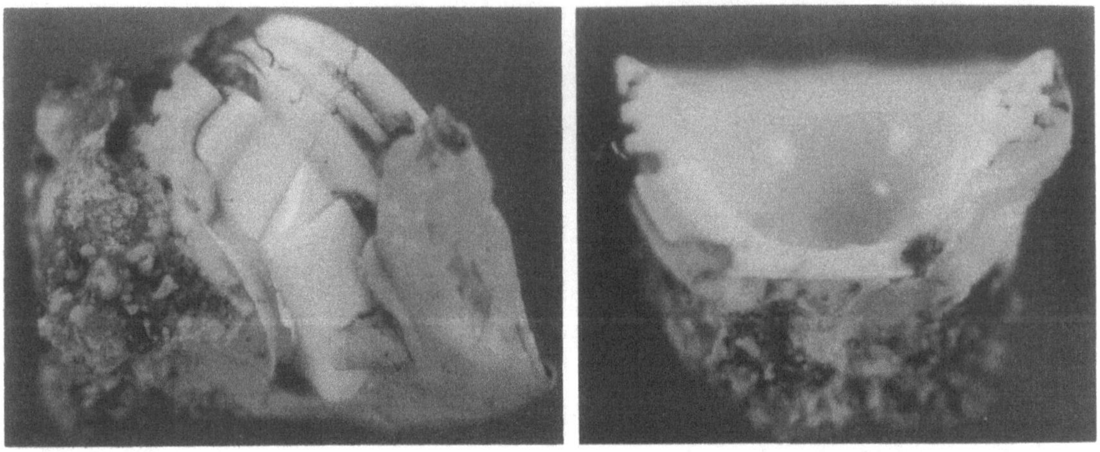

a b

Fig. 13. Brittle fracture (a) and wear (b) of a polyethylene terephthalate acetabular prosthesis

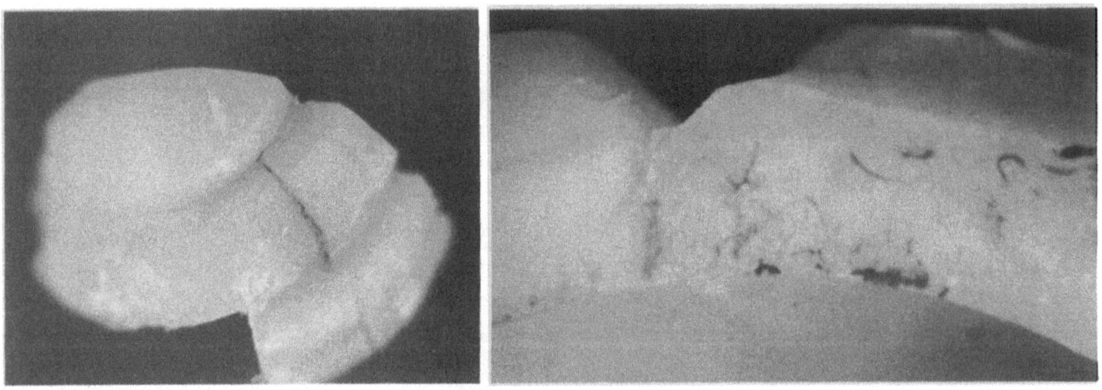

a b

Fig. 14. Fatigue fracture of an UHMW polyethylene acetabular prosthesis. Crack propagation occurred along the grooves in the implant

of plastics in industry and in the home, the basic mechanisms of polymer degradation have become well known. They include thermal degradation, chemical and biological degradation, as well as changes resulting from exposure to radiation. Several of these factors may act concurrently [11].

The chemical resistance of polymers varies widely, from the practically inert Teflon on the one hand to the highly unstable epoxy resin on the other (Fig. 8a). The moisture or water uptake of a polymer provides an indirect index of its chemical resistance (Fig. 8b).

The thermal stability of polymers depends largely on their molecular structure. The softening temperature of a given polymer will further limit its range of applications. Polyethylene, for example, may undergo a change of shape at only 60 °C. Thermal stability is also greatly influenced by the nature of the medium. Oxidizing media are particularly harmful. We tested the chemical and thermal stability of polyoxymethylene by boiling it in Ringer's solution for 160 days. The relation between tensile strength and strength at 2% strain served as the criterion for a change in mechanical properties. As Fig. 9 shows, the polyoxymethylene underwent no embrittlement under these conditions, and its strength was virtually unchanged.

Mechanical degradation is mainly a problem with the semi-crystalline polymers. A constant mechanical stress may rupture the polymeric chains in the weaker, noncrystalline regions (Fig. 10).

No changes in the polyoxymethylene could be seen either grossly or microscopically in endoprostheses that had been implanted for periods of 24 and 52 months (Fig. 11).

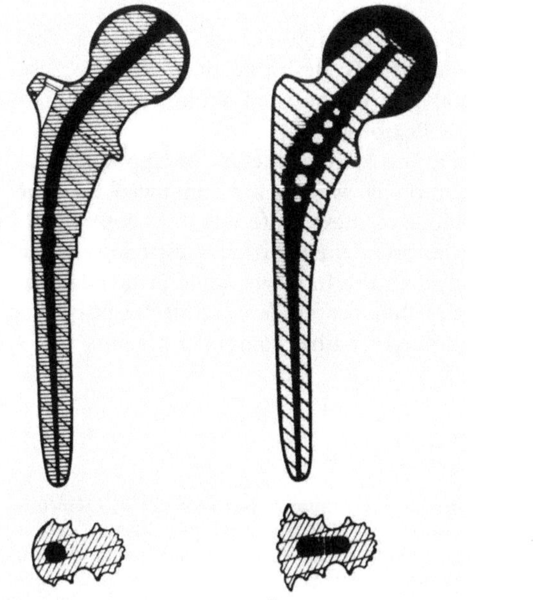

a b

Fig. 15. Structure of the "isoelastic" prosthesis. **a** 1973 model; **b** 197[illegible] model

The ultraviolet stability of polymers is often poor. UV irradiation stimulates additional cross-linking of the molecular chains, leading to embrittlement of the material. This mode of degradation is of little importance for implants, however.

Resistance to ionizing radiation is also highly polymerspecific. Sterilization by γ-rays is contraindicated for Teflon, polymethylmethacrylate, polyoxymethylene and polypropylene (Fig. 12), as it will cause embrittlement. Radiation therapy with cobalt-60 that does not exceed a dosage of 10,000 gCy (rad) is destructive only to Teflon.

The mechanisms by which polymers undergo degradation in the human body are not yet completely understood. This is illustrated by the embrittlement and excessive wear of polyester sockets exposed to the mechanical, biochemical and thermal stresses of the physiologic milieu (Fig. 13 a, b), as well as by the fatigue fractures, excessive wear and additional cross-linking (em-

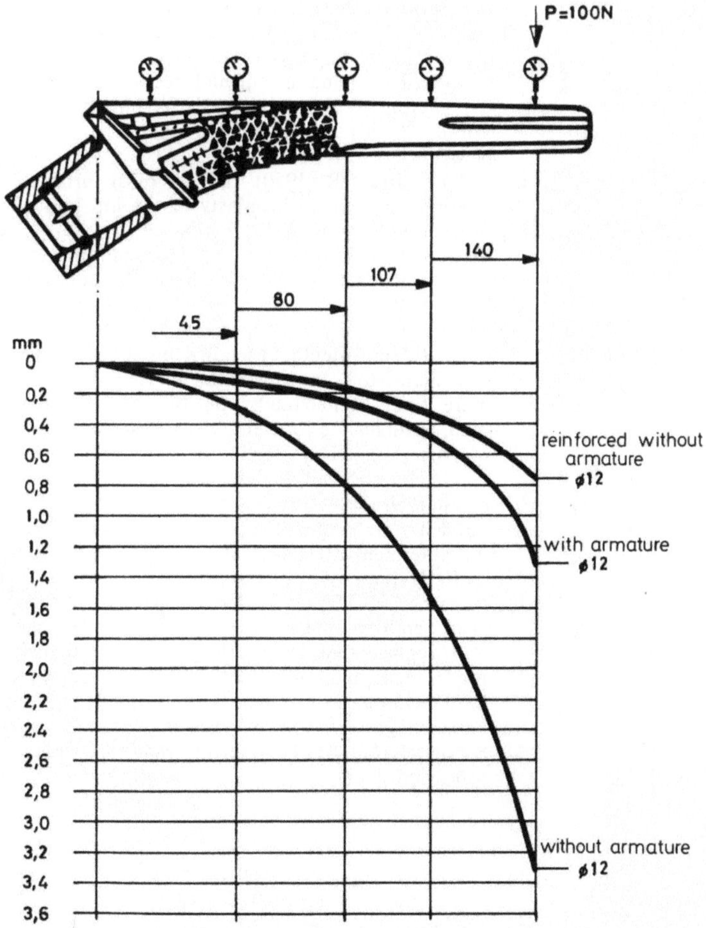

Fig. 16. Elasticity of the prosthetic stem. The experimental setup and load are indicated. Stem diameter = 12 mm

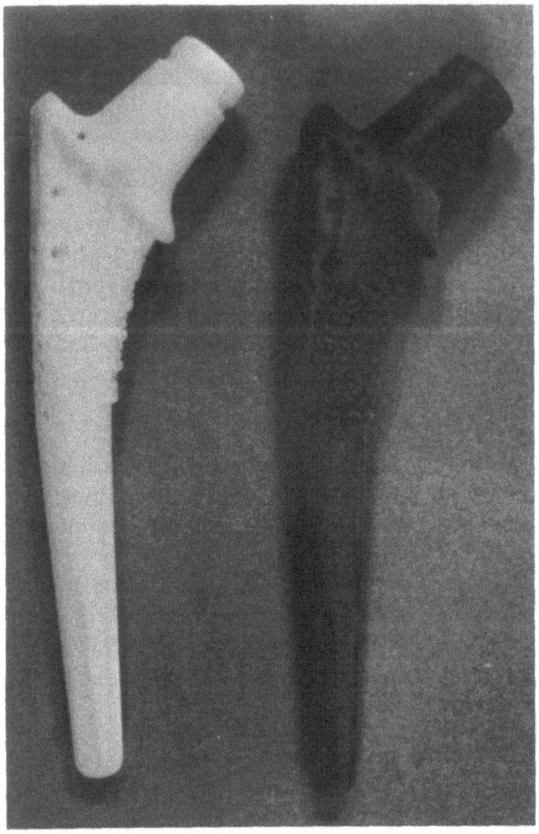

Fig. 17. Plastic prosthesis. *Left:* with metal armature. *Right:* carbon fiber-reinforced

brittlement) that have been observed in polyethylene sockets (Fig. 14a, b). Gamma-ray sterilization may be a factor in the latter instance.

The "isoelastic" hip prosthesis consists of an outer shell of polyoxymethylene that is reinforced by an internal metal armature. This armature can be stiffened or left flexible wherever needed, without altering the external shape of the prosthesis (Fig. 15). Clinical experience has shown that the first model of 1973 was too elastic in the area of the neck, collar and proximal stem and consequently loosened in that region [8–10]. For the 1975 model, the armature was made more rigid in that area, though the neck was left somewhat flexible. As mentioned earlier, polyoxymethylene can also be reinforced by carbon fibers (Figs. 16 and 17). This is not necessarily desirable, however, because the distal part of the stem should have a high degree of flexibility.

Given the state-of-the-art of applied polymer technology, we are are convinced that the applications of these materials in endoprosthetics can be broadened further – especially when one considers the improvements in mechanical properties that are made possible by polymer-metal or polymer-fiber composite systems.

References

1. Bourgeois R, Wagner J, Burny F (1973) Détérmination des propriétés mécaniques locales des os longs à l'aide de micro-éprouvettes. Acta Orthop Belg [Suppl] 1 39:25
2. Charnley J (1966) Total prosthetic replacement of the hip joint using a socket of high density polyethylene. Center for hip surgery, Wrightington Hospital, publication 1
3. Charnley J (1979) Low friction arthroplasty of the hip. Springer, Berlin Heidelberg New York
4. Geret V, Rahn BA, Mathys R et al. (1979) A method for testing tissue tolerance for improved quantitative evaluation through reduction of relative motion at the implant tissue interface. In: Winter G (ed) Advances in biomaterials. Wiley, New York, p 351
5. Judet J, Judet R (1950) The use of an artificial femoral head for arthroplasty of the hip joint. J Bone Joint Surg [Br] 32:166
6. Mathys R (1973) Stand der Verwendung von Kunststoffen für künstliche Gelenke. Aktuel Traumatol 3:253
7. Mathys R sen, Mathys R jun (1974) Die Grenzflächen (Metall-Metall, Metall-Kunststoff, Kunststoff-Kunststoff. In: Hartmann F (Hrsg) Biopolymere und Biomechanik von Bindegewebssystemen. Springer, Berlin Heidelberg New York S 401
8. Morscher E, Mathys R (1974) La prothèse totale de hanche isoélastique fixée sans ciment. Premiers résultats cliniques. Acta Orthop Belg 40:639
9. Morscher E, Mathys R (1975) Erste Erfahrungen mit einer zementlosen isoelastischen Totalprothese der Hüfte. Orthop. 113/4:745
10. Morscher E, Mathys R, Henche HR (1976) Isoelastic endoprosthesis – A new concept in artificial joint replacement. In: Schaldach M (ed) Engineering in medicine, vol 2. Advances in hip and knee joint technology. Springer, Berlin Heidelberg New York
11. Schnabel W (1981) Polymer Degradation. Hanser, München Wien

The Use of Carbon as an Implant Material*

W. Hüttner and K. J. Hüttinger

Introduction

Carbon was introduced as a biomaterial more than 10 years ago. A pioneer in this area was Bokros [1], who developed artificial heart valves that have been implanted in many thousands of cardiac patients [2]. They are produced by depositing silicon-alloyed carbon on a prefabricated graphite substrate. Similar carbon products are currently being tested for use as percutaneous implants and dental anchors. Both pyrocarbons and glassy carbon are being proposed and tested for the latter application [3, 4]. Carbon fibers are being woven into tissue form and used as replacements for ligaments, tendons and portions of the abdominal wall [5–7], and carbon fiber-reinforced composites are being tested as internal bone plates in experimental animals [8–10].

Since the mid-1970s, much research work in the Federal Republic of Germany, with funding from the Ministry of Research and Technology, has been directed toward utilizing the advantages of carbon, such as biocompatibility, chemical inertness, controllable mechanical properties and excellent tribologic properties, specifically for the production of components for total hip replacements. Work is currently being done on carbon fiber-reinforced polymers with matrices of epoxy resin [11] and triacine resin [12, 13] for the stems of femoral endoprostheses, and carbon fiber-reinforced carbons are being developed for the fabrication of pure-carbon components [14, 15]. A high-strength, isotropic carbon and a carbon/silicon carbide composite have been developed for use as gliding components in artificial joints [14, 16, 17]. Progress on the carbon/silicon carbide composite made it possible to start the clinical testing of double-cup prostheses in 1980 [18, 19].

* Supported by Federal Ministery of Research and Technology (MT 290 and MT 03)

In the present paper we shall discuss the properties of the pure carbon materials and the endoprosthetic components fabricated from them, based upon the latest results of research and development in that area.

Gliding Components Made from Carbon/Silicon Carbide and Isotropic Carbon

Figures 1 and 2 show the structure of the high-strength, isotropic carbon (ISO-C) and the carbon/silicon carbide composite (C/SiC) in polarized light. ISO-C displays very small anisotropic regions in a hard matrix that appears isotropic. The porosity of the material is 6%. In the case of C/SiC, the hard, wear-resistant, isotropic SiC is combined with anisotropic, lubricating graphite. Each phase permeates the other completely; the porosity is less than 0.5%.

The mechanical properties of both materials are summarized in Table 1. Figure 3 shows the fatigue strength of the materials under a cyclic bending load. ISO-C has a static strength of 140 N/mm² and an E-modulus of 2.4 kN/mm²; C/SiC has a bending strength of 220 N/mm² and a much higher E-modulus of 140 N/mm².

The fatigue strength of ISO-C is 70–75% of its static strength, while that of C/SiC is 75–80%. In all cases the dynamic bending strength under cyclic loading remains constant after 10^4 load cycles, i.e., no further decline of

Table 1. Mechanical Properties of IsoC and C/SiC

		IsoC	C/SiC
φ	g/cm³	1.8	1.7
$\sigma_{st.}$	N/mm²	140	220
$\sigma_{dyn.}$		70–75% $\sigma_{st.}$	75–80% $\sigma_{st.}$
E	kN/mm²	2.3	140

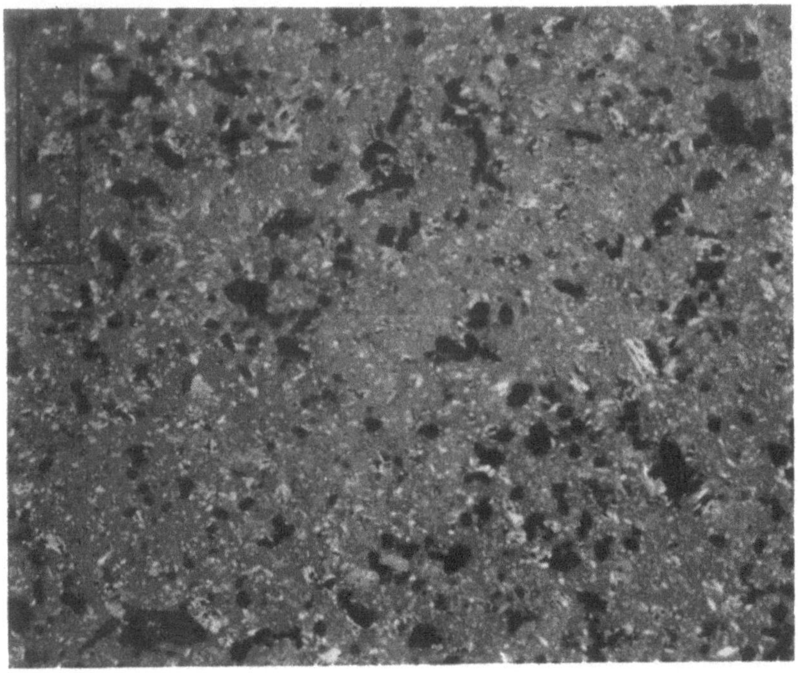

Fig. 1. Structure of the isotropic carbon (ISO-C) in polarized light

dynamic strength is observed with increasing load cycles. These results are independent of the test medium (air, distilled water, physiologic saline).

The tribologic properties of the materials were evaluated by the ring-on-disk method. Figure 4 shows the depth of penetration and coefficient of friction for the combinations of ISO-C on C/SiC and C/SiC on C/SiC as a function of the contact pressure per unit area [20]. As the contact pressure rises from 5 to 37 N/mm², both the friction coefficient and depth of penetration show a linear increases. C/SiC on C/SiC shows more favorable tribologic properties than C/SiC

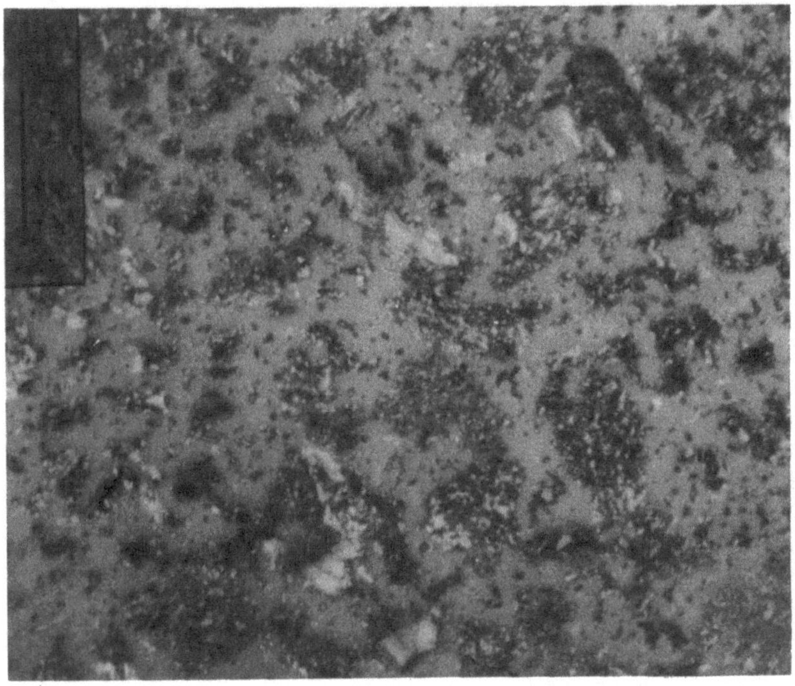

Fig. 2. Structure of the carbon-silicon carbide composite (C/SiC) in polarized light

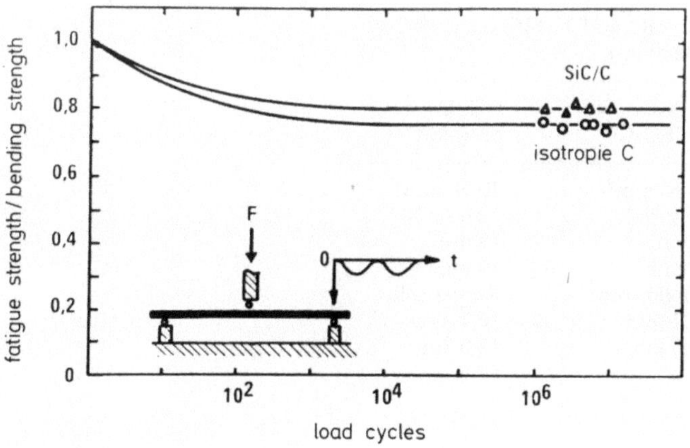

Fig. 3. Fatigue strength of the carbon materials ISO-C and C/SiC under a cyclic bending load

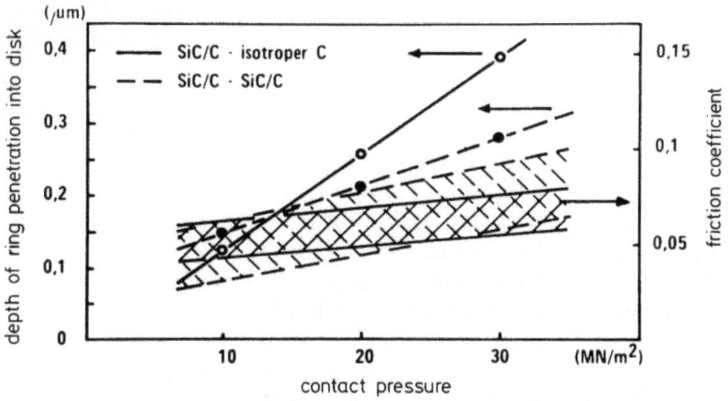

Fig. 4. Depth of penetration and friction coefficient of ISO-C on C/SiC and C/SiC on C/SiC as a function of specific contact pressure (ring-on-disk method). — C/SiC-isotropic C; - - - C/SiC-C/SiC

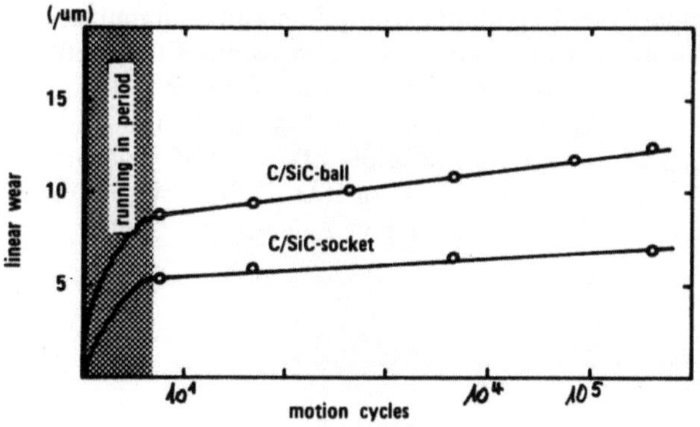

Fig. 5. Wear behavior of the C/SiC double-cup prosthesis (ball-in-socket test; contact pressure 37 N/mm^2; play between cup and socket 0.15 mm; media: distilled water, Ringer's solution)

on ISO-C. The results for a contact pressure of 20 N/mm^2 in a test medium of Ringer's solution are shown in Table 2.

The results of ball-in-socket measurements with the combination C/SiC-C/SiC on a simplified hip-joint similator at contact pressures of 37 N/mm^2 are shown graphically in Fig. 5. Running-in wear is complete after $0.2 \cdot 10^6$ load cycles, and the wear volume is equal to 0.03 $\mu m^3/10^6$ cycles. Distilled water and physiologic saline were the test media.

In Fig. 6 the wear of material combinations used in conventional prostheses is compared to that of C/SiC. The same ball-in-socket test setup was used at loads of 2500 N and $1 \cdot 10^6$ to $4 \cdot 10^6$ motion cycles. These measurements enable a direct comparison of the different material combinations and clearly indicate that C/

Table 2. Tribologic Properties of ISO-C on C/SiC and C/SiC on C/SiC at a Contact Pressure of 20 N/nm² (Ring-on-Disk Method)

Test conditions: ring on disk	C/SiC on ISO-C	C/SiC on C/SiC
Contact pressure	20 N/mm²	20 N/mm²
Oscillating frequency deflection	2 Hz/±30°	2 Hz/±30°
Ring inside diam.	13 mm	13 mm
Ring outside diam.	19 mm	19 mm
Lubricating medium	Ringer solu.	Ringer solu.
Travel per cycle	16.7 mm	16.7 mm
Travel per test	12.0 km	12.0 km
Duration of test	87 h	87 h
Results		
Depth of penetration per 10^7 cycles	4.3 μm	3.7 μm
Depth of penetration per 10^5 m travel	2.7 §m	2.2 μm
Coefficient of friction	0.06–0.05	0.07–0.05

SiC on C/SiC is subject to far less wear than the other combinations.

Wear tests of double-cup C/SiC-on-C/SiC prostheses run on the Munich I hip-joint simulator yielded comparable results. The test load was 2500 N, and the duration of the tests was $3 \cdot 10^6$ cycles. Running-in wear was complete after $0.5 \cdot 10^6$ cycles. After that point no additional wear was measurable. The surface roughness values (Ra values) after $0.5 \cdot 10^6$ cycles were 0.18 μ for the socket and 0.29 μ for the femoral cup. A 1.5 cm-long scratch placed in the equatorial area of the femoral cup after the first load cycles did not adversely affect the wear behavior of the system.

The extraordinary wear resistance of C/SiC at high interfacial pressures and low gliding speeds is derived from two properties. The first essential property is the two-phase composition of the material, the hard SiC forming on phase and the soft graphite the other. The hard phase provides a firm articulating surface that can bear loads, and particles that are worn from the hard phase can be absorbed by the soft graphite phase, thereby avoiding a self-potentiating wear process. The second favorable property has to do with the layered structure of the carbon lattice. The orientation of the graphite layers parallel to the gliding surface enables the formation of a solid lubricating film and a minimization of surface energy, thereby lowering the coefficient of friction. One such film is shown in Fig. 7. The graphite lubricating film is so thin that the underlying structure of the C/SiC is clearly visible. In the case of ISO-C, the isotropic regions form the hard phase, while the smaller aniso-

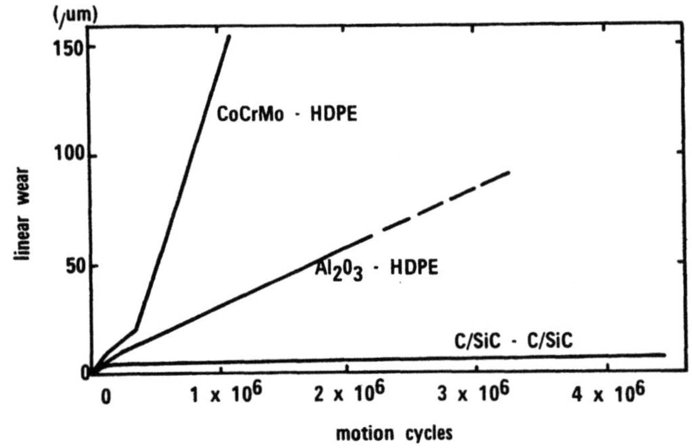

Fig. 6. Wear behavior of various material combinations for cup prostheses as tested by the ball-in-socket method

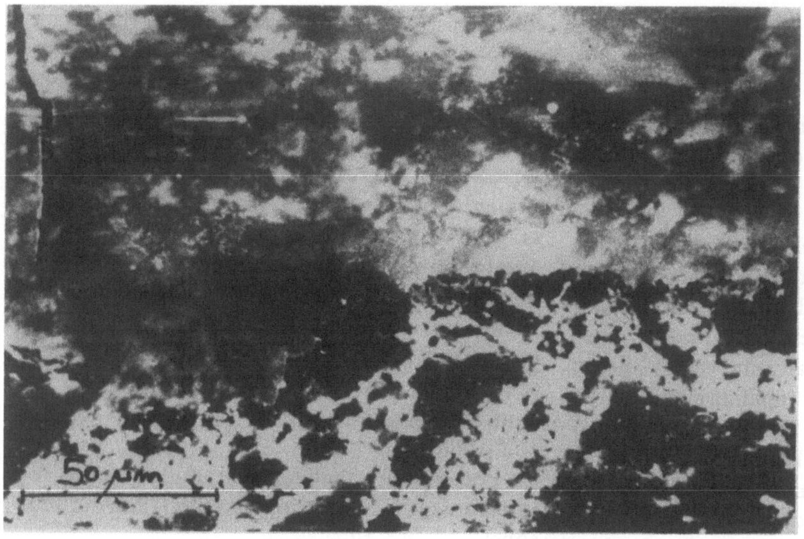

Fig. 7. Scanning electron micrograph of the solid graphite lubricating film on a C/SiC surface following friction testing under dry conditions

Table 3. Static and Dynamic Strength of Double-Cup Prostheses under Compressive Shock Loading

No of load cycles before static testing	7.39×10^6	48.81×10^3	80×10^3
Max. dynamic load (kN)	50	40	30
Static load (kN)	112	96.2	50
Fracture	cup	cup (microcrack after cycling) socket	cup

tropic regions and the pores constitute the soft phase. The interrelationship between the phases is like that described for C/SiC. These properties of C/SiC and ISO-C also explain why, contrary to general opinion, it is possible to have sliding interfaces composed of the same material, as the results for C/SiC demonstrate.

The fatigue resistance of the C/SiC double-cup prostheses was tested on the Munich I hip-joint simulator in accordance with the procedures specified by preliminary standards. The prostheses withstood the requisite load of 5 ± 4 kN for $5 \cdot 10^6$ cycles at a frequency of 25 Hz without failure.

We were also interested in determining the response of the C/SiC double-cup prostheses to sudden compressive loading. There were no standard procedures available for testing this property, and so a special *in vitro* test had to be devised [21]. Dynamic loading of the prostheses was followed by static loading to fracture. The onset of the fracture was detected by means of acoustic emission signals. The dynamic strength values were measured at maximum loads of 30, 40 and 50 kN. At 30 kN the number of load cycles was limited to $80 \cdot 10^3$. At 40 kN a fracture of the femoral cup was observed after $48.81 \cdot 10^3$ cycles, and at 50 kN the test was terminated after $7.39 \cdot 10^6$ cycles (Table 3). It should be noted that a dynamic strength of 40 kN is equal to about 50 times the human body weight, and that the corresponding number of load cycles, $48.81 \cdot 10^3$, is roughly equivalent to 133 years of subjecting the joint once daily to a 40 kN load. The static strengths range between 50 and 112 kN. Generally the femoral cup was the component that fractured, because the bone cement used as the adhesive began to flow under the high loads and caused tensile stresses to be exerted on the cup.

Prosthetic Stems Made from Carbon Fiber-Reinforced Carbon (CFRC)

The idea of using fiber-reinforced composition as a basis for the fabrication of endoprosthetic stems is a logical one, for it is possible to vary the strength and stiffness values of such materials over a wide range, and thus to adapt them to specific physiologic requirements.

The processes involved in the manufacture of CFRC composite systems are shown schematically in Fig. 8. Generally the carbon fibers are given a desired directional orientation by weaving, winding and/or laminating and then are fixed with an organic binder by pressing or some other technique. This is followed by the controlled thermal breakdown of the organic binder to carbon. At this point the product generally has a porosity of 10–30%, and its density must be increased until the desired porosity is obtained. This is usually done by the chemical gas-phase deposition of carbon into the porous structure or by impregnation with organic binders followed by controlled pyrolysis. A special process used to bind commercial mixtures of polyaromatics (e.g., coal-tar pitch) yields relatively dense CFRC composites even after the first pyrolysis. This is achieved by hot-pressing the composite at temperatures up to 700 °C [22].

Figure 9 shows a photomicrograph, taken in polarized light, of a CFRC composite that is unidirectionally reinforced at right angles to the direction of its fibers. The strength and stiffness ranges of the composite are shown in Fig. 10. The corresponding ranges for titanium alloys, cobalt-base alloys and bone are also shown for comparison. The bending strength of the composite ranges from 150 to 1500 N/mm², and its E-modulus from 25 to 280 kN/mm². It should be noted that strength and stiffness always correlate for a given fiber orientation, i.e., high strength implies a high E-modulus and vice-versa. The wide range of variation is due mainly to differences in the spatial orientation and percentage content of the fibers. CFRC composites always have a higher E-modulus than the corresponding carbon fiber-reinforced polymers (CFRP), because the carbon matrix itself can contribute significantly to the stiffness of the composite [23].

For endoprosthetic stems, unidirectional reinforcement is inadequate for the following reasons:

a) Stems are subject to tensile, compressive and shear loads that act in various directions and partially overlap.
b) The E-modulus is invariant with unidirectional reinforcement. Thus, a reinforcement must be devised in which the carbon fibers have at least a biaxial orientation within the x-y plane.

In Table 4 the torsional and bending strength properties of CFRC and CFRP composites having identical reinforcement in the x-y plane are compared. The properties of the CFRC materials are quite similar for both the bi- and triaxial fiber orientation. This particularly applies to the torsion properties. Similar results are reported in the literature [9]. The torsion strengths are approximately 30 N/mm²,

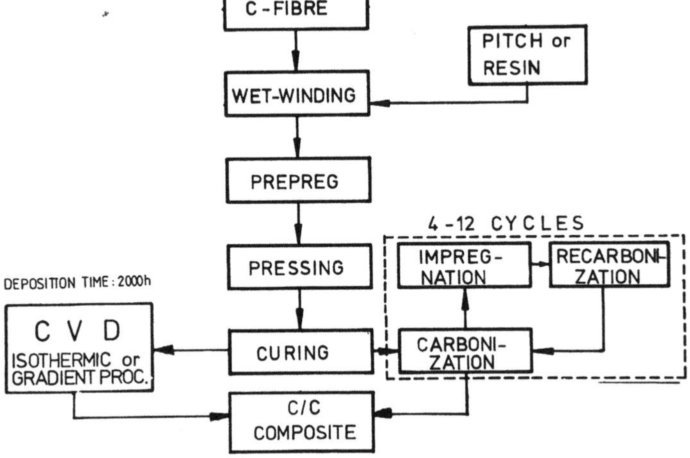

Fig. 8. Processes involved in the manufacture of carbon fiberreinforced carbon (CFRC) composites

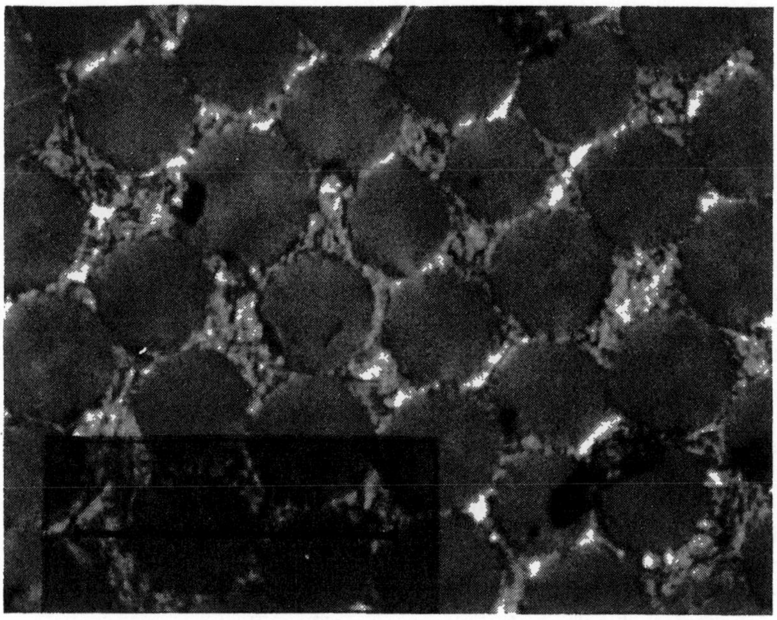

Fig. 9. Structure of a CFRC composite unidirectionally reinforced perpendicular to the direction of its fibers

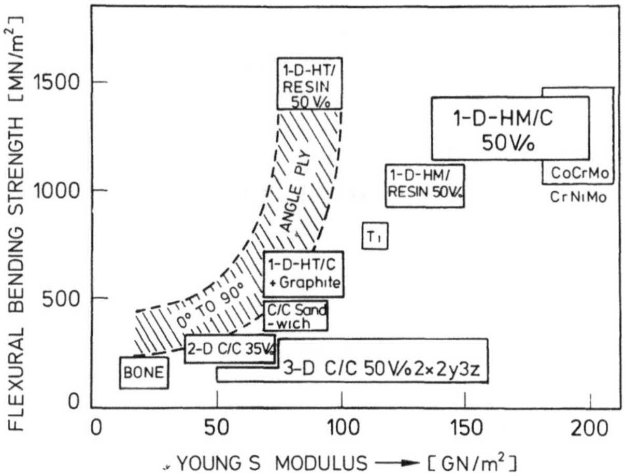

Fig. 10. Strength and stiffness spectrum of CFRC and CFRP composites

Table 4. Mechanical Properties of Selected Carbon Fiber-Reinforced Composite Materials

		CFRC (triaxial)	CFRC (biaxial)	CFRP (triaxial)
Torsion strength	(N/mm²)	29.9	31.1	76.8
Twist angle to failure	(°)	9.75	12,3	24
Shear modulus	(kN/mm²)	3.1	2.6	2.7
Bending strength	(N/mm²)	283	248	605
Strain to failure	(%)	1.6	1.5	2.1
Bending modulus	(kN/mm²)	42.9	43.7	39.5

and the shear moduli are 2.6 and 3.1 kN/mm², respectively. The bending strengths reach values of 248 and 283 N/mm², and the associated bending moduli are approximately 43 kN/mm², or about ⅕ the value of cobalt-base alloys.

The stiffness values measured for a triaxially reinforced CFRP composite are comparable to those for the CFRC composites, but the torsion strength of 76.8 N/mm² and bending strength of 605 N/mm² are more than twice the corresponding values for the CFRC materials. These differences are due entirely to the properties of the polymeric matrix.

The fatigue behavior of the materials under torsion and bending loads is represented by the Woehler curves in Fig. 11. Under a cyclic bending load, the fatigue limits are 65–70% of the static strength. No significant differences are apparent between the two materials. The fatigue limits under a dynamic, alternating torsion load are 60–65% of the static torsion strength for the CFRP composite and 65–70% for CFRC. The Woehler curves are comparable to those for unreinforced carbon materials. After more than 10^4 alternating load cycles, the ratio of dynamic to static strength remains constant. Thus, no further fatigue is observed at a constant load level.

In view of the intended use of CFRC composites in the fabrication of endoprosthetic stems, it is important that the fracture characteristics of these materials also be explored. Although the CFRC composites are made up of two brittle components, they are pseudoplastic at room temperature and do not fail catastrophically. Figure 12 shows experimental stress-strain curves measured under torsion and bending loads. In no case is a catastrophic failure observed. Complete destruction requires extreme twist angles up to 180° or strains up to 5% under bending loads. This is roughly comparable to the yield point of metallic materials. The pseudoplastic properties of the materials are illustrated in Fig. 13, which shows a piece of biaxially reinforced CFRC composite through which nails have been driven. No fracture or delamination occurred. However, the degree of pseudoplasticity depends upon the type of carbon fibers used, the type of reinforcement employed, and the final treatment temperature during processing [24–27].

The development of a human stem is not yet complete, and so the results presented here are the most current available. So far strength tests have been performed on stems that correspond in design to the "Munich standard femur" [28]. The stems were analyzed with regard to their strain properties at various embedding levels and subjected to fatigue testing. The test setup and stem placement were based upon rec-

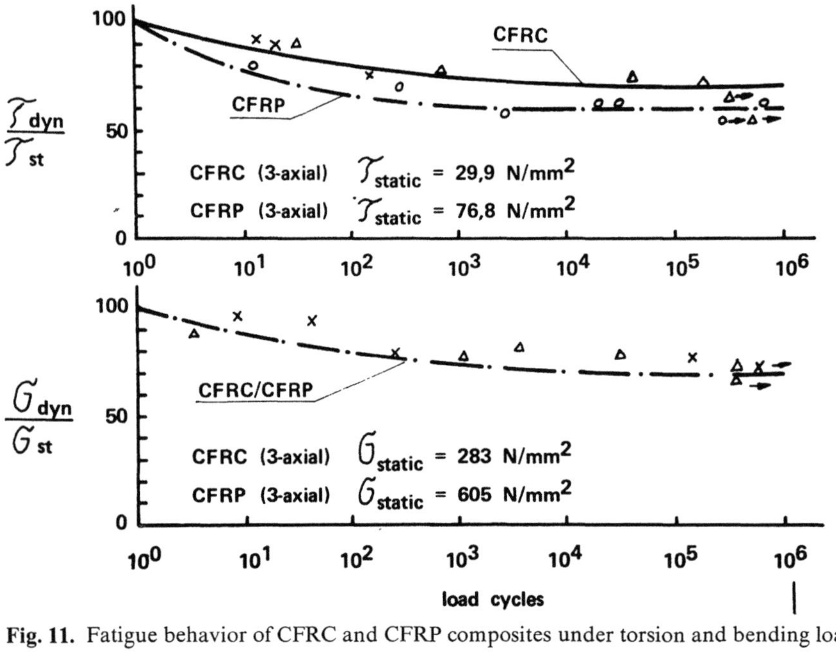

Fig. 11. Fatigue behavior of CFRC and CFRP composites under torsion and bending loads

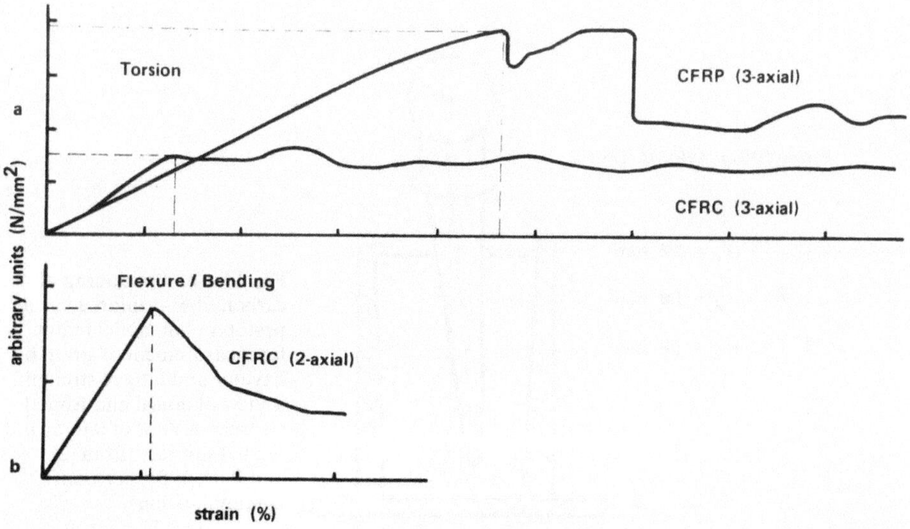

Fig. 12. Stress-strain curves of CFRC andCFRP composites under **a** torsion and **b** bending loads

ommendations from the Biomechanics Laboratory of the University of Munich (Plitz, 1981, personal communication). Details of the setup are shown in Fig. 14. For fatigue testing the stem is embedded 50 mm below the level of the collar. The minimum recommended load for this test is 1.7 ± 1.4 kN, and the stem is angled 5° laterally with respect to the vertical load axis. For the strain analyses, the stem is embedded at three different levels: $H_1 = 22$ mm below collar level, $H_2 = 58$ mm, and $H_3 = 86$ mm. Six strain gauges spaced 18 mm apart are applied to all four sides of the stem (frontal, dorsal, lateral, medial).

In the CFRC stems, the strain peaks on the lateral side are relatively independent of the embedding level (Fig. 15); they are located in the region of the calculated maximum bending moments (gauge position 2–3). On the dorsal side, however, a strong linear deflection is measured when the stem is embedded at H_3 (86 mm below collar) compared to H_2 and H_1. This is due to a lengthening of the moment arm and the correspondingly higher torsion moment.

Figure 16 shows the strain behavior of stems embedded at H_2 and H_3 for graduated loads from 0.5 to 4.6 kN. Again it is seen that the strain pattern on the lateral side of the stem is independent of embedding level. The locations of the compressive and tensile strain peaks also show little variation, although, as expected, they become more prominent as the load is increased. In the normal load range of 0.5 to 1.5 kN, no pronounced strain peaks are apparent anywhere along the stem. A quasi-neutral point is observed between gauge positions 4 and 6. It is also noteworthy that the distal tip of the stem (gauge position 6) shows no strain despite the increasing load.

Figure 17 shows the strain measured on the lateral side of five different CFRC stems subjected to a constant load of 5 kN. The CFRC stems are all identical in design but have different fiber structures. The design is responsible for the basic strain pattern, i.e., tensile stress between gauge positions 1 and 4, zero stress at po-

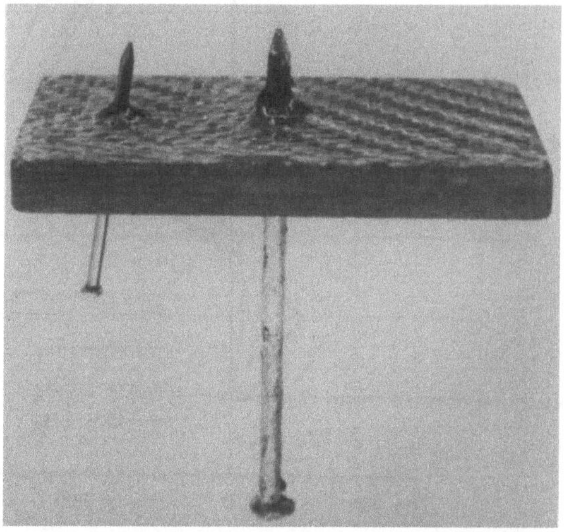

Fig. 13. Demonstration of the pseudoplastic behavior of CFRC composites

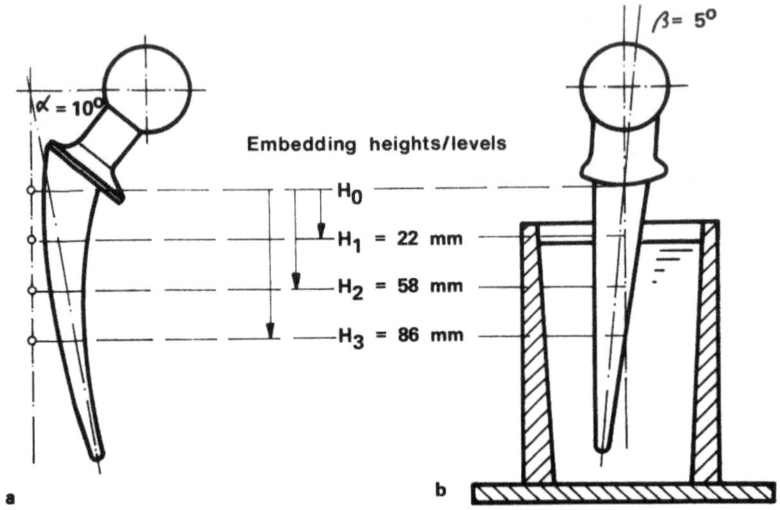

Fig. 14a, b. Positioning of carbon fiber-reinforced stem prototypes in model femur for measurement of strain behaviour and fatigue strength. **a** View of dorsal and frontal surfaces. **b** View of lateral and medial surfaces (from [28] and Plitz, 1981, personal communication)

sitions 4 and 5, and compressive stress between positions 4 and 6, while the different fiber structures determine the magnitude of the deformations. These varying fiber structures lead to differences of up to 17% in the region of the lateral strain maxima.

On the front surface of the stem, differences in fiber orientation have even more pronounced effects (Fig. 18). Parallel to the stem axis, it is possible to level off strain peaks and thus avoid critical torsion stresses. Perpendicular to the stem axis, it is even possible to design a stress-free stem. This shows that the critical torsion moments that are associated with loosening of the prosthetic stem need have no adverse effects on the stem. Parallel investigations on CFRP stems yielded essentially the same results.

The results of hip-simulator fatigue tests on a selected type of CFRC stem are summarized in Table 5. The dynamic tests were performed in a graduated fashion, with the basic load of 1.7 ± 1.4 kN being increased 3-fold to 5.1 ± 4.2 kN. After a total of 7 million load cycles the test was terminated, at which stage

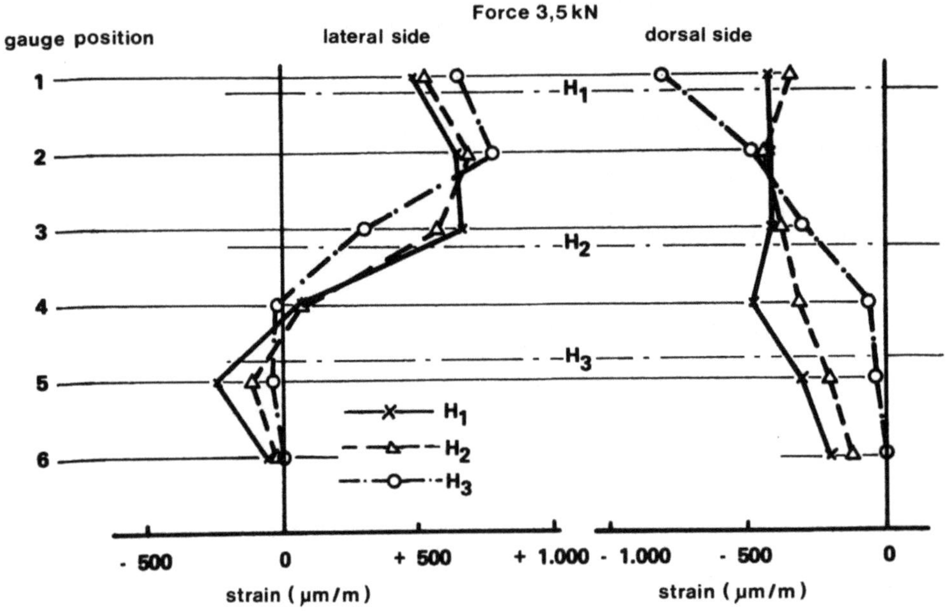

Fig. 15. Strain along the lateral and dorsal sides of the stem as a function of embedding level

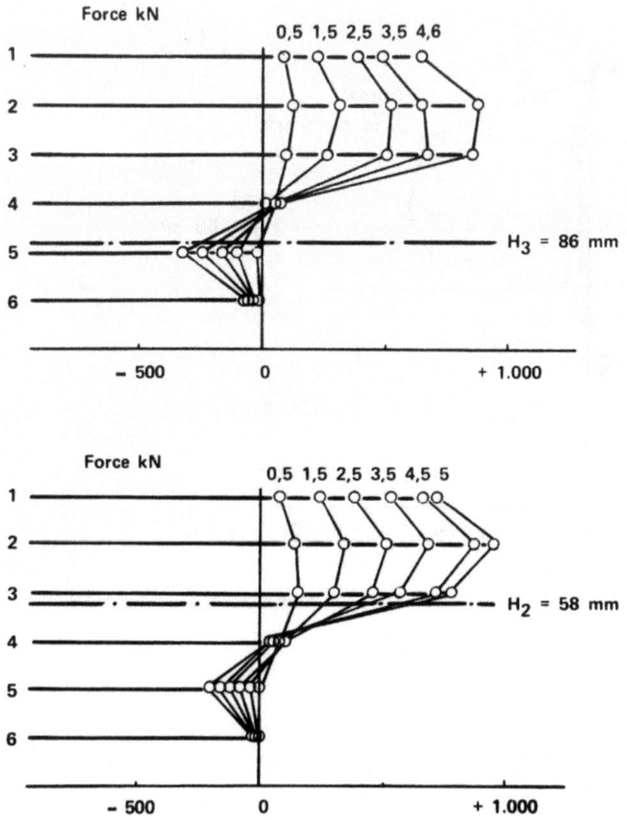

Fig. 16. Lateral stem strain under incremental loading for embedding levels *a* H_2 [sic] and *b* H_3 [sic]

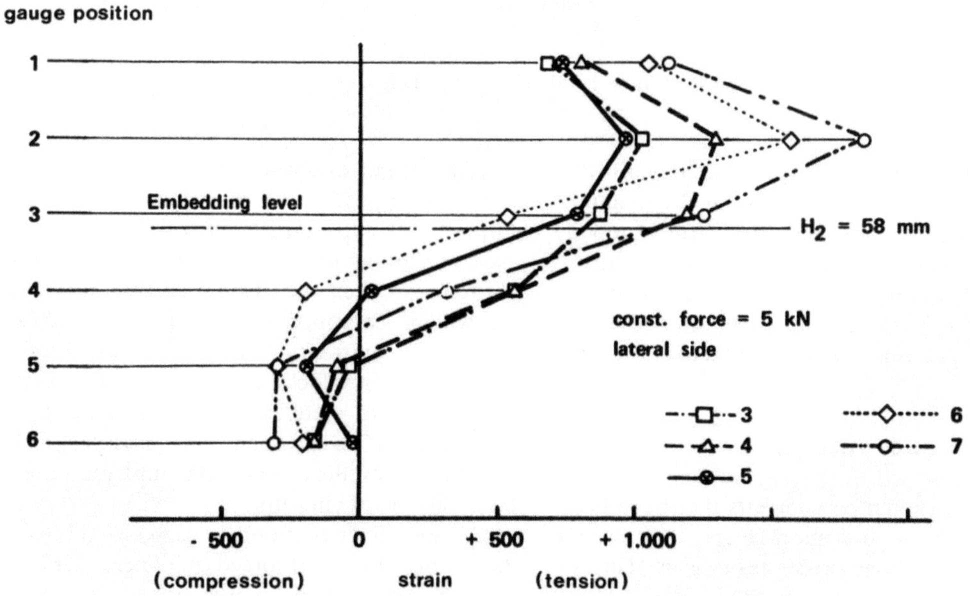

Fig. 17. Strain along 5 CFRC stems with different fiber structures under a constant load of 5 kN

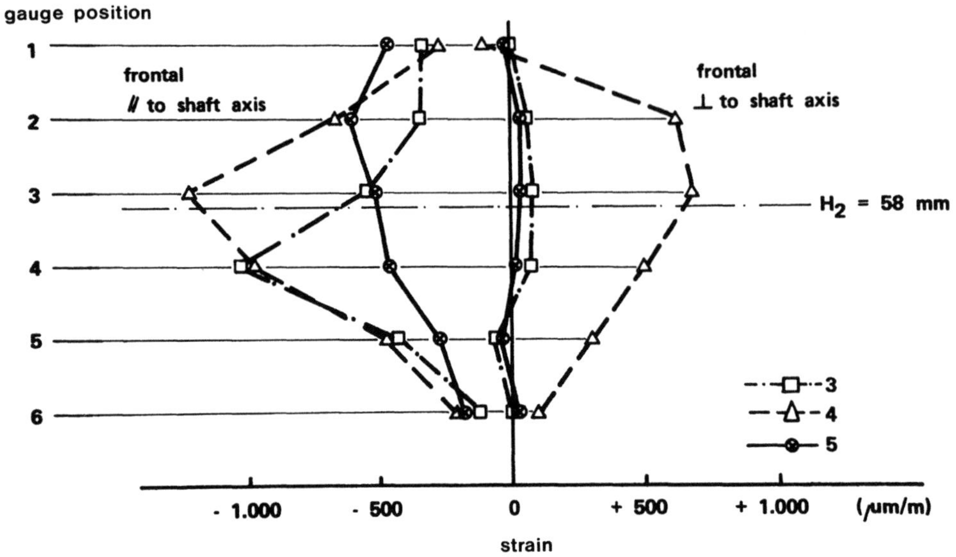

Fig. 18. Strain along the front side of the stem parallel and perpendicular to the axis of CFRC prototype stems with various fiber orientations

Table 5. Results of Hip-Joint Simulator Tests of CFRC Stem Prototypes

1. Load to failure, static (n = 10)	24 ±0.3 kN		
	load	No cycles	
2. Load, dynamic[a] (each n = 1)	1.7 ±1.4 kN	3×10⁶ plus	no failure and no plastic deformation
	2.2 ±1.8 kN	1×10⁶	
	2.25±2.1 kN	1×10⁶	
f = 10 Hz	2.55±1.8 kN	4×10⁶ plus	
	3.4 ±2.8 kN	1×10⁶ plus	
	4.25±3.5 kN	1×10⁶ plus	
	5.1 ±4.2 kN	1×10⁶	

[a] Fatigue tests were performed in Lab. für Biomechanik, Univ. München

the CFRC stem showed no permanent deformation or other damage. So far the dynamic load to failure has not been fully tested, although fatigue data indicate that an upper limit of 12–14 kN is reasonable. This would correspond to a mean load level of 6±5.7 to 7±6.7 kN at a constant initial load of 0.3 kN.

Summary and Outlook

The carbon gliding components that have been developed show good mechanical stability and promising tribologic properties *in vitro*. The coefficients of friction are low (0.05–0.07) and independent of the medium. Wear is minimal or negligibly small, and durability is excellent. The clinical testing of these materials was started with double-cup prostheses. A transitional phase is planned in which prosthetic stems constructed of proven cobalt-base and titanium alloys will be equipped with heads made of C/SiC. Tests are currently being done to determine whether the "self-locking cone" used to attach Al_2O_3 heads to metal stems can also be used with the C/SiC components. Meanwhile, work is continuing on the cement-free implantation of the C/SiC prosthetic cup.

Carbon fiber-reinforced carbons (CFRC) and carbon fiber-reinforced polymers (CFRP) have been developed for use in the fabrication of endoprosthetic stems. Main emphasis is placed on the CFRC stems, because the chemical inertness of the carbon precludes eventual changes of material properties within the body. The CFRC stems show high fatigue strengths, even when tensile and compressive stresses are accompanied by large torsion moments. The ability to modify the strain behavior of the component makes it possible to avoid critical stress situations while altering the stiffness of the stem. A special feature of the CFRC stems is the essential independence of strain patterns on the embedding level of the stem. In practical terms this means that the peaks of tensile and compressive strain always remain localized in the same areas of the stem even if loosening occurs.

Some optimization and development remain to be completed before clinical testing may begin. In the short term this includes statistical analyses of stability, applying the principle of construction to other stem designs, combining the CFRC stems with heads made of C/SiC (all-carbon prosthesis), and conducting stress analyses of the bone-CFRC stem system. Longer-term studies must be done on the excellent shock-absorbing properties of carbon fiber-reinforced composites, which are far superior to those of metals, and how they alter the effects of micromovements between the implant and bone. Another crucial point is quality control and the associated need for failure analyses so that lifetime predictions can be made.

References

1. Bokros JC (1977) Carbon biomedical devices. J Carbon 15:353–371
2. Bokros JC (to be published) Carbon in medical devices. In: Vinvenzini P (ed) Ceramics in surgery. Elsevier, Amsterdam
3. Jenkins GM, Grigson CJ (1979) The fabrication of artifacts out of glassy carbon for biomedical applications. J Biomed Mater Res 13:371–394
4. Grenoble DE, Voss R (1976) Materials and Designs for implant industry. Biomater Med Devices Aritf Organs 4 (2): 133–169
5. Jenkins DHR, Forster IW, McKibbin B, Ralis ZA (1977) Induction of tendon and ligament formation by carbon implants. J Bone Joint Surg [Br] 59:1
6. Fitzer E, Hüttner W (1977) Preparation of pyrocarboncoated carbonfibers for the use in ligament replacement. Extended Abstracts 13th Biennial Conf. on Carbon, Irvine, Calif. 1977, 180
7. Neugebauer R, Claes L, Helbing G, Wolter D (1979) The replacement of the abdominal wall by a carbon cloth on rabbits. Prep. 11th Int. Biomat. Symp., 5th Ann. Meeting Soc., Biomat., Vol 3, Clemson, South Carolina, 28. 04.–01. 05. 1979
8. Woo SL, Akeson WH, Coutts RD, Matthews JV, Amiel D (1974) Potential application of graphite-fiber and methylmetacrylate resin composites as internal fixation plates. J Biomed Mater Res 8:321–338
9. Fitzer E, Hüttner W, Claes L, Kinzl L (1980) Torsional strength of carbonfiber-reinforced carbon for the application as internal bone plates. Carbon 18:383–387
10. Claes L, Kinzl L, Neugebaur R (1981) Experimentelle Untersuchungen zum Einfluß des Plattenmaterials auf die Entlastung und Atrophie des Knochens unter Osteosyntheseplatten. Biomed Techn 26/4:66–71
11. Scheer W (1980) Kohlenstoffaserverstärktes Epoxidharz – ein Werkstoff für Humanimplantate, Verarbeiten und Anwenden kohlenstoffaserverstärkter Kunststoffe. VDI-Verlag Kunststofftechnik, Düsseldorf
12. Gohl W (1982) Kohlefaserverstärkter Zweikomponenten-Werkstoff für Knochenersatz. Forschungsbericht BMFT-FB-T82-036, April 1982, Fachinformationszentrum Karlsruhe
13. –
14. Brückmann H, Hüttinger KJ (1980) Carbon, a promising material in endoprosthetics, Part 1: The Carbon materials and their mechanical properties. Biomaterials 1:67–72
15. Böder H, Rose PG (1980) Produkte aus Kohlenstoff für medizintechnische Anwendungen, Preprints Carbon '80, 3. Int. Kohlenstofftagung, Baden-Baden, 30. 06.–04. 07. 80, S 676–679
16. Brückmann H, Keuscher G, Hüttinger KJ (1980) Carbon, a promising material in endoprosthetics, Part 2: Tribological properties. Biomaterials 1:73–81
17. Brückmann H, Hüttner W, Mäurer H-J, Hüttinger KJ (1981) Lösen Kohlenstoffe die Werkstoffprobleme hochbelasteter Endoprothesengelenke? Sprechsaal, 114. Jahrgang, 2/1981
18. Rettig H, Weber U, Hüttner W (1981) Alloarthroplastik des Hüftgelenkes unter Einsatz von Kohlenstoff als Implantatmaterial. Rheumamedizin 3/4: 100–102
19. Rettig H, Weber U, Nietert M (1983) Experimentelle und klinische Erfahrungen mit Kohlenstoff-Hüftendoprothesen. In: Morscher E (Hrsg) Die zementlose Fixation von Hüftendoprothesen. Springer, Berlin Heidelberg New York Tokyo
20. Timoshenko S (1934) Theory of elasticity. Mc Graw Hill, New York
21. Hüttner W, Keuscher G, Müller K (to be published). In vitro impact tests of carbon/siliconcarbide double cup prostheses. In: Vincenzini P (ed) Ceramics in surgery. Elsevier, Amsterdam
22. Brückmann H (1979) Entwicklung und anwendungsspezifische Untersuchung von Kohlenstoff-Werkstoffen für Endoprothesen am Beispiel des künstlichen Hüftgelenkes. Dissertation, Universität Karlsruhe

23. Fitzer E, Hüttner W (1981) Structure and strength of C/C-composites. J Phys. D Appl Phys 14:347–371
24. Hüttner W (1980) Parameterstudien zur Herstellung von kohlenstoffaserverstärkten Kohlenstoff-Verbundkörpern nach dem Flüssigimprägnierverfahren. Dissertation, Karlsruhe
25. Fitzer E, Hüttner W, Manocha LM (1980) Influence of process parameters on the properties of C/C-composites with pitch as matrix precursor. Carbon 18:291–295
26. Fitzer E, Geigl KH, Hüttner W, Weiss R (1980) Chemical interactions between the carbonfiber-surface and epoxy resins. J Carbon 18:389–393
27. Jortner J (1977) Sheer deformation of 3D carbon/carbon-composites. Prep. 13th Biennial Conf. on Carbon, Irvine, Calif. 1977, 443
28. Ungethüm M (1978) Technologische und Biomechanische Probleme der Hüft- und Kniealloarthroplastik. In: Aktuelle Probleme der Chirurgie und Orthopädie, Bd 9. Huber, Bern

Ceramic Materials for Implants

A. Zeibig

Introduction

Of the many high-quality ceramic materials that have been developed, only a few are considered suitable for use in implants. At present the selection is limited to the high-purity, chemically stable oxides. In addition to maximum biocompatibility, which depends on chemical parameters, crystalline structure and other physical properties, there are several additional criteria that must be satisfied by potential implant materials:

- high mechanical endurance for maximum functional reliability and longevity in the body,
- formability to exacting tolerances for the spherical components of artificial joints,
- extremely high-quality surface finish for components that articulate with other artificial or natural members.

Given the current interest in implants with load-bearing capabilities, the discussions that follow will be limited to implants which must function under large mechanical loads while attached to the skeleton. We must expect such implants to perform safely under high-stress transients (up to 50 times the body weight) and to withstand a total of more than 10^7 normal load cycles in physically active individuals.

High-purity aluminum oxides, known also as "bioceramics," are the only materials known that might be capable of satisfying the complex range of medical and technical requirements. Clinical trials are already being conducted with solid and porous bioceramic coatings, including coatings of the "bioactive" type. As yet, however, none of these coatings has demonstrated significant success in terms of a clinically reliable application for load-bearing implants.

Aluminum Oxide as a Bioceramic Material

To the best of our knowledge, the idea of fabricating implants from high-purity, sintered aluminum oxide was first mentioned in a German patent application of 1932. Since then, initial expectations with regard to biocompatibility have been confirmed by numerous investigations (Hulbert et al., 1970; Predeck et al., 1972; Boutin, 1972; Heimke et al., 1973; Plenk Jr., etc.). The use of bioceramic femoral heads has made it possible to reduce wear rates significantly in total hip systems. The factor $1/5$ is generally recognized for the conventional combination of a metal head with a polyethylene socket (Ungethuem et al., 1978; Scales; Semlitsch et al., 1975). The results of long-term mechanical tests and the first long-term implantations of a ceramic-on-ceramic system indicate that this factor can be reduced to about $1/10$, assuming the use of high-quality materials and the closest possible tolerances between the articulating components (Boutin, 1977; Mittelmeier, 1976).

The production of bioceramic materials is a somewhat complicated process that involves many steps. When designing implants, it is important to realize that sintering, which is done at a temperature of about 1700 °C, causes up to a 20% shrinkage in the linear dimensions of the components. This means that the desired final dimensions, surface geometry (2–3 μm) and surface finish ($\leqq 0.03$ μm) can be achieved only by subsequent working of the surface. Given the extreme hardness of the material, which is one reason for its excellent wear resistance, this working can be done only with diamond tools or diamond polishing agents. For technical reasons, the required degree of surface precision and surface finish can be obtained only with axially-symmetrical and spherical design forms.

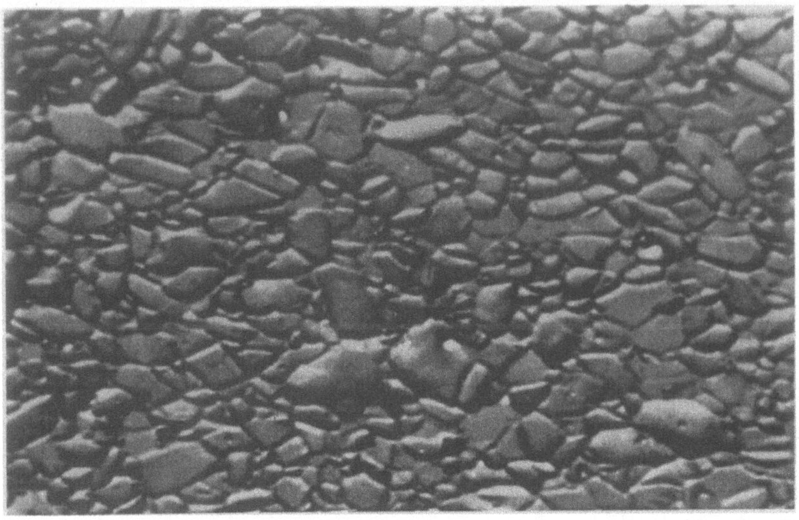

Fig. 1. Crystal structure of the bioceramic material (Al_2O_3 99.7%). Mean crystal size 3–4 μm

The crystal structure (Fig. 1) and bond strength of the individual crystallites have advantages that are well known: chemical inertness, high biocompatibility, high mechanical strength and wear resistance, workability and precision finish. They also have one major disadvantage, however: The bioceramic material, like all ceramics, is brittle. This means that it cannot undergo elastic or plastic deformation in response to mechanical loads. In this respect the bioceramics differ sharply from metals and polymers. Under an increasing external mechanical load, a short range of proportional elastic deformation is followed by complete, spontaneous failure as soon as the material-specific load limit is reached.

Tailoring the Design to the Material

When we compare the bending and tensile strength of a bioceramic with its compressive strength (Fig. 2), we find that the latter is greater by about a factor of 10. By exploiting this

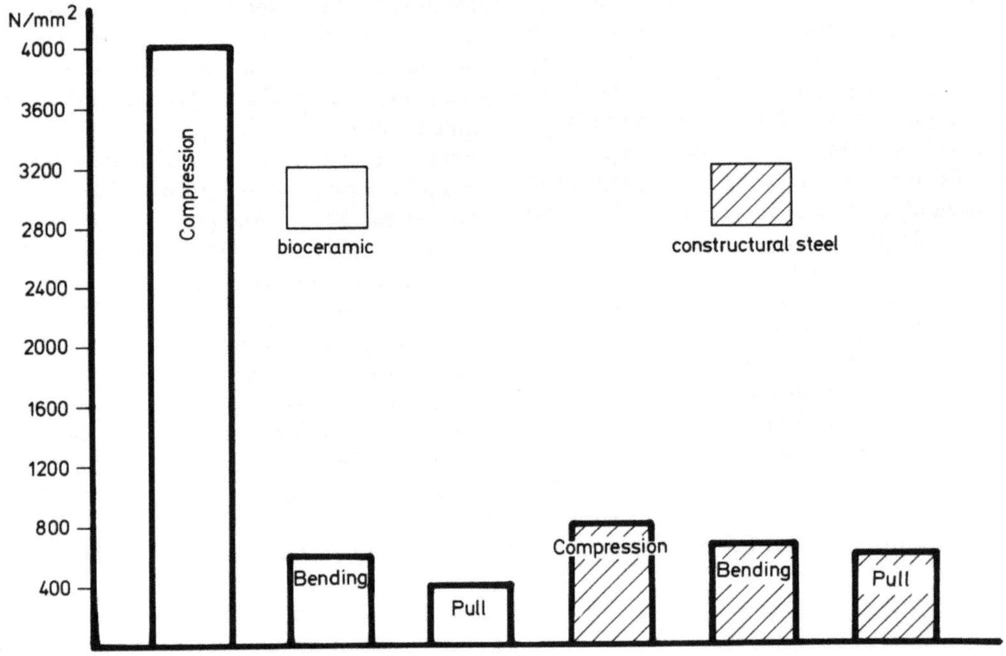

Fig. 2. Comparison of the compressive, bending and tensile strengths of bioceramic and structural steel

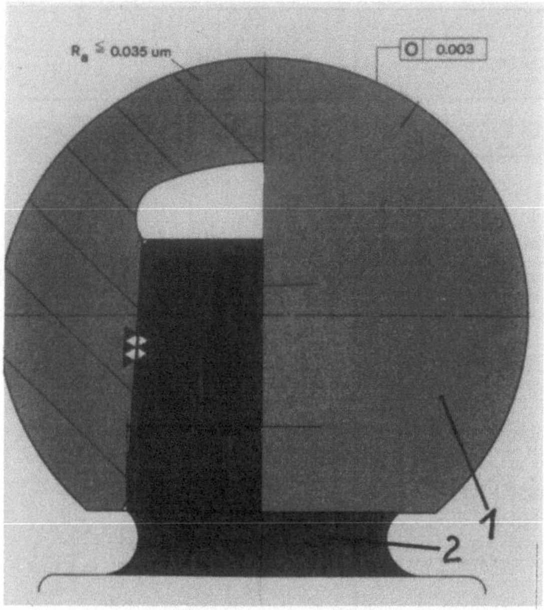

Fig. 3. Attachment of bioceramic femoral ball (*1*) to metal stem (*2*) using the self-locking cone

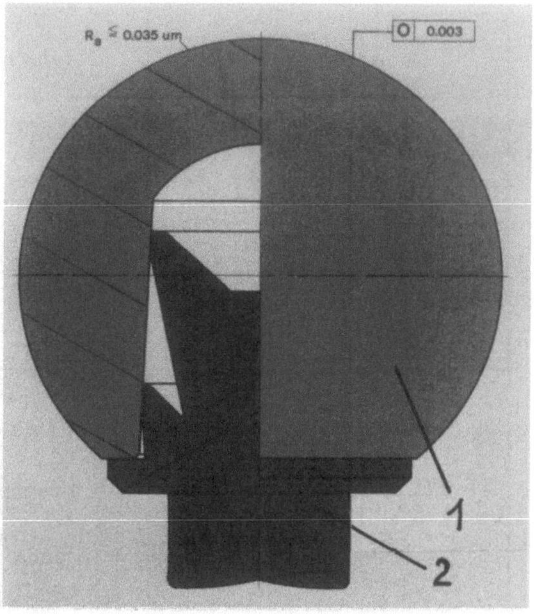

Fig. 4. Attachment of bioceramic femoral ball (*1*) to metal stem (*2*). The axial load component is absorbed by a supporting plate

property and still satisfying biomechanical demands, it is possible to develop highly advantageous and economical implant designs, as the following examples illustrate:

Femoral Ball: A very popular total hip system has been devised in which the bioceramic femoral ball is attached to the metal intramedullary stem by means of a "self-locking cone" (10% taper) (Fig. 3). The ball is held securely in place by friction, which must be balanced by internal, circumferential forces within the ball. The axial load capacity of the system is limited by the finite tensile strength of the material (tangential stress within the recess of the ball). On the other hand, if the ball is provided with a supporting plate that can absorb the axial load component (Fig. 4), then the high compressive strength of the material can be utilized to increase substantially the total load capacity of the stem-ball system.

Femoral Head Cup Arthroplasty: For surface replacement arthroplasty of the femoral head, a relatively thin shell is all that is needed to ensure good tribologic function. This principle (Wagner) makes optimum use of the high compressive strength of the ceramic. Because the external mechanical load on the cup is a compressive stress of specific distribution that is directed toward the center of the cup, a wall thickness of only 1–2.5 mm is sufficient. The total external load capacity is 30,000 N, and internal pressure tests conducted routinely for each device indicate a pressure level of 100 bar (Fig. 5).

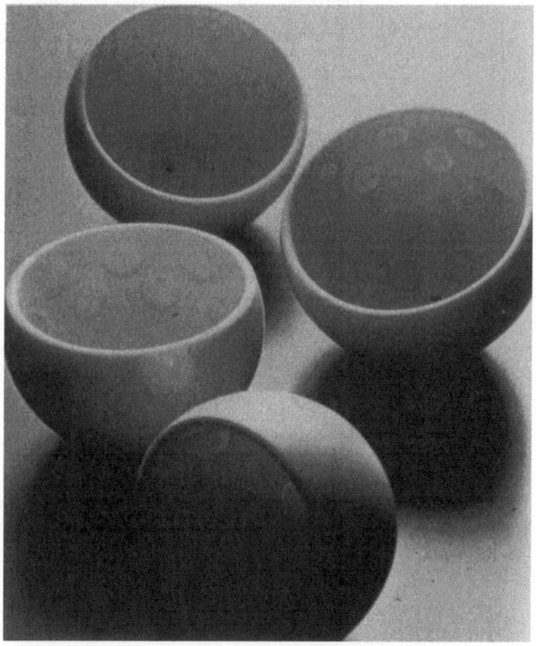

Fig. 5. Bioceramic femoral cups (Wagner type); wall thickness 1–2.5 mm

Testing	Type of control	Results
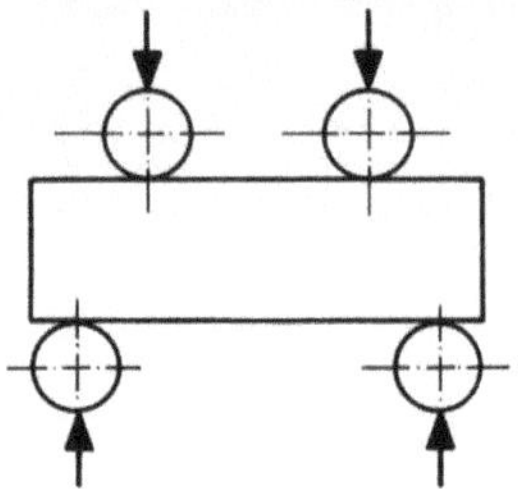	duzing production	tensile strength $\delta_B \geqq 500$ N/mm^2
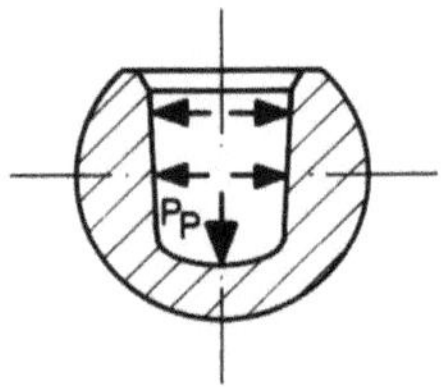	of individual (100 %)	internal pressure 1250 / 1000 bar
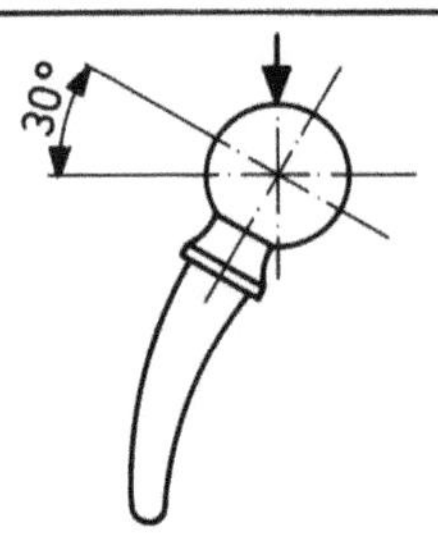	spot - check (of different types)	40 000 N 5000 ± 4000 N 2×10^6 cycles
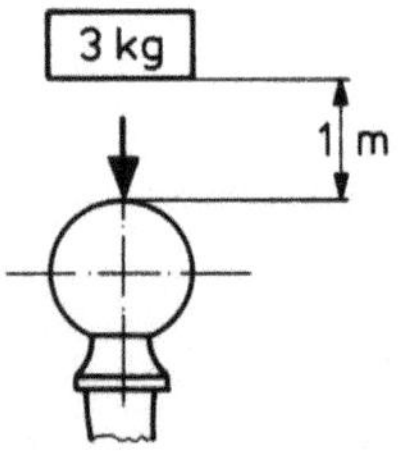	spot - check (of different types)	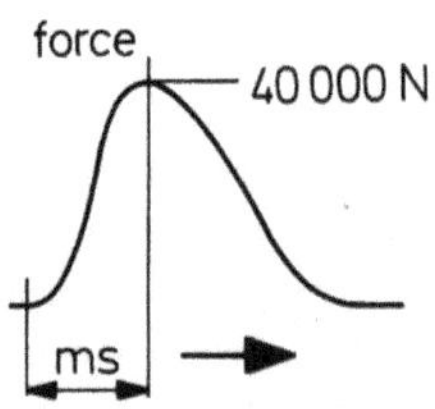
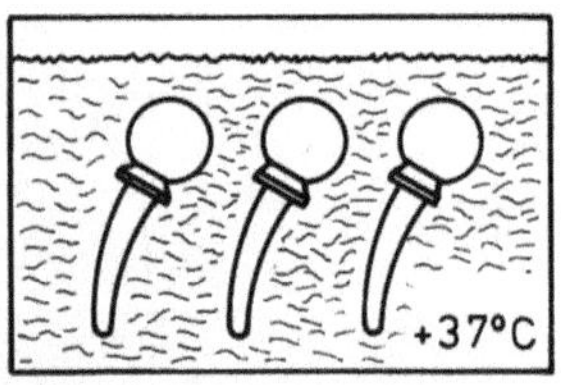 Ringer - solution	spot - check (of different types)	5000±4000 N $\leqq 10^7$ cycles period of testing $\leqq$ 5 years

Fig. 6. System for testing and verifying mechanical strength properties of bioceramic femoral balls 32 mm in diameter

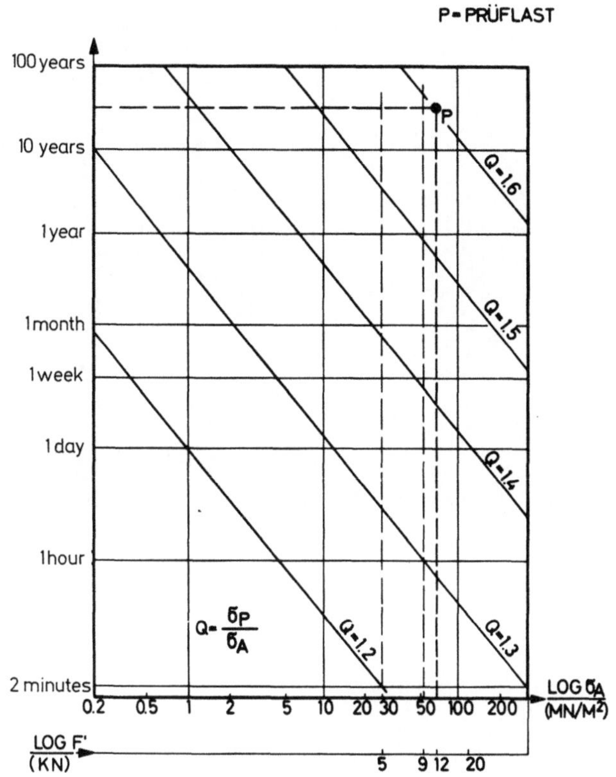

Fig. 7. Longevity data on bioceramic femoral balls 32 mm in diameter; test data for demonstrating a useful life of 30 years

Time-Volume Dependence of Strength Properties

For the development, design, testing and successful clinical use of bioceramic implants, it is not enough to work only with strength data available in material handbooks, specifications and standards. It is necessary to consider more specialized material characteristics and statistical data such as concentrated load-bearing capacity, static and dynamic load endurance, crack propagation velocity, and microcorrosion behavior. In the case of the femoral ball designed for attachment to the self-locking cone, it has been shown (Maier et al., 1982) that the fatigue strength value used in calculations should be only about 60% of the strength value measured with standard specimens. A knowledge of the functional implications of this "time-volume effect" on material strength is extremely important for the proper design of test systems (Fig. 6), for the quality control of prosthetic components, and for ensuring a minimum longevity of 30 years (Fig. 7).

Illustrative Implant Designs

Implant designs for use in orthopedic surgery may be classified into three main groups:

The design of implants for cementless fixation is based upon the principle of the conical sleeve attachment (Fig. 8 a, b). Specifics on the use of this principle for humeral and femoral prostheses have been described in various papers (Salzer et al., 1975; Mathejovsky, 1973). Reversing this principle leads to the well-known acetabular component design in which fixation is achieved by means of anchoring pegs (Fig. 9) (Boutin, 1972; Salzer et al., 1974) or by means of external threads (Mittelmeier, 1976; Griss et al., 1975). In all cases a solid primary press-fit must be achieved at the time of insertion. High-precision instruments are used to shape the bone and ensure an optimum fit.

The cement fixation of bioceramic implants is a well-known technique that requires no further explanation. The principal advantage of bioceramic over polyethylene in cement fixation is its significantly higher heat capacity and ther-

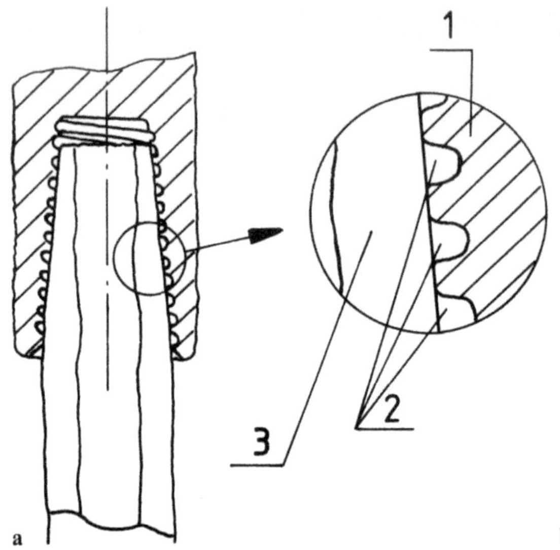

a

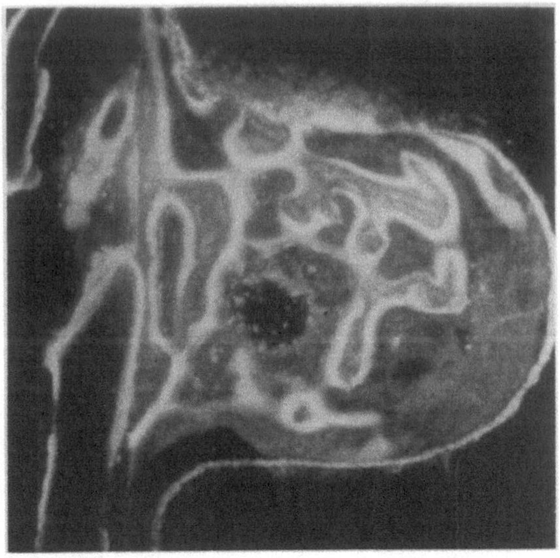

b

Fig. 8. **a** Principle of the conical sleeve attachment. *1* Endoprosthesis, *2* space for new bone, *3* cortical bone. **b** Histologic demonstration of new bone formation in the ingrowth grooves of the implant (tetracycline labeling)

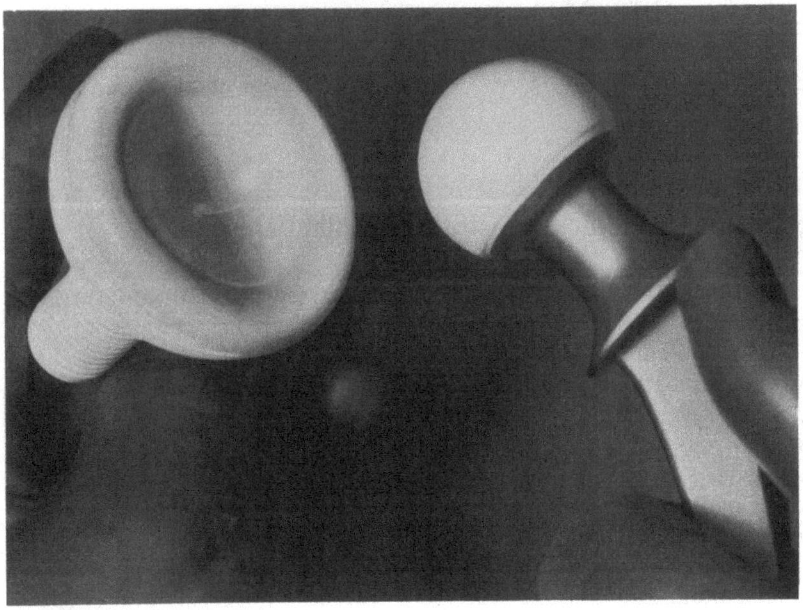

Fig. 9. Bioceramic acetabular component with anchoring pegs and ceramic- on-metal design for femoral endoprosthesis

mal conductivity. As a result of this, heat generation during polymerization of the cement should not present a problem under conditions of a thin cement mantle and large implant surface, as in the case of surface replacement systems.

The third group of bioceramic implants is by far the most widely used. This consists of implants that are not directly attached to the bone, such as the various femoral ball designs with diameters from 32 to 54 mm. Functionally, it does not matter whether the metal component supporting the ball is attached with or without cement, as long as the preparations for implantation and the implantation itself do not place undue stresses on the bioceramic component, as may result from hot sterilization due to differences in thermal expansion of the metal and bioceramic, impact loading, or damage to the metal cone during insertion and positioning of the metal stem.

Conclusion

The results and experience of 10 years' research and development and more than 5 years' clinical use prove that finely-crystalline, high-purity aluminum oxide has significantly improved endoprosthetics in a number of areas. It is by no means a universal material, however. It yields the desired results only when there is a careful coordination between medical and technical requirements, material properties and manufacturing processes. We estimate that since 1975–76, more than 50,000 bioceramic implants have already been supplied for clinical use. This number underscores the importance that bioceramics have achieved in the clinical setting, while demonstrating the great responsibility that is borne by the manufacturer and user in terms of the quality of the implants and their functional reliability.

References

Boutin P (1972) Arthroplastic totale de la hanche par prothèse en alumine frittée. Rev Chir Orthop 58:229–246

Boutin P (1977) L'arthoplastie totale de la hanche par prothèse en alumie. Résultats de 150 cas d'ancrage direct de la pièce acétabulaire. Int. Orthop 1:87–94

Griss P, Heimke G, Andrian-Werburg H v (1975) Die Aluminiumoxidkeramik-Metall-Verbundprothese. Eine neue Hüftgelenktotalendoprothese zur teilweise zementfreien Implantation. Arch Orthop Unfallchir 81:259–266

Heimke G, Beisler W, Andrian-Werburg H v, Griss P, Krempien B (1973) Untersuchungen an Implantaten aus Al_2O_3-Keramik. Berichte der Dtsch. Keram. Ges. 50:4–8

Hulbert SF, Young FA, Mathews RS, Klawitter JJ, Talbert CD, Stelling FH (1970) Potential of ceramic materials as permanently implantable skeletal prosthesis. J Biomed Mater Res 4:433–456

Maier HR, Krauth A, Stärk N, Zeibig A (1982) Long life ceramic-metal hip joints. In: Winter GD, Gibbons DF, Plenk H Jr (eds) Biomaterials 1980. Wiley & Sons, New York Chichester

Mathejovsky Z (1973) Results of arthroplasty in tumors affecting the hip. Arthroplasty of the hip. Thieme, Stuttgart, p 226

Mittelmeier H (1976) Anchoring hip endoprostesis without bone cement. In: Schaldach M, Hohmann D (eds) Engineering in medicine, vol 2. Advances in artificial hip and knee joint technology. Springer, Berlin Heidelberg New York

Plenk H (1982) Biocompatibility of ceramics in joint prostheses. In: William DF (ed) Biocompatibility of orthopedic implants – vol 1:269–295 CRC incorp. Boca Raton

Predecki P, Auslaender PA, Stephan JE, Mooney VL, Stanitski C (1972) Attachment of bone to threaded implants by ingrowth and mechanical interlocking. J Biomed Mater Res 6:401–412

Salzer M, Locke H, Engelhardt A, Zweymüller K (1975) Keramische Endoprothesen der oberen Extremität. Kongreßband. Z Orthop 113:458–461

Salzer M, Zweymüller K, Locke H, Plenk H Jr, Punzet G (1975) Biokeramische Endoprothesen. Med Orthop Techn 95:40

Scales JT, Wright JKW (1980) The evaluation of wear of total hip prostheses. In: Winter GD, Leary GL. The evaluation of biomaterials, p 141. John Wiley & Sons

Semlitsch M, Willert HG, Dörre E (1975) Neue Werkstoffpaarung Al_2O_3-Keramik/Polyäthylen zur Verminderung des Polyäthylenabriebs bei Gelenkpfannen von Hüftendoprothesen. Med Orthop Techn 95:143–144

Ungethüm M, Hinterberger J, Plitz W (1978) Tribologica. Properties of Al_2O_3-ceramica. In: Hastings, Williams (eds) Advances in biomaterials. Mechanical properties of biomaterials. Wiley, London

A Metal-Ceramic Composite Designed for Cementless Fixation to Bone

H. Scharbach

The question of material is central to all considerations on the development of a cementless skeletal implant system that has good long-term stability. Even the best implant design, operating technique and postoperative management cannot ensure success if the bone-replacement material fails to meet the many specific demands that are placed upon it. Material is the major determinant of biological adaptation, solid bony integration and longevity of the implant.

On the other hand, it would be presumptuous to assume that lifeless matter can mimic perfectly the function and structural properties of living bone – especially when the selection is limited to single materials. The biological and electrical weaknesses of metals, the brittleness and low bending strength of ceramics and graphite, and the relatively poor longevity of polymers are well known. A sizable gap exists between the essential requirements of an implant material and the capabilities of the single materials that are currently available. A bone implant that can distribute stresses to the bone in a largely normal fashion and can be implanted without bone cement must satisfy at least the following minimum criteria:

1. High static and dynamic load capacity 2. High toughness 3. Good formability and/or workability 4. Good longevity (no swelling, deformation or decomposition)	metal core
4. Good longevity (no swelling, deformation or decomposition) 5. High corrosion resistance 6. Surface adaptability 7. High hardness and good tribologic properties (for joints) 8. High electrical resistance 9. Biocompatibility and/or bioactivity	ceramic coating

The overworked concept of "isoelasticity" was intentionally omitted from this list, because it would be unrealistic to demand it of a bone-replacement material. The elasticity of bone is subject to much variation depending on the individual, the skeletal region (even within the same bone), and the direction in which loads are applied. We believe it is far simpler and more realistic to achieve an approximate isoelasticity through design features.

Fusion of Classic Materials

The only way to satisfy all the criteria listed above is by combining classic materials into a composite system. Metal and ceramic have been chosen for this purpose. Requirements 1–4 are met by certain stainless steels and special alloys, while properties 4–9 are characteristic of certain glasses or ceramic materials. However, two further conditions must be satisfied if the composite is to function properly:

a) The metal must form the main body of the implant and provide the necessary load-bearing capacity, while the ceramic is applied externally as a coating that will participate in all biochemical and electrical interactions with the host tissue.
b) An extremely high-strength bond must be created between the core and coating.

This, then, was the objective of a research project that was started in 1973 by the Pfaudler-Werke Corp. in collaboration with Dr. A. Engelhardt and which, since 1977, has been funded by the West German Ministry of Research and Technology. The result of the nine-year project is a material with the trade name Osteoceram: a metal/glass ceramic composite that is tailored specifically to the needs of skeletal implantation [1].

Metal Core

From the many types of stainless steels and special alloys available, it was possible to select those which showed the greatest promise in terms of their coefficient of expansion and chemical reactivity toward the glass ceramic, and which also featured a high static and dynamic strength and toughness. Selected ferritic chromium steels and austenitic CrNiMo steels are suitable for implants and implant components that can be coated over their entire surface. Even more favorable are certain cobalt- and nickel-base alloys (cast or wrought), which function well even when partially coated.

Mechanical and metallographic control studies have shown that the short-term heating necessary for the coating process has virtually no effect on the strength of the substrate.

Coating Technique and Bond Strength

All physical properties of the multi-layer composits depend directly on the strength of the

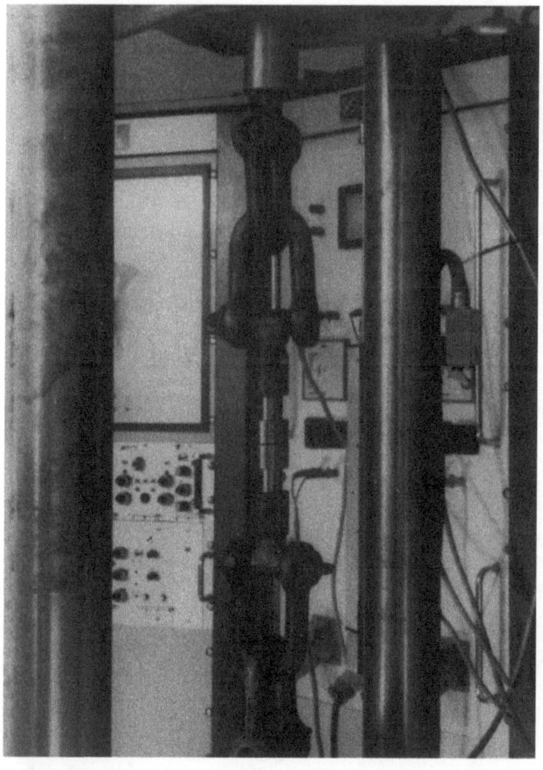

Fig. 1. Tensile test of two stainless steel specimens bonded together by glass ceramic

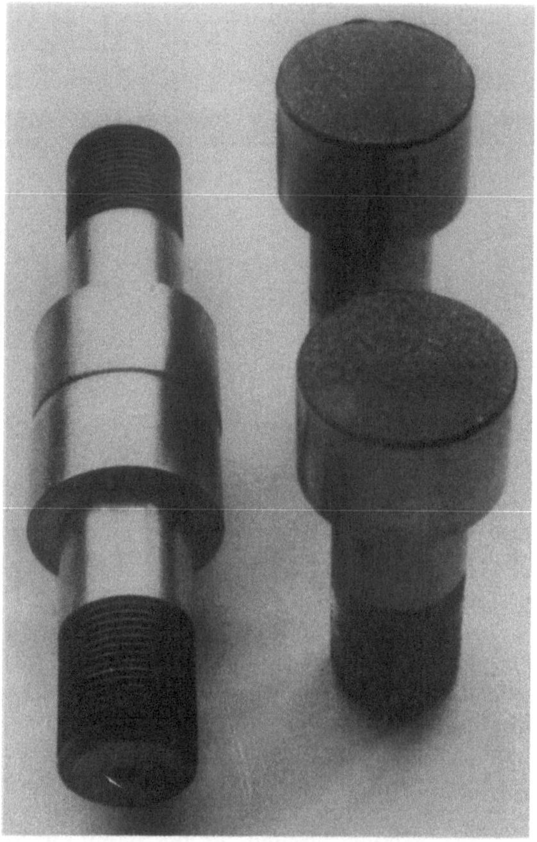

a b

Fig. 2. The ceramic-bonded specimen **a** before tensile testing and **b** after testing

bond between the layers, which is why priority is placed on the coating technology and resulting adhesion. Considering the basic contrast between the materials to be bonded together – a tough, crystalline metal on the one hand and a brittle, amorphous ceramic on the other – one can well appreciate the difficulty of this undertaking.

The adhesion is mediated by a layer of specially developed glass ceramic whose redox behavior, thermal expansion and surface tension are carefully matched to those of the metal core. This material, in the form of a finely-milled powder, is sintered onto the metal substrate at 900–1000 °C, creating a powerful adhesive force as high as 100 N/mm². This is several times greater than the adhesive strength of the best polymeric adhesives and surpasses even the tensile strength of the ceramic itself, which is between 50 and 60 N/mm². A tear-apart test of two stainless steel specimens bonded together

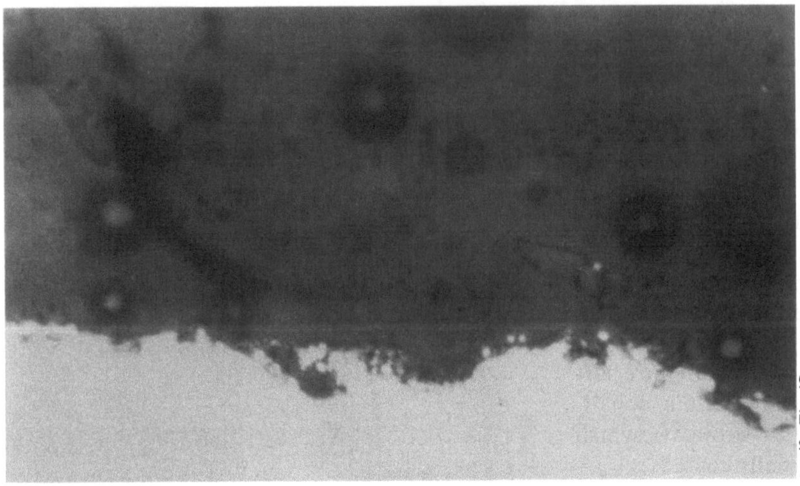

Fig. 3. Micrograph of a ground section showing the intimate mechanical interlocking produced by the glass-steel reaction (×700)

by the adhesive ceramic (Fig. 1) makes this clear. Fig. 2a shows the bonded specimens prior to testing, and Fig. 2b shows them after testing. The composite specimen did not separate at the metal-ceramic interface, as expected, but within the ceramic itself.

The extreme strength of the bond results from high-temperature reactions in the interfacial zone which lead to a partial chemical breakdown of the metal substrate, enabling true chemical bonding to take place at an atomic level. The ground section in Fig. 3, magnified 700 times, shows the high degree of interlocking produced by the glass-steel reaction, which serves to enhance the bond produced by chemical adhesion. This powerful bond gives the glass ceramic applications that previously were reserved for steel alone.

Glass Ceramic Coating

At least one coating layer is sintered onto the adhesive layer. The coating consists of a biocompatible glass ceramic that is chemically and thermodynamically stable. Oxides of the elements Si, Zr, Ca, Mg, Na, K and Li are best for this purpose.

The glass ceramic coating, too, is matched to the stainless steel core in terms of expansion coefficient and elastic modulus in such a way that large compressive stresses are generated during cooling. Owing to this prestressing, the coating will be able to withstand momentary temperature rises (Δt) up to 160 °C and will not fracture under mechanical loads before the elastic limit of the metal core is exceeded. This elastic impaction gives the ceramic coating a bending fatigue strength which far surpasses that of the unbonded ceramic. This has been confirmed with a specially developed rotary bending machine, under dry conditions as well as in physiologic saline [2].

The high electrical resistance of the Osteoceram layer (10^{12} Ωcm) has two advantages:

a) The coating cannot short-circuit, and thus disrupt, the piezoelectric and ferromagnetic signal patterns that aid in regulating bone formation.
b) It prevents all forms of electrochemical corrosion that might cause dissolution of the metal.

The ceramic coating varies in thickness from 0.2–2 mm, is nonporous, and is completely impermeable to liquids and gases. Hence, it keeps the metal substrate safely isolated from potentially disruptive biochemical processes.

Glass Ceramic Coating with Exceptional Load-Bearing Capacity

Osteoceram-N is a high-strength variant of the Osteoceram coating. By adding nucleating agents to the ceramic and by following the sin-

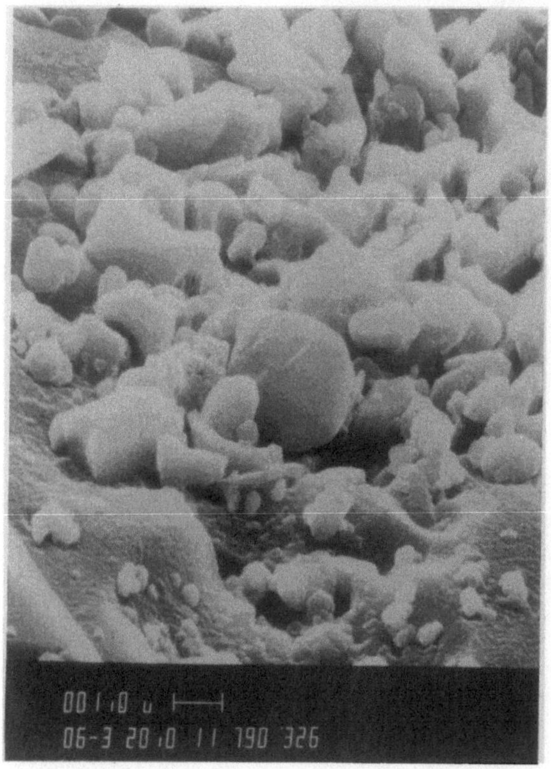

Fig. 4. Electron micrograph showing the crystalline structure of Osteoceram-N

tering process with a special heat treatment, a controlled crystallization of the coating is achieved. The high crystal content of the ceramic greatly increases the impact strength and wear resistance of the coating. The electron micrograph in Fig. 4 shows the crystalline structure of Osteoceram-N under very high magnification [3]. The material is designed primarily for use in articulating surfaces.

The best tribologic properties are achieved by combining Al_2O_3 with Osteoceram-N, owing to the different hardnesses of the articulating components and their markedly hydrophilic character. Fig. 5 shows the actual prosthesis: an Al_2O_3 ball combined with an Osteoceram-N-lined socket.

Surface Finish

Where bioinertness is needed but no bony contact is expected, the glass ceramic coating may be given a smooth, high-gloss surface finish (Osteoceram-G).

To enhance load transfer between the bone and implant, the surface can be made as rough as desired by chemical or mechanical treatment (Osteoceram-R).

If a grinding or cutting action is needed for implantation, hard, bioinert crystals may be embedded in the ceramic coating. This type of finish is useful, for example, in a self-tapping anchoring screw (Fig. 6).

If bony ingrowth is desired as a means of securing implant fixation, the ceramic can be given a spongy structure with a 100–500 μm pore size (Osteoceram-S, Fig. 7).

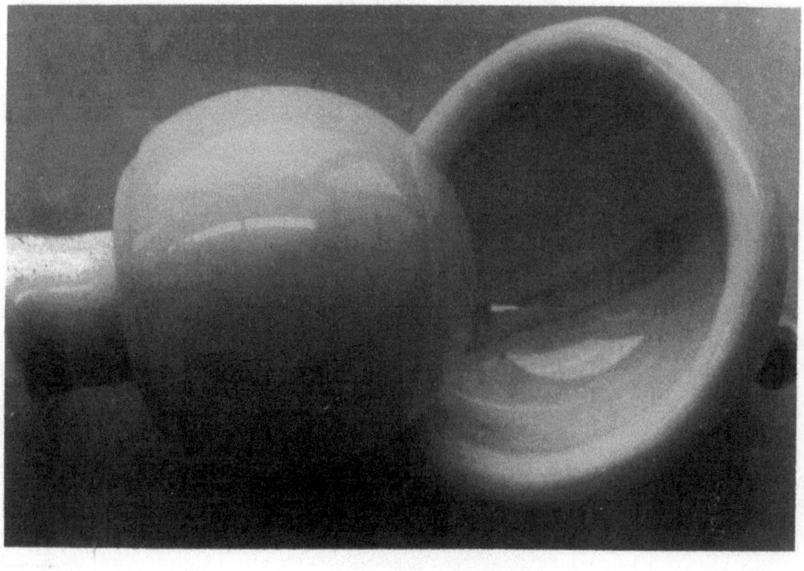

Fig. 5. Al_2O_3 ball and Osteoceram-N-lined socket with lubricating groove

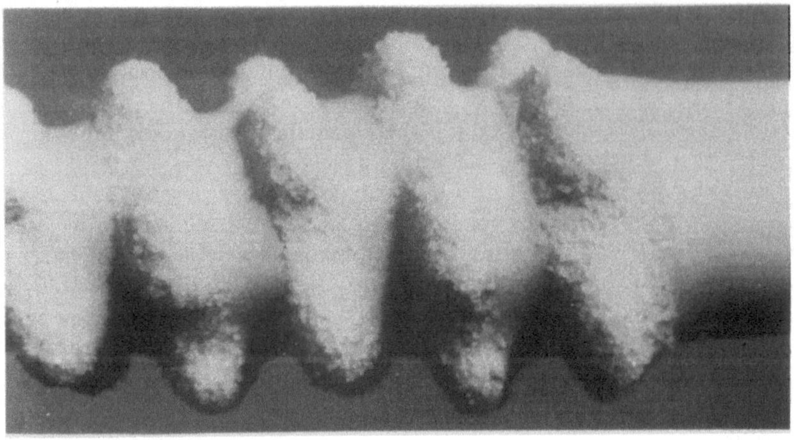

Fig. 6. Self-tapping anchoring screw

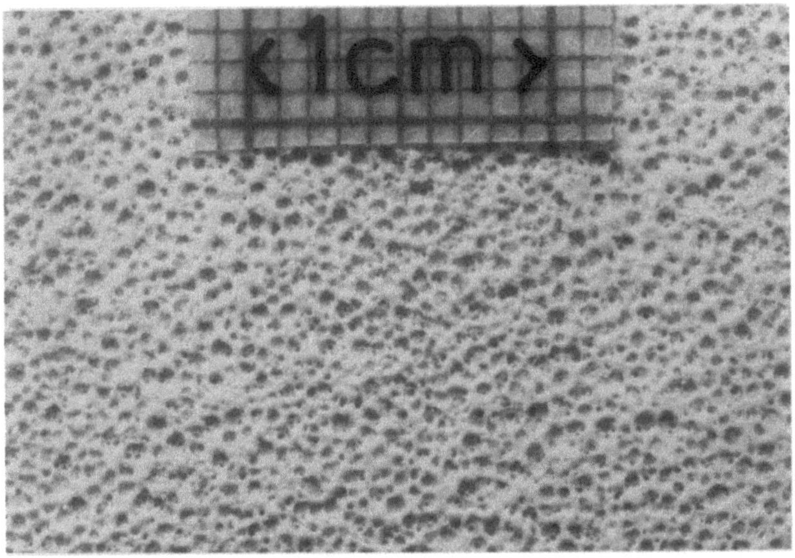

Fig. 7. Spongy structure with pore sizes of 100–500 μm

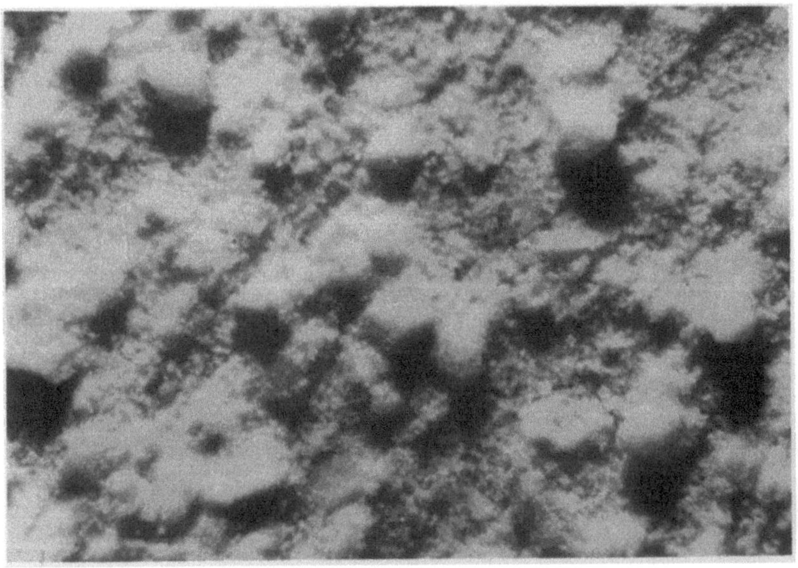

Fig. 8. Tricalcium phosphate added to an Osteoceram coating

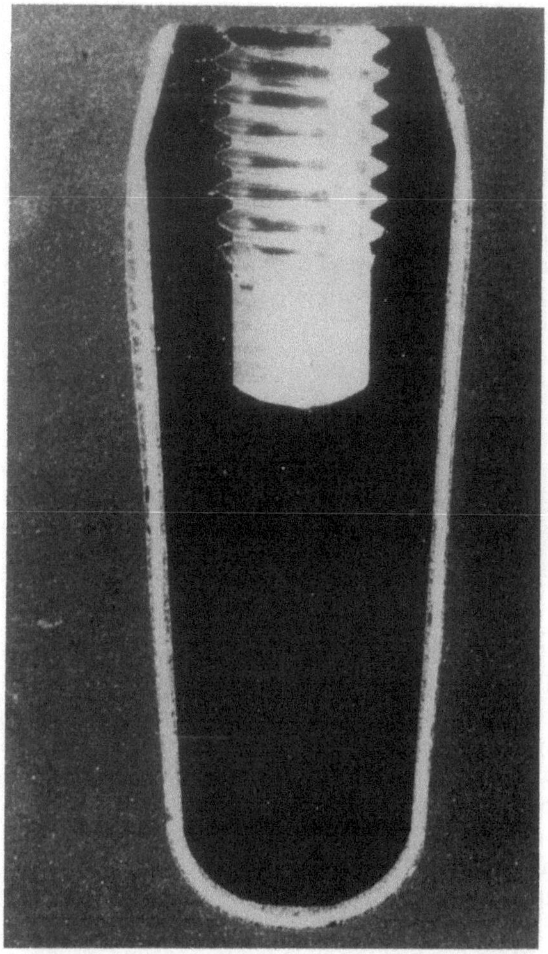

Fig. 9. Cross-section of a dental root implant with a metal core and 250-μm thick Osteoceram-P coating

Bioreactive Coating

The Osteoceram coating that is fused to the metal core can in turn serve as a substrate for bioreactive substances such as bioglasses or calcium phosphates (Osteoceram-P).

These substances, with their controlled solubility, are believed to exert a mineralizing effect on the surrounding bone [4]. Fig. 8 shows a light micrograph of an Osteoceram layer to which bioreactive tricalcium phosphate has been added.

Figure 9 shows the magnified cross-section of a dental root implant. The threaded socket is surrounded by a metal core, which in turn is coated with a layer of Osteoceram-P 250 μm in thickness.

The photo in Fig. 10 shows various types of Osteoceram specimens and implants.

Clinical Testing

Cylindrical Osteoceram specimens were implanted into the femurs of 186 rabbits for periods up to 120 weeks. According to Engelhardt and Kraft, direct bone-implant contact with no intervening connective tissue was observed after 6 weeks at the latest. No inflammatory or neoplastic reactions were noted [5]. Figure 11, taken from that series, reveals extensive, direct bone contact at the smooth implant surface after 164 days.

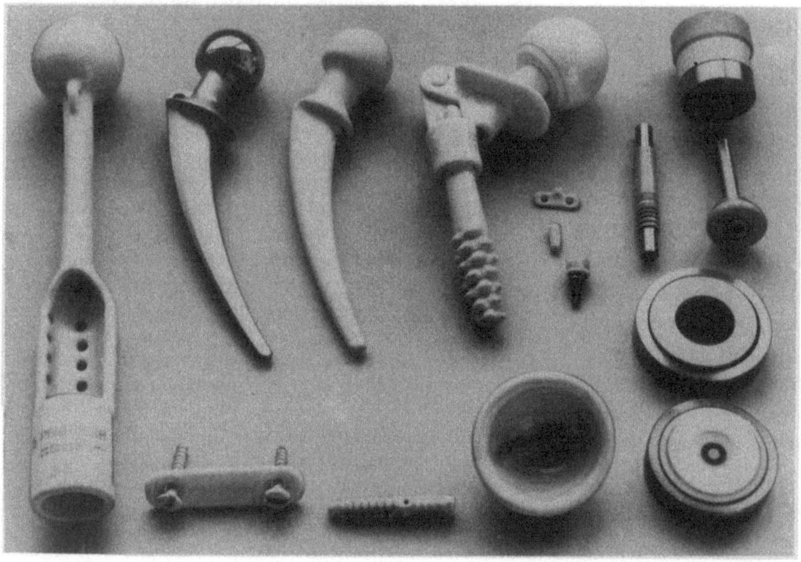

Fig. 10. Various Osteoceram specimens and implants

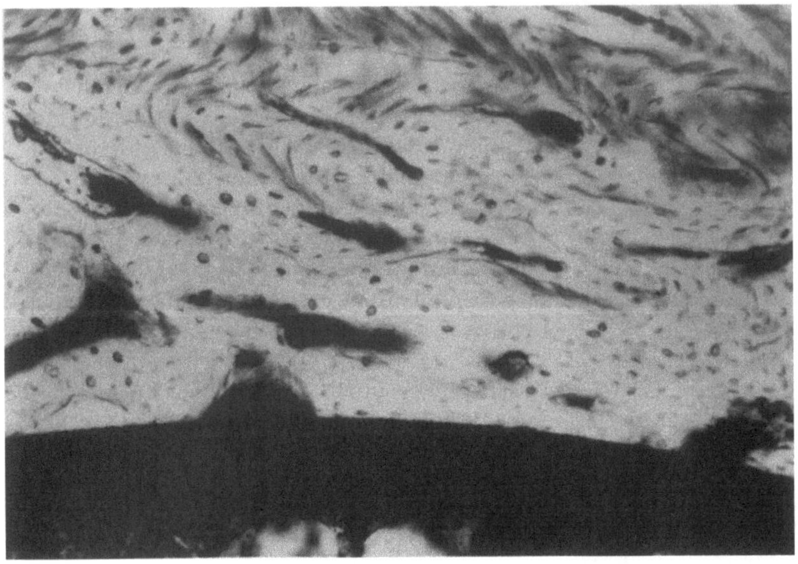

Fig. 11. Extensive, direct bone contact at a smooth implant surface (rabbit femur, 164 days)

Supplementary *in vitro* tests with fibroblasts and *in vivo* tests for toxicity and carcinogenicity were conducted by Komitowsky at the German Cancer Research Institute in Heidelberg. No pathologic changes or abnormalities of cell growth were found. In addition, Osteoceram implants have been successfully used in 7 cases to bridge tumor resection defects in the humerus and hip area.

Over a follow-up period of up to 7.5 years, there has been no failure of bony fixation in any of the endoprostheses despite frequent conditions of high stress. The same applies to the first total hip prostheses of Engelhardt and Grell.

Evaluation of Biologic Behavior

Owing to the biocompatibility of its components, its high thermodynamic and chemical stability, and its electrical neutrality, Osteoceram was expected to have a bioinert behavior. However, this assessment fails to appreciate the biologic character of the material and requires differentiation, for the broad range of alloplastic materials that the body accepts without an immune reaction but nevertheless encapsulates in fibrous tissue can lay claim to the same attribute. The Osteoceram surface, on the other hand, allows intimate bony contact to develop and must be regarded as bioactive in the positive sense, regardless of the mode of action of any bioglasses or phosphates that are additionally applied.

Summary

The bone implant material Osteoceram ideally combines the best properties of metals with the specific advantages of glass ceramic while avoiding their disadvantages. This is accomplished by utilizing the metal as a load-bearing substrate to which the bioactive ceramic is applied as a coating. A high bond strength between these components is an important prerequisite.

The shape of the metal substrate and the surface finish of the glass ceramic coating can be varied over a very large range, which makes the Osteoceram system suitable for a great many skeletal implant applications. So far the excellent clinical results obtained in various skeletal regions give cause for much optimism.

References

1. Engelhardt A (1982) Endlich eine ausgereifte Total-Endoprothese. Ärztl Prax XXXIV. Jahrg. vom 26. 01. 82 8:226
2. Steinmann N, Grell H (1978) Korrosionsprüfeinrichtung für eine Umlaufbiegemaschine. Studienarbeit an der Fachhochschule Aalen, 27. 03. 78
3. Scharbach H (1965) Nucerite, ein neues Email für hohe mechanische und chemische Beanspruchungen in der Verfahrenstechnik. Werkstoffe Korrosion 16. Jahrg. 1:20–23
4. Riess G (1978) Klinische Erfahrungen mit Trikalziumphosphatimplantaten. Quintessenz 29, Referat Nr. 5767
5. Engelhardt A et al. (1976) Trends in the development of permanent ceramic implants. In: Schaldach M (ed) Engineering in medicine, vol 2. Advances in artificial hip and knee joint technology. Springer, Berlin Heidelberg New York

Titanium and Titanium Alloy Prostheses with Porous Fiber Metal Coatings *

P. Ducheyne, M. Martens, P. De Meester and J. C. Mulier

Introduction

In an effort to improve the long-term reliability of permanent implants, several new techniques have been investigated for the skeletal fixation of the components. Independent work at various laboratories has shown mechanical interlocking by bone ingrowth into porous coatings to be one of the most promising techniques in this regard [4, 8, 10, 11, 13].

By and large, the short- and medium-term results of hip prostheses are satisfactory. Therefore, interest in new prosthetic designs and materials has been shifting toward the analysis of long-term performance. It has been found that a multidisciplinary approach involving specific, long-term experimental studies is required. More limited approaches to the problem will do little to advance the general state of the art [2, 9].

With regard to the "ingrowth" fixation of prostheses, our studies have encompassed various interdisciplinary aspects. All were investigated specifically in relation to the eventual clinical use of total hip prostheses. Figure 1 shows the interrelationship between 9 factors: (1) pore size and porosity, (2) the mechanical properties of the porous coating and metal substrate, (3) bonding between the substrate and coating, (4) the biocompatibility of the porous structures, (5) bone-bonding capability under functional loading, (6) design and primary implant stability, (7) stress distribution in the substrate-coating-tissue complex, (8) the viability of the surrounding bone, and (9) the stimulation of bone growth.

* Acknowledgments: The metal fibers used in some of the experiments presented were kindly furnished by Bekaert NV, Zwevegem. Data on metal ion levels were furnished by Dr. J. Helsen and Dr. G. Willems. This study was funded in part by Zimmer Inc., Warsaw, U.S.

Porous fiber metal coatings have a number of advantages. The present paper will deal mainly with those relating to mechanical and elastic aspects [10], biocompatibility [11] and the properties of fiber metal coatings [8]. First, however, we shall examine briefly the types of porous ingrowth structures that will be discussed. Figure 2 shows a scanning electron micrograph of a porous structure with a 10% density that is composed of titanium fibers 2 cm long and 50 µm in diameter. Figure 3 shows a sintered bond between adjacent 100-µm-thick Ti fibers that were sintered for 2 hours at 1250 °C. Figure 4 shows bone ingrowth into an aggregate of 100-µm fibers (50% density) that was implanted in the trabecular bone of the femoral epiphysis of a dog for 12 months.

Mechanical and Elastic Properties of Porous Fiber Structures

There are at least six reasons for using thin (50–100 µm), straight metal fibers for the fabrication of porous coatings:

1. Unlike polymeric coatings, metal coatings are able to form strong bonds with metal substrates.
2. A porous fiber structure contains an interconnecting network of interspaces or channels that have a uniform mean diameter. Porous ceramic or metallic power structures have much smaller interconnecting pore sizes (Fig. 5).
3. For any given density and pore size, fiber metal structures are stronger and more fracture-resistant. As Table 1 shows, the strength ratio between the porous and dense form of the material is markedly higher for fiber metal structures than for other porous materials of equal density. This can be explained by the effect of the pores on the structure. In the case

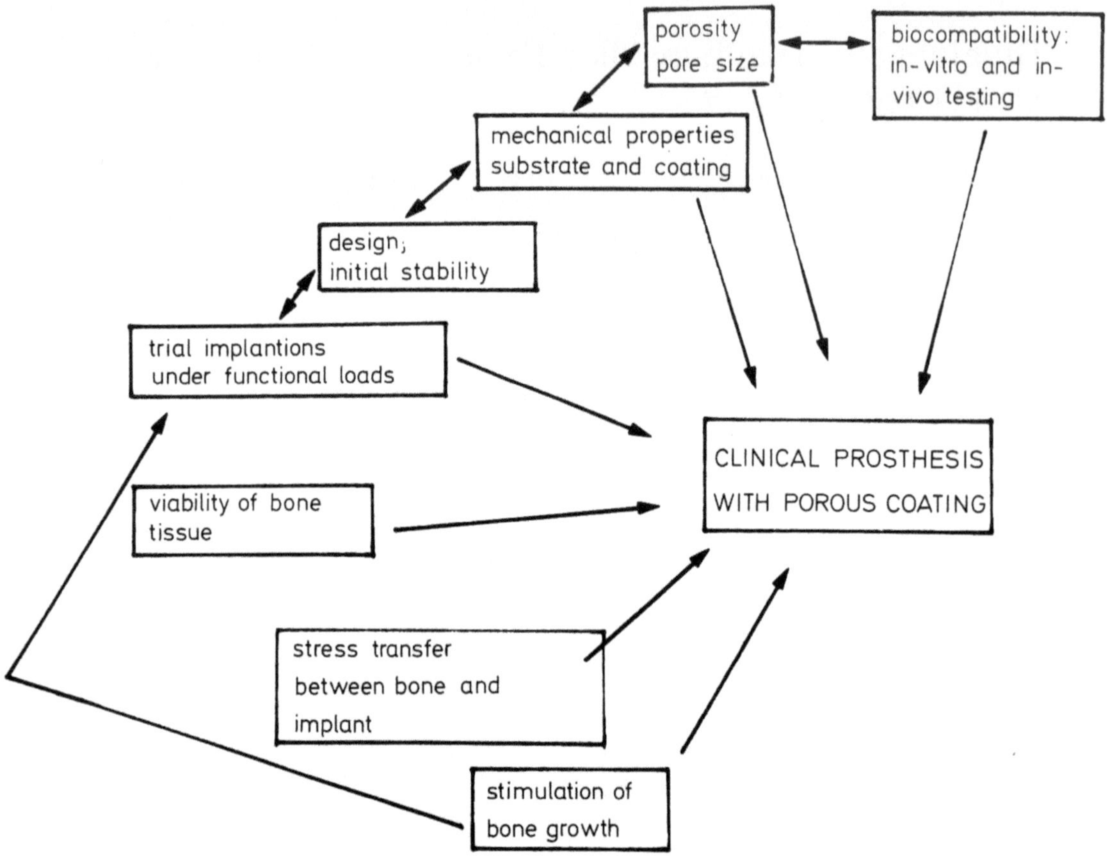

Fig. 1. Interrelationship between various factors and the clinical use of porous coatings

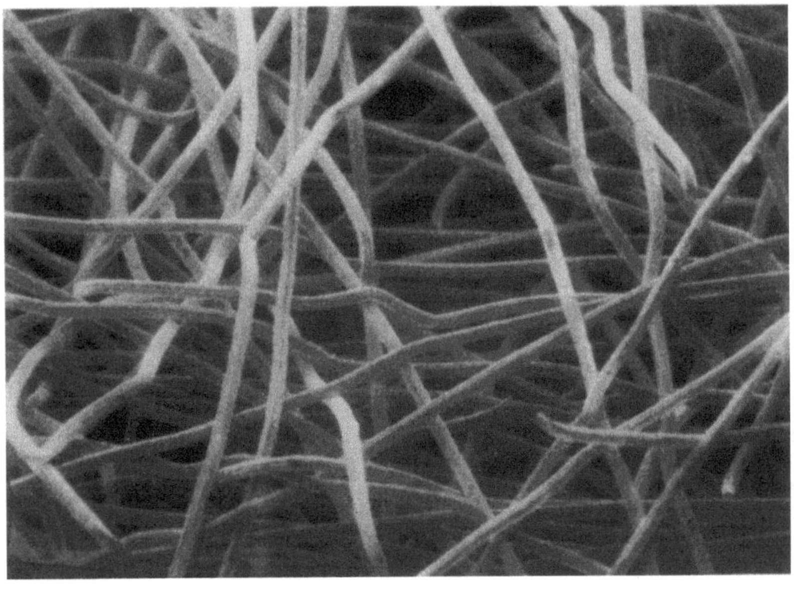

Fig. 2. Scanning electron micrograph of a fiber metal structure with 90% porosity (50×)

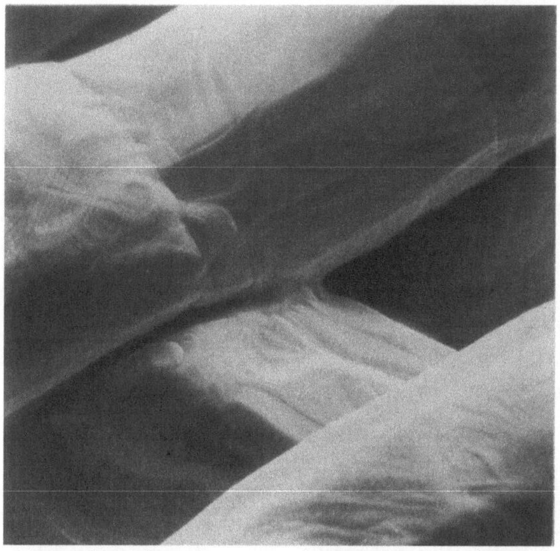

Fig. 3. Scanning electron micrograph of a sintered bond (500×)

of powders, the pores create stress concentrations to a much greater extent than in the fiber materials. The fibers making up the porous material may be considered to function as individual structural members [6, 7].

4. The elasticity of porous fiber or wire structures closely matches the elasticity of the surrounding bone. Porous structures made of stainless steel fibers 50 and 100 μm in diameter have an E-modulus of 20 and 2 GPa, respectively, as measured under tension and compression. The values for fiber titanium structures have not yet been measured over a comprehensive range of densities. However, available measurements show the same general tendency as that for stainless steel. The values stated above are entirely comparable to the elastic moduli of cortical bone (~17 GPa) or trabecular bone (0.1–1.7 GPa).
5. A press fit is easily achieved with implants having porous wire coatings, since the coating can be elastically deformed. After press fitting, the coating remains an open structure.
6. With sintered porous structures composed of fibers 50–100 μm in diameter, the risk of tearing or detaching thin fibers during handling and insertion is negligible [5, 12].

Biocompatibility Aspects: Corrosion Testing and Metal Ion Release

Implants with porous coatings have an increased area of contact with surrounding body fluids and tissues. Recent data [11] indicate that even in short-term models, the presence of a metal implant (e.g., made of stainless steel AISI 316L) leads to an increase in the plasma levels of iron and chromium. This emphasizes the importance of biocompatibility aspects. Two questions are of interest in this regard:

1. The possibility of rapid corrosion due to the large number of voids and crevices in the porous material.
2. The question of whether the rate of metal ion release is influenced by the greatly increased surface area.

We have investigated three porous fiber materials: (1) porous stainless steel AISI 316L, (2) porous stainless steel AISI 316L coated with a 5-mm layer of monochloroparaxylene, and (3) fiber titanium. *In vitro* corrosion tests were done using either the potentiostatic anodic polarization (p.a.p.) method or time-potential measurements. Solid and porous specimens of known surface area were immersed in buffered Hank's solution at 37 °C, in which the oxygen concentration was maintained in the physiologic range.

Table 1. Ratio of Strength Values between the Porous and Nonporous Forms of Various Materials

Material	Density (%)	Ratio of strength values (%)
Annealed stainless steel fibers AISI 316L,	50	18
50 μm in diameter	65–70	35–40
Cast Co-Cr alloy powder	70	17
Al_2O_3	50	12
	70	21

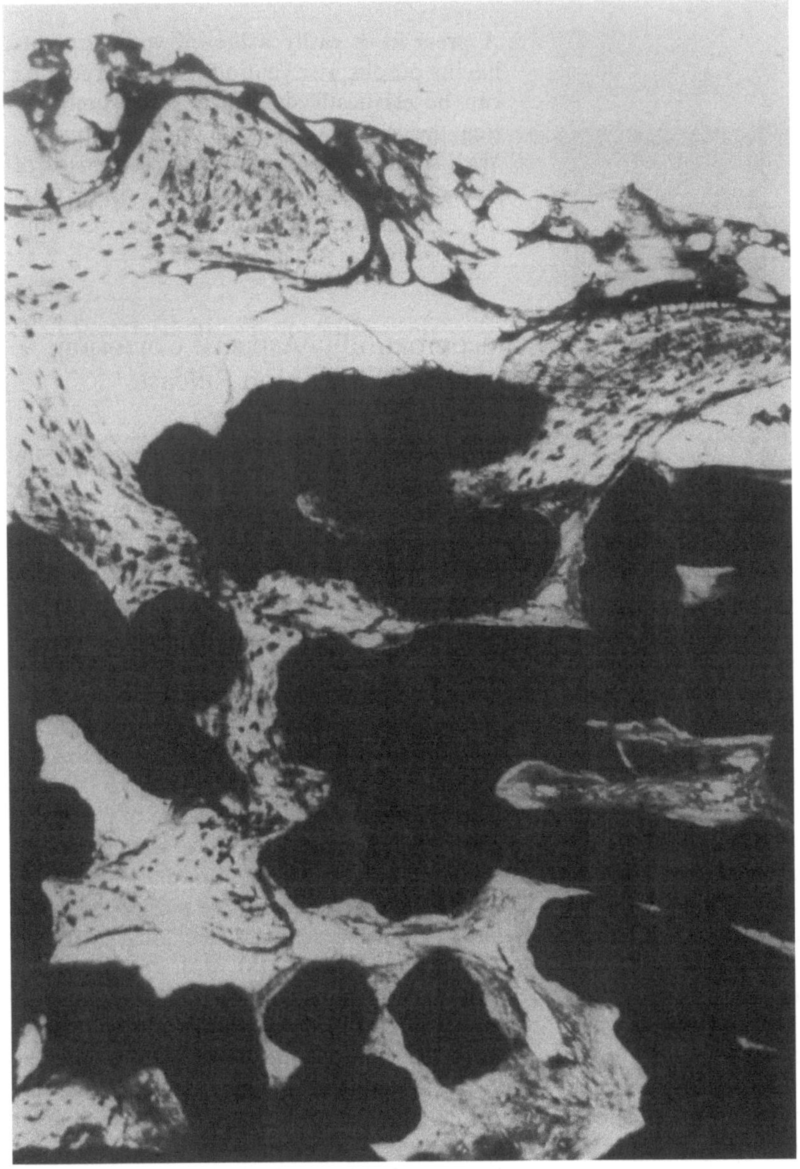

Fig. 4. Bone ingrowth into porous titanium (150×)

Figure 6 shows the results of the polarization test for stainless steel specimens. Some of the specimens were nonporous, while the remainder had a 50% porosity (fiber diameter 100 μm). The current density of the porous specimens was calculated by dividing the measured current by the apparent surface area of the base of the equivalent flat cylinder. In the pressed porous specimens, the passivity breakdown potential is markedly lower than that of the solid specimens, with breakdown occurring at E = 500 mV and 850 mV, respectively. It does not appear that the passivity breakdown was associated with a selective rupture of the sintered bonds, for scanning electron microscopy showed signs of a generalized attack. SEM analysis of specimens retrieved from p.a.p. testing immediately after passivity breakdown showed no evidence of corrosion. It is likely, therefore, that the failure had its onset within the interior of the porous structure. All these observations in stainless steel point to critical circumstances. Thus, if unfavorable conditions were to arise within the porous structure, such as an oxygen lack, corrosion might well develop *in vivo*. Based upon these findings, we have rejected porous stainless steel

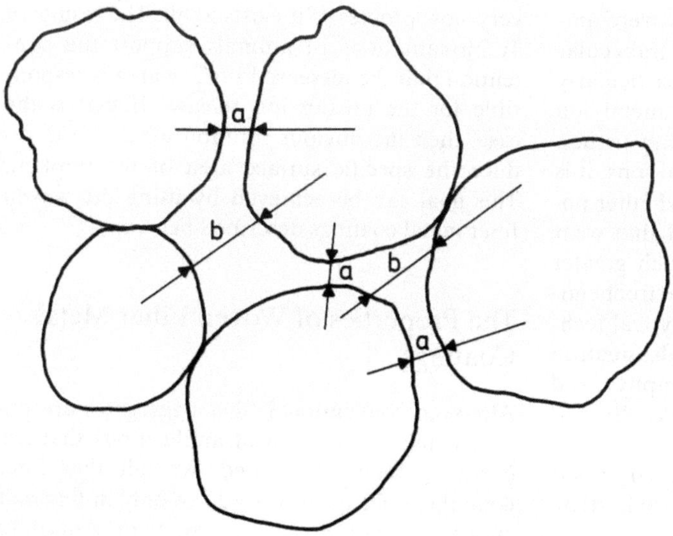

Fig. 5. Porous powder structure. The interconnecting channels **(a)** are smaller than the pores **(b)**

for patient use. Of course, it might be possible to coat the metal fibers uniformly with a layer of impermeable material. This would be one way of avoiding direct contact between the stainless steel and the body environment. We tried a thin polymeric coating for this purpose but had disappointing results [3]. Perhaps the coating was not applied evenly or was prone to damage. We finally concluded that monochloroparaxylene was not a suitable coating material for porous stainless steel implants.

The behavior of porous titanium is fundamentally different from that of stainless steel. Figure 7 shows the average polarization values for porous Ti. No passivity breakdown was observed in the range of potentials investigated. In addition, the potential-time measurements showed no long-term corrosion effects of any kind. With regard to fiber metals, it appears unlikely that circumscribed or generalized corrosion would be a problem in porous titanium implants.

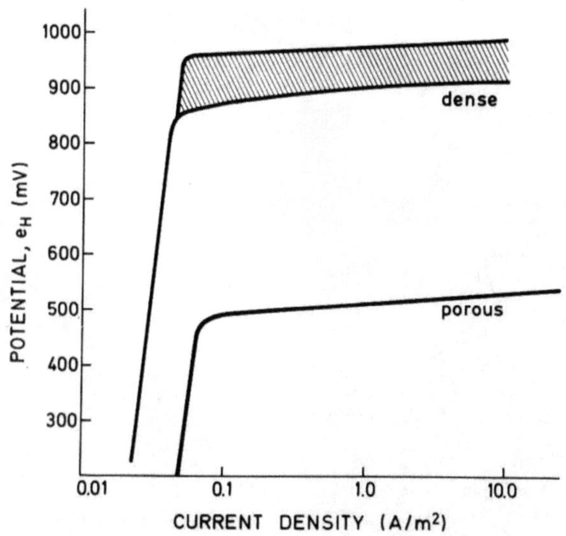

Fig. 6. Potential current density for solid and porous stainless steel AISI 316L

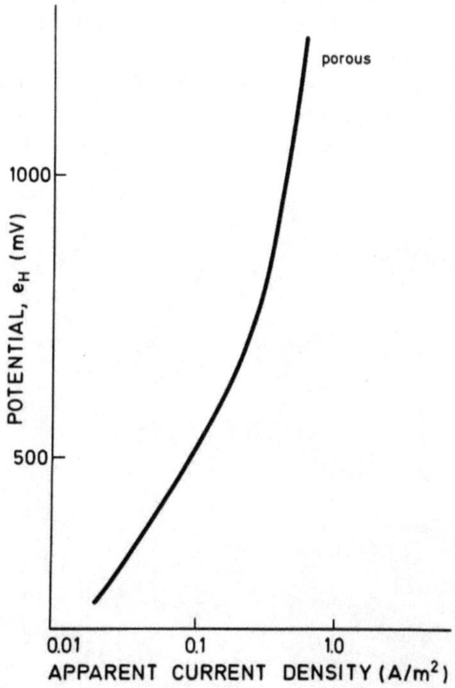

Fig. 7. Potential current density for porous titanium

For corrosion testing, specimens were implanted for 6 and 12 months in the trabecular bone of canine epiphyses. We were particularly interested in determining the trace metal ion levels that accumulated in surrounding tissues. When considering the release of metal ions, it is important to realize that all metals, whether porous or nonporous, release ions, and that wear processes probably account for a much greater proportion of this release than do electrochemical phenomena. Three different analytical techniques were used to evaluate ion levels: neutron activation analysis, pulse polarography, and atomic absorption spectrophotometry. Preliminary data indicate the following:

1. There is no significant difference in tissue nickel levels between solid and porous stainless steel.
2. Titanium levels in the vicinity of the solid Ti specimens are either unmeasurable (< 15 ppm) or very low (37 or 50 ppm).
3. A definite increase is found in the vicinity of porous Ti specimens: Around these porous bodies, which have about 40 times more specific surface area than the solid specimens, the Ti concentration ranges from undetectable values to 1812 ppm (average = 636 ppm). While we cannot yet account for the large scatter of these data, the relatively high level of Ti in adjacent tissues is nonetheless apparent.

A comparison between the Ni and Ti analysis of tissues surrounding porous metals shows that the transport of Ti from the implant site is a very slow process, if it exists at all. The results of Ti implantations in animals support the contention that the increased surface area is responsible for the greater ion release. If that is the case, then the obvious solution would be to reduce the specific surface area of the implant. This goal can be achieved by using the woven fiber metal coatings described below.

The Properties of Woven Fiber Metal Coatings

Although conventional fiber aggregates are excellent for certain clinical applications that are currently being developed, we felt that fiber coatings could be improved not only in terms of specific surface area but also with regard to other characteristics. This led to the development of our woven design for fiber metal coatings. A monolayer woven fiber metal coating is shown in Fig. 8. Two different pore types can be distinguished: type 1, representing the distance between two parallel fibers, and type 2, representing the maximum distance between the fiber and metal substrate. The latter pore type allows interlocking of the bone tissue and fibers, thus enabling fixation by ingrowth.

The following characteristics of the woven fiber coatings merit special discussion:

1. The pore size is uniform and perfectly controllable.
2. Any pore size, even large pores, can be produced without compromising the strength,

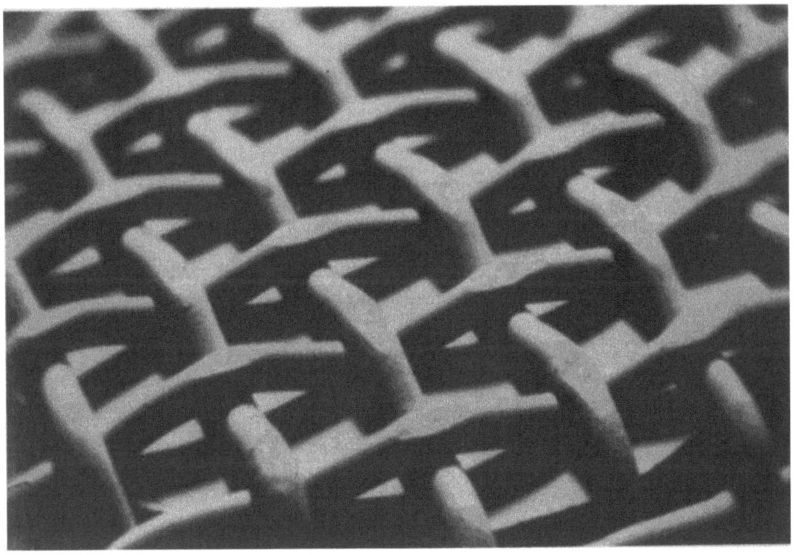

Fig. 8. Scanning electron micrograph of a woven fiber metal coating (16×)

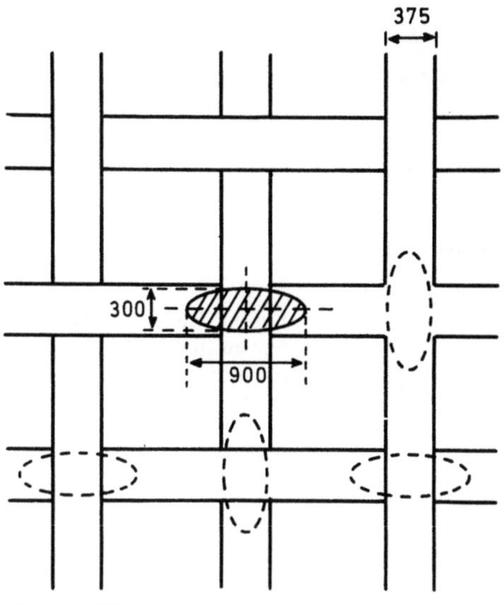

Fig. 9. Elliptical contact areas between a woven fiber coating and its substrate

ductility or structural integrity of the porous material.

3. Uniform bonding can be achieved between the fiber coating and substrate. Reproducible, elliptical contact areas are fashioned by cold-working the woven fiber mesh (Fig. 9) before pressure-sintering it onto the metal substrate. Figure 10 shows the change in type-2 pore size as a function of contact area between the fiber coating and substrate for various fiber thicknesses. The curve shows that for a given fiber thickness, the size of the type-2 pores decreases as the contact area is increased. For a 20% contact area, the type-2 pore size is 150 μm for a Ti mesh with 16 fibers per inch. The fibers themselves are 0.5 mm in diameter (16–500 mesh). The type-1 pores measure 1.1 mm. The actual bond between the substrate and coating is produced by sintering. Figure 11 shows the metallurgical transition from a Ti-6%Al-4%V substrate to a Ti fiber mesh (16–500). A metal-to-metal bond is apparent. The average strength of the bonds after sintering (2 hrs at 800 °C and 4.1 MPa pressure) is 277 MPa. This is excellent compared to that of the pure titanium starting material. Commercial-purity titanium, with the lowest impurity content, has an ultimate tensile strength of 350 MPa.
4. The sintering method employed causes minimal change in the static and dynamic strength and fracture resistance of the substrate metal. We particularly investigated the alloy Ti-6%Al-4%V. As with most metals used in orthopedic surgery, normal sintering temperatures greatly reduce the strength, fracture resistance and/or fatigue limit of the material. Thus, the conventional sintering of a porous coating onto the stem of a femoral endoprosthesis yields a device that is highly susceptible to fatigue fracture. Ti-6%Al-4%V alloy is ordinarily sintered at approximately 1200 °C. These temperatures yield a structure that is brittle at room temperature and has a large grain size (0.5–3 mm). No heat treatment is known that can reverse this process.

By using pressure as an activator during sintering, it is possible to lower the sintering temperature significantly. The pressure sintering of fiber titanium coatings onto a Ti-6%Al-4%V substrate has been successfully done at

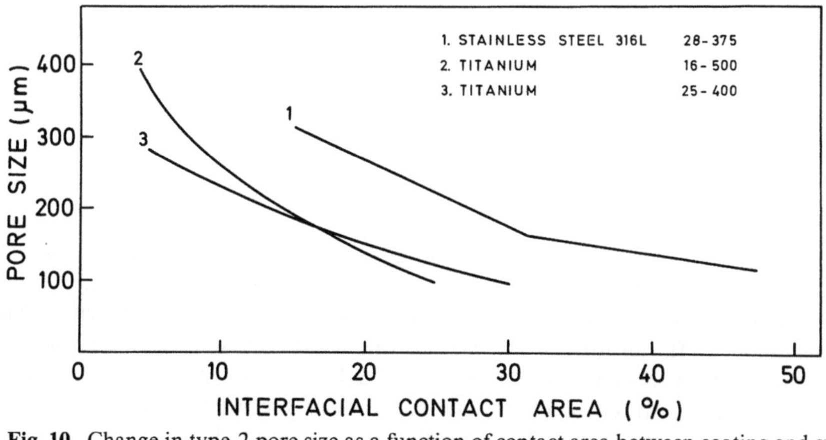

Fig. 10. Change in type-2 pore size as a function of contact area between coating and substrate

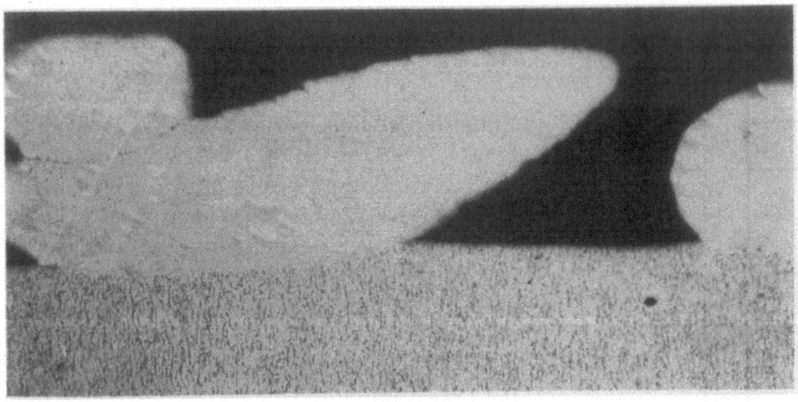

Fig. 11 Bond between woven fiber titanium coating and Ti- 6%Al-4%V substrate

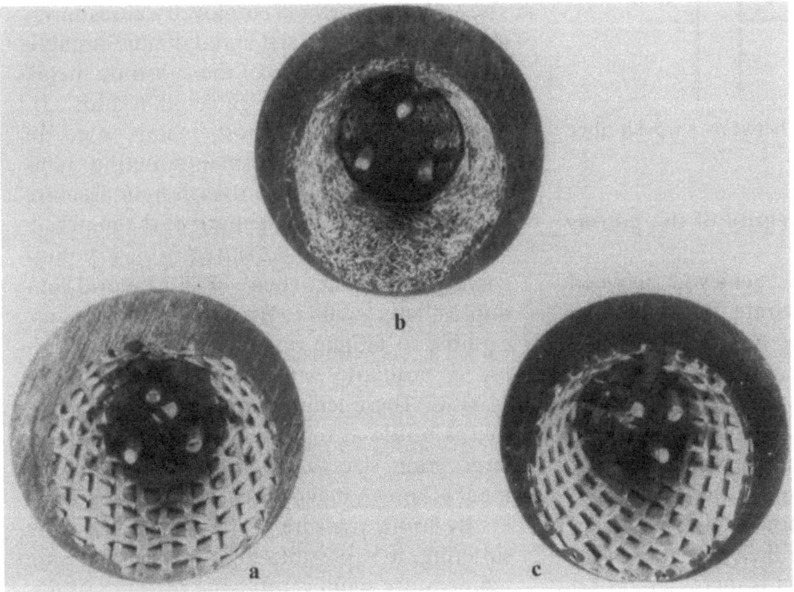

Fig. 12. Femoral cups for surface replacement in dogs. **a** Irregular fiber coating and **b, c** woven fiber coatings

Table 2. Change in Certain Mechanical Properties of the Alloy Ti-6%Al-4%V Produced by Sintering for 2 hrs at 900 °C

	Before (annealed condition)	After
Fracture elongation (%)	13.0	13.8
0.2% yield stress (MPa)	1029	906
Tensile strength (MPa)	1134	1016
Fatigue limit (MPa)	–	760

temperatures of 800–925 °C. These temperatures are below the $\alpha+\beta$ to β transition temperature (975 °C), and so the embrittling transition structure is avoided. The growth of grain size at these temperatures is minimal. A typical average grain size after sintering is 15 μm. The change in certain mechanical properties is shown in Table 2. Static strength is decreased by about 10%, and the fatigue limit probably follows the same trend. Ductility is unaffected. By sintering at 1200 °C, it would be reduced from 13 to 4% elongation.

5. The specific surface area of the woven fiber metal coatings is limited. This is best illustrat-

ed by examining the coated implants themselves. Figure 12 shows the interior of femoral cups for surface replacement arthroplasty in dogs. The thickness of the irregular fiber coating and of the monolayer woven coating is 0.6 mm. While surface area is increased by a factor of 8 with the irregular fiber coating, it is increased by a factor of 1.5 with the woven mesh. The fiber coatings in question have a smaller specific surface area than the specimens used in the biocompatibility tests (40-fold increase). Nevertheless, the woven design will always produce a smaller increase in specific surface area than an irregular fiber aggregate.

Conclusions

The following conclusions may be drawn on the basis of the data presented:

1. Titanium is preferable to stainless steel as a material for the fabrication of porous fiber metal coatings.
2. The fiber metal approach yields implant materials with good strength and elasticity. These properties enable smooth intraoperative handling, including an easy press fit with little risk of particle detachment.
3. Woven fiber titanium meshes can be pressure-sintered onto Ti-6%Al-4%V substrates to produce a high-strength bond between coating and substrate. The mechanical properties of the substrate metal are affected little by the sintering process. The specific surface area of the woven fiber metal coating is relatively small.

The properties discussed in the present article justify the use of porous titanium materials in total hip prostheses.

References

1. Black J, Smith GK, Woodman JL (1977) The role of implant surface area in corrosion in vivo. First European Conference "Evaluation of biomaterials", Strasbourg, France
2. Ducheyne P (1981) Editorial. Research priorities in biomaterials. The experience from metals. Biomaterials 2:66–67
3. Ducheyne P (to be published) In vitro corrosion study of porous metal fibre coatings for bone ingrowth. Biomaterials
4. Ducheyne P, Martens M, Aernoudt E, Mulier J, De Meester P (1974) Skeletal fixation by metal fiber coating of the implant. Acta Orthop Belg 40:799–805
5. Ducheyne P, Heymans L, Martens M, Aernoudt E, De Meester P, Mulier JC (1977) The mechanical behaviour of intracondylar cancellous bone of the femur at different loading rates. J Biomech 10:747–762
6. Ducheyne P, Aernoudt E, De Meester P (1978) The mechanical behaviour of porous austenitic stainless steel fibre structures. J Mat Sci 13:2650–2658
7. Ducheyne P, De Meester P, Aernoudt E, Martens M, Mulier JC (1980) Elastic and mechanical properties of porous metal fibre structures allowing bone ingrowth. In: Hastings GW, Williams DF (eds) Advances in biomaterials. Wiley & Sons, Chichester
8. Galante JO, Rostoker W, Lueck R, Ray R (1971) Sintered fiber metal composites as a basis for attachment of implants to bone. J Bone Joint Surg [Am] 53:101–114
9. Hench LL (1981) Guest editorial. J Biomed Mater Res 15:3–7
10. Hulbert SF, Young FA, Mathews RS, Klawitter JJ, Talbert CD, Stelling FH (1970) Potential of ceramic materials as permanently implantable skeletal prostheses. J Biomed Mater Res 4:433–456
11. Klawitter JJ, Hulbert SF (1971) Application of porous ceramics for the attachment of load bearing internal orthopaedic applications. J Biomed Mater Res 5/1:161–229
12. Reilly DT, Burstein AH (1974) The mechanical properties of cortical bone. J Bone Joint Surg [Am] 56:1001–1022
13. Welsh P, Pilliar RM, McNab I (1971) Surgical implants; the role of surface porosity in fixation to bone and acrylic. J Bone Joint Surg [Am] 53:963–977

Tissue-Ingrowth Implant Fixation by a Soft Porous Coating

Ch. A. Homsy

Thank you for extending me the honour of your invitation to share with you the results of the past 14 years of work on the problem of tissue-ingrowth implant fixation by a soft porous coating.

It is well known that the process of healing around an implant which is non-porous leads to the formation of a capsule. It is also well known that the capsule forms around the mantle of acrylic cement used to stabilize endoprostheses and is a factor in the occurence of loosening [1]. Our objective from the beginning was to develop a coating which could be fixed to an endoprosthesis such that tissue could grow into the coating and thereby stabilize the implant with respect to surrounding tissue.

In making such an implant, we had to understand that all materials have a potential for being not-tolerated by the body depending upon whether they release, through chemical reaction, chemical entities that can react with the surrounding body tissue.

We developed in 1969/1970 an efficient *in vitro* protocol that allowed us to distinguish those materials which had high potential for biocompatibility with the body [2]. This involved exposing the candidate materials to a pseudobódy fluid which was held at elevated temperatures in order to take advantage of time/temperature superposition to model long-term implantation at body temperature. The fluid could be examined by tissue culture or by physical-chemical techniques to identify anything that has moved into the fluid from the test material.

This technique allowed us to identify materials that were of high probability of total compatibility with the body. From this list we selected the PTFE Polymer and graphite fiber initially, and more recently the use of aluminium oxide, to prepare a composite material to which we gave the name PROPLAST[1] [3, 4, 5]. The essential features of this material are: biotolerance provided by the ingredients; very carefully controlled pore geometry, involving a range of pore size suitable for tissue ingrowth; a very high void percentage, greater than 75%; and appropriate interpore openings. Also, the material has a low modulus of elasticity, or softness, analogous to soft tissue in order that the early tissue fibers growing into the material will not be traumatized by shearing micromotion between the material and adjacent tissue. And finally, the material exhibits a very special surface activity which accommodates protein precipitation to provide a substrate for fibrosis and an extremely high specific surface area which is also believed to be a key to rapid fibrosis.

The scanning electron photomicroscope shows the very complex pore morphology of the material where the PTFE represents a matrix upon which resides either the graphite or aluminum oxide. PROPLAST material exhibits a low modulus, so as not to traumatize early ingrowing soft tissue from shear motion and also to maintain a resiliency to absorb shock in impact applications such as endoprosthesis stabilization. The low modulus also allows a uniform distribution of load from the endoprosthesis to the surrounding tissue by accommodating the unavoidable irregularities of the prepared medullary cavity (Fig. 1).

Study on the use of PROPLAST has extended over the past 14 years and initially, in 1968/1969, involved *in vitro* tests for biocompatibility followed by extensive animal implant studies to confirm this biocompatibility. There have been, continuing to today, animal prototype studies to demonstrate efficacy in specific applications and also to suggest operative technique refinements. In 1970 precommercial clinical trials were begun with a PROPLAST coating stabilized im-

1 PROPLAST is a registered trademark of VITEK, Inc., Houston, Texas, USA. US patents 3.992,725 and 4.129,470. And patents worldwide.

plant for the replacement of the condyle of the temporomandibular joint [6]. Recently, papers have been presented in the U.S. indicating that large numbers of such implants have been successful when followed between 5 and 9 years postimplantation.

In 1972 clinical trials began with blocks of PROPLAST I, the initial grey form, which could be carved at the operating table for restoration of facial contour. This material became commercially available in the U.S. in 1974 and in Western Europe in 1976. The enthusiam for its use led to the availability of preformed shapes for common procedures such as mentoplasty, rhinoplasty and zygomatico-maxillary augmentation. Long-term follow-up of such implants to 8 years post-surgery have confirmed their safety and effectiveness [7].

These uses for the material were documented for the FDA in 1977. Almost 400 patients were followed for as long as 5 years and an extremely low complication rate ascertained. This led to the decision of the FDA to consider the PROPLAST material for facial applications as a "Standard" material, which means that safety and effectiveness have been demonstrated.

When used as a fixation coating on an endoprosthesis, tissue grows into the material and then, as cyclical micromotion occurs, as it must occur in any loaded implant, the coating yields, yet stabilizes the implant, much in the manner of the periodontal membrane around the tooth root. This is nature's solution to attaching a mechanically loaded element to a bony bed. Also, the interface eliminates concern for the difference in modulus of elasticity between the material of the endoprosthesis stem and the surrounding bony tissue. In effect we have recognized that fibrous tissue will always form around an implant. We have used the porous

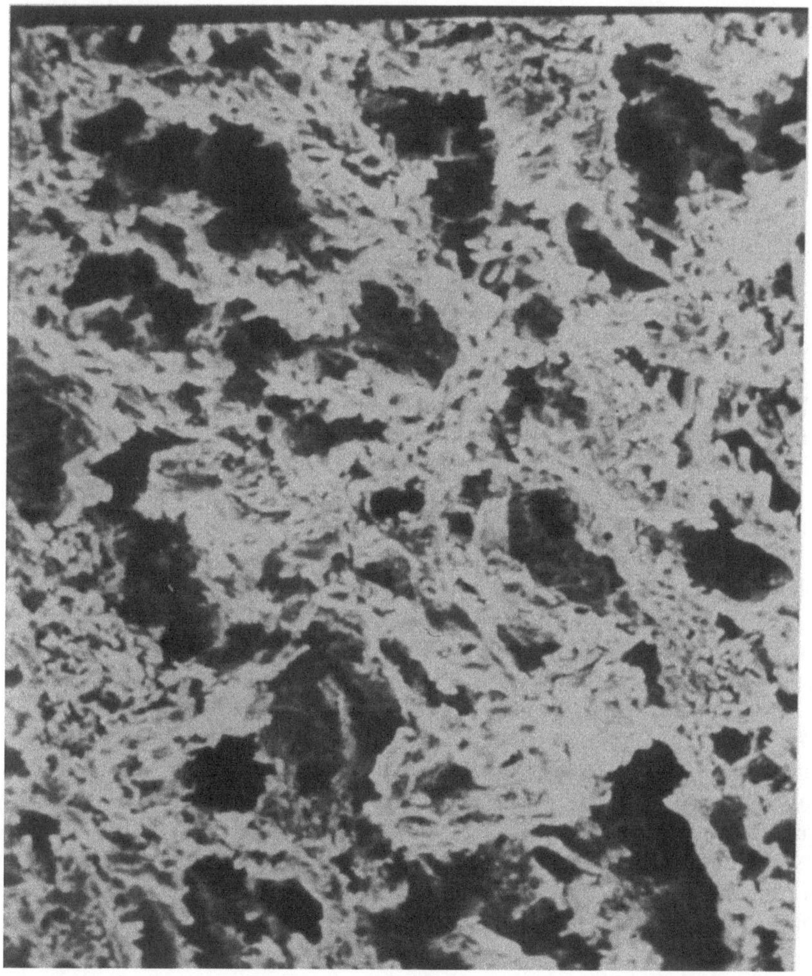

Fig. 1. Scanning electron micrograph of the porous PROPLAST material ($\times 64$)

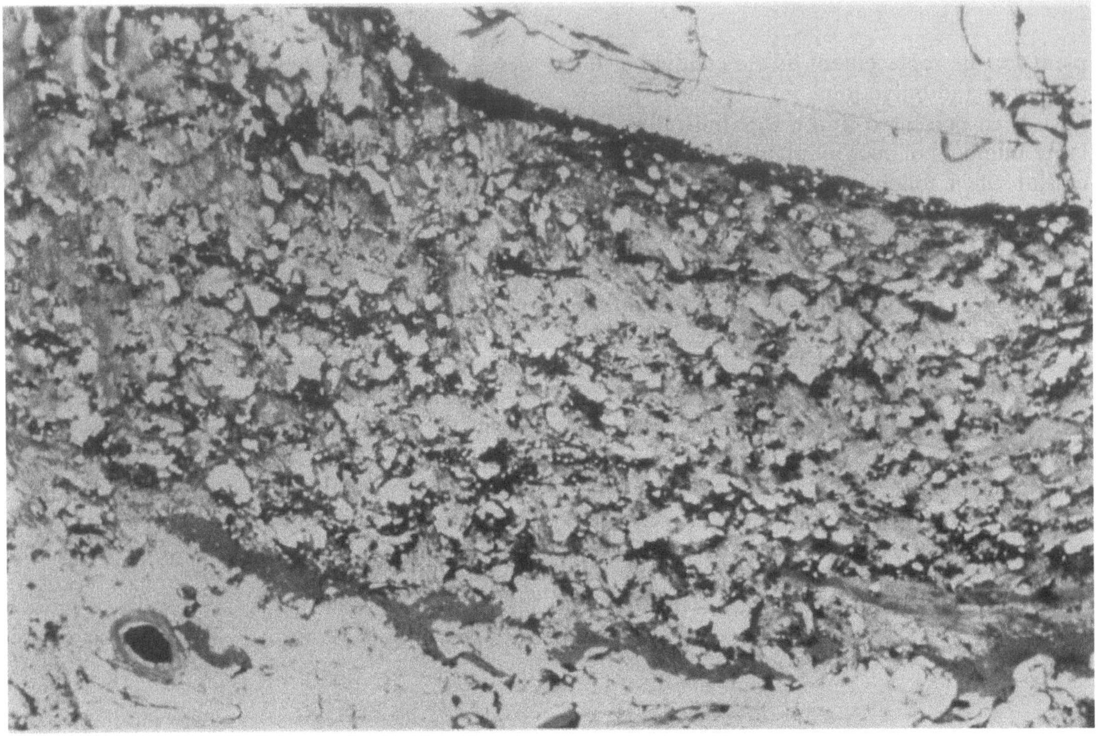

Fig. 2. Histologic section of the PROPLAST coating of a canine femoral head prosthesis 3 weeks postoperatively showing complete infiltration of the coating by fibrous tissue and consequent connection of the implant to the adjacent tissue

coating of PROPLAST to place that fibrous tissue in a location where it can be useful to us.

In 1968 we began dog implantation studies using a femoral head endoprosthesis. As early as 3 weeks, when the proximal femur was decalcified and the cortical bone incised down to the metal of implant, reflection of the cortical bone showed that the 1-mm coating of PROPLAST stayed with the cortex, while a thin layer of the material remained with the metal of the prosthesis to which it was fused.

The histopathology at 3 weeks confirmed the 1-mm coating to be completely filled with loose fibrous tissue (Fig. 2).

At 16 months there was a maturation of this tissue, but it was still essentially fibrous tissue with good vascularity.

At 5½ years this histopathology picture remains essentially the same. Very recently we have recovered from a baboon a cranial defect patch which has been implanted for 8½ years. In this instance there was a substantial percentage of osseous tissue within the PROPLAST, as would be expected in applications where micromotion, caused by cyclical loading, would be not important.

From the work of Rhinelander in which a segment of a dog ulna has been replaced with a block of PROPLAST, it has been well shown that fibrous tissue ingrowth into the implant was rapid and richly vascularized (Fig. 3). A recent paper by Rhinelander et al. shows the rapid growth in fixation strength of Schneider rods carrying PROPLAST coatings when compared with rods that are uncoated. The strength of attachment was found appropriate for endoprosthesis fixation [9].

We have, on one occasion, been able to directly measure the force needed to remove a F. Thomson type endoprosthesis stabilized by the PROPLAST coating, which had been in a patient for 3 years. Resection was necessary because of protrusio acetabuli. The force needed to remove the implant was approximately 160 kg, which is consistent with animal data. With the removal of such an implant, one sees that the separation between the implant and tissue has occurred within the coating, with a por-

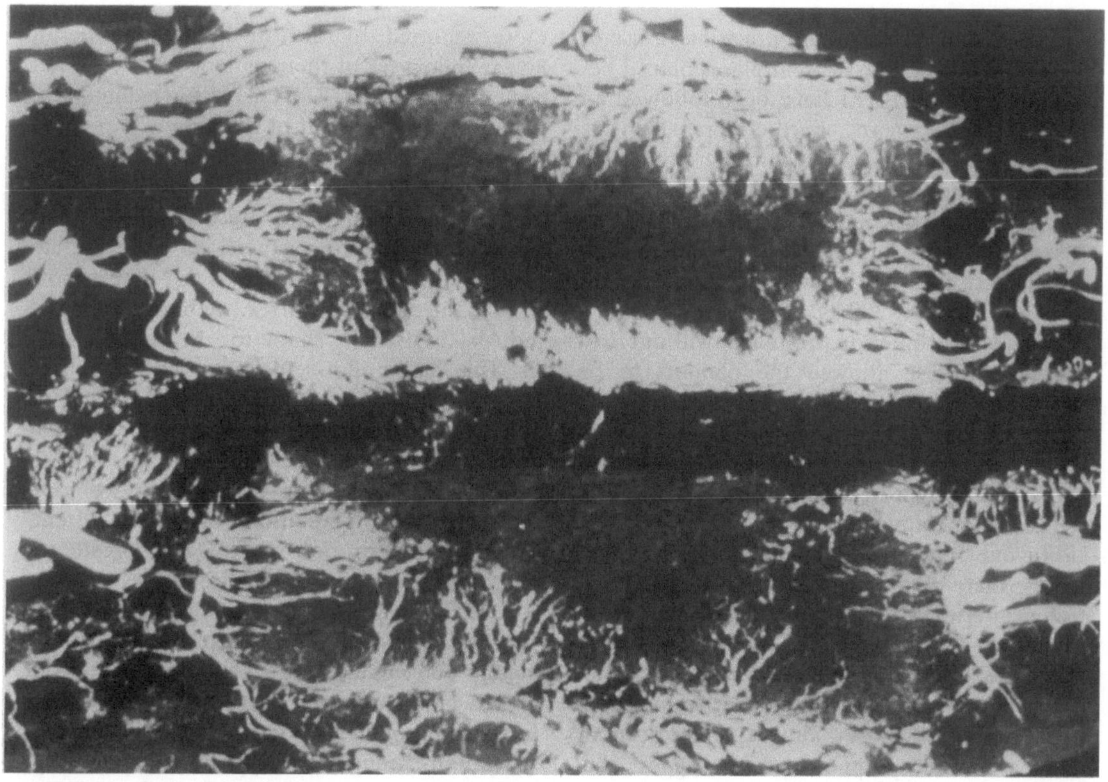

Fig. 3. Dog ulna replaced with a block of PROPLAST. 12-weeks postoperatively. Fibrous tissue ingrowth was rapid and richly vascularized

tion of the coating retained on the implant and the remainder of the coating retained within the medullary canal and easily removed by curettage. In the usual instance with such prostheses, 8 to 12 sharp blows with the mallet on the punch dislodged the implant. The PROPLAST coating now used for endoprosthesis stabilization exhibits two times the strength of the material used in these studies (see below).

Since April of 1978 we have conducted a careful clinical evaluation of the use of the coating to stabilize Aufranc-Turner geometry femoral components of total hip implants. Between April 1978 and December 1981, 90 patients received a total of 99 components. The majority of these implants were placed by 3rd- and 4th-year orthopedic residents in our teaching institution under the guidance of senior staff. In our institution all patients under 55 years of age requiring total hip arthroplasty have been required to receive a PROPLAST-coated implant since April 1978, because of the concern for long-term problems with acrylic cement. The older patients were offered acrylic cement implants, since at our institution it is necessary to teach both techniques.

The protocol evolved gradually over the study period. From 4/78 to 2/79 an initial group of 14 implantations were carried out with imprecise instrumentation and limited implant sizes and by an anterior approach requiring hand rasping only to develop the canal. These have been followed an average of 3.5 years. The anterior approach continued to be used until 2/80 in a second group of 47 implants as the instrumentation became more precise and a larger number of stem sizes became available. These have been followed an average of 2.5 years. Then, the posterolateral approach with trochanteric release was adopted in order to ensure the best possible exposure for the cementation of the acetabulum. This allowed us to introduce the use of the ASIF intramedullary reamer, which enabled an accurate match between medullary cavity and stem size to be achieved. Further improvement in the precision of hand rasps for the development of the metaphyseal canal also was achieved; the transtrochanteric approach allowed maximum precision in use of these. The third group of 38 implants placed between 12/79 and 12/81 have been followed an average of 1.5 years. Furthermore, for this group of 9 patients the coating strength had been doubled to 20 kg/cm² ultimate tensile strength and 10 kg/cm² shear strength. The surface area of these Aufranc-Turner stems was approximately 50 cm². Therefore, fixation strength was approximately 300 kg.

The initial anterior approach without trochanteric release allowed the patients to be handled as cemented cases in terms of initiating weight bearing at approximately 3 weeks. With the adoption of the transtrochanteric approach, substantial weight bearing was deferred until 6 weeks postoperatively.

In our June, 1982, review of these 99 implants, there are 19 deletions. One infection, 1 technical error, 3 unavailable for review, 12 lost to follow up. We consider 11 implants of the series to be failures, although not all of these implants have been revised. We count them as failures because there are radiographic indications and/or clinical symptoms which suggest that they will eventually come to revision.

The majority of the failures, 8 out of 11, demonstrate features indicating that the implants were not press-fitted at implantation. These were initially loose and subject to macromotion and never became stabilized. Subsidence of these implants was apparent between 5–10 weeks postsurgery with the development of pain.

In 1 of the 11 cases the onset of failure was clearly late and corresponded to patient trauma causing a substantial posterior torque to be applied to the head of the implant. The radiographic evidence and appearance at resection indicate that the small proximal cross-sectional area of the Aufranc-Turner stem allowed the stem to rotate within the relatively soft cancellous bone to which it was attached by the tissue ingrowth.

The remaining patients, all of whom have been meticulously followed, show stability of the implant, no subsidence, and a satisfactory clinical course. In following these 68 patients, pain and function parameters according to the six-point scale of Charnley have been used to measure remission of pain and the improvement in function over time [10]. We have compared improvement in these parameters against those reported by Griffith & Charnley in an 8-year follow up of their patients who received cemented implants. The curves for reduction in pain and improvement of function in our study essentially match those obtained from the referenced literature.

In order to eliminate late instability caused by weak surrounding cancellous bone and to place the tissue ingrowth coating as close as possible to the endosteal cortex, we have developed the ANAFORM™ [2] shape for the endoprosthesis. This shape allows the ingrowth fixation to be accomplished to strong endosteal cancellous bone and cortical bone. It stabilizes the implant against rotational torque (Fig. 4).

Since the beginning of this year we have completed 27 implantations using this system. Recently in Europe, ANAFORM prostheses have been successfully implanted in several centers. The system provides the following features:

ANAFORM shape which provides approximately 100 cm² of ingrowth surface area and corical bone support; 2-mm PROPLAST coating which provides 10 kg/cm² of shear strength; a fixation strength of approximately 600 kg; highly refined instrumentation and implantation protocol to allow simple, rapid and uniform press-fit implantation; three stem sizes to accommodate m/l isthmus width between 10 mm and 17 mm; three neck lengths for each stem size; and optional antibiotic infusion container which allows 14 cc of antibiotic solution to impregnate the coating where indicated, such as in revision cases.

The implantation procedures are quite straightforward. A template is used to define the line of the neck osteotomy. The template also is used to locate the axis for reaming the medullary canal using guided intramedullary reamers of the ASIF type. The reamers are sequentially increased in size according to the operative protocol. This protocol directs when the appropriate reamer size, corresponding to one of the three stem sizes, has been reached.

Next, the hand rasp of corresponding size is used to develop the cavity in the metaphyseal canal. Special straight reamers are used, if necessary, to trim the endosteal cortex proximomedially at the calcar and proximolaterally.

---

2 Trademark of VITEK, Inc., Houston, Texas, USA. Patents pending worldwide

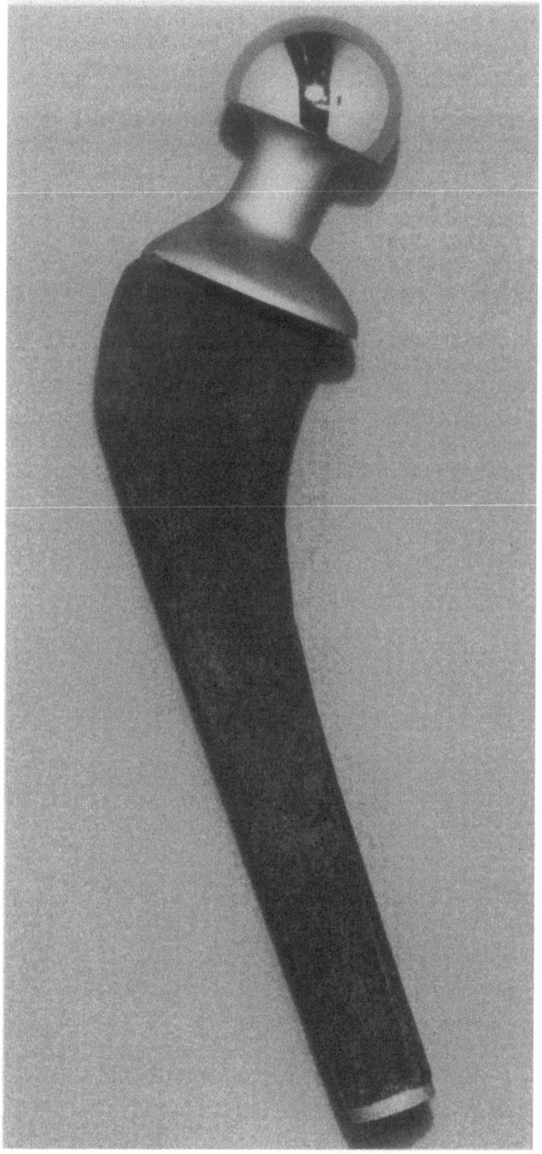

Fig. 4. PROPLAŠT-coated ANAFORM endoprosthesis made by VITEK (Houston)

When trochanteric release is not used, the straight reamers are particularly helpful for developing the lateral proximolateral cavity geometry. Full seating of the hand rasp confirms the correct preparation of the medullary cavity.

The insertion of the implant by hand according to the design of the system will be possible only to approximately 10 mm from the neck osteotomy level. Then the implant is gently seated with the mallet to produce a very firm uniform press-fit fixation for stability and tissue ingrowth in the early postoperative weeks. Because of the compliance of the PROPLAST coating, one can carry out the final seating manoeuver without concern for trauma to the shaft of the femur.

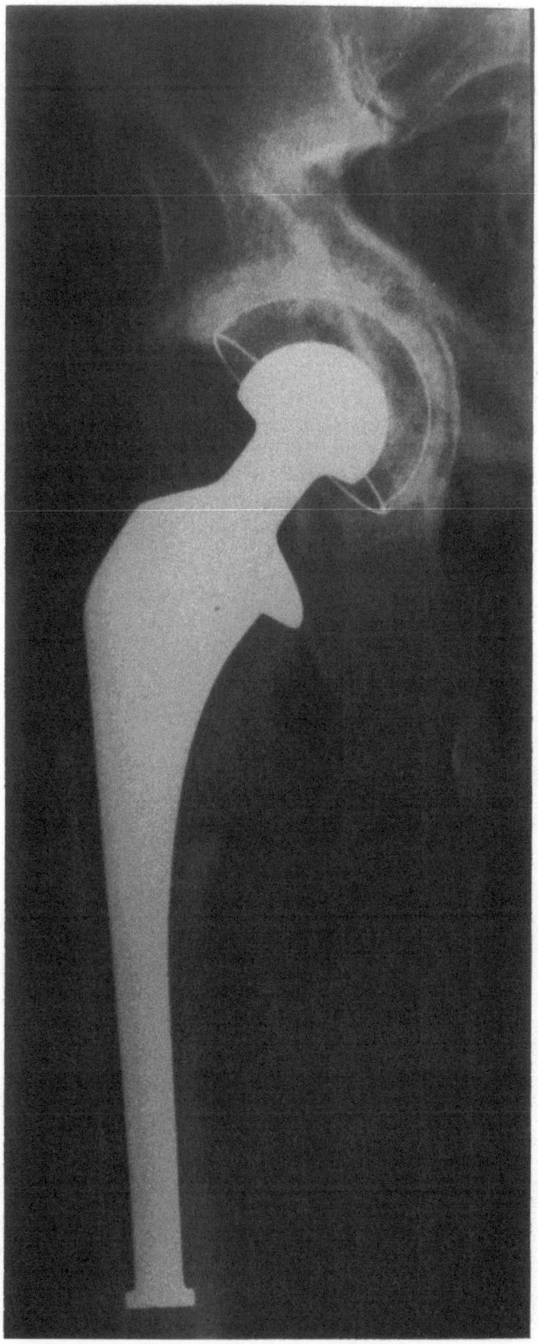

Fig. 5. Postoperative X-ray of a PROPLAST-ANAFORM prosthesis implanted in Holland. The 2-mm PROPLAST coating is radiolucent (by courtesy of Dr. W. Runne)

References

1. Homsy CA, Tullos HS, Anderson MS, Di Ferrante NM, King JW (1972) Some physiological aspects of prosthesis stabilization with acrylic polymer. Clin Orthop 83:317–328
2. Homsy CA (1970) Biocompatibility in selection of materials for implantation. J Biomed Mater Res 4:341–356
3. Homsy CA (1982) Biocompatibility of perfluorinated polymers and composites of these polymers. Chapter 3. In: Williams DF (ed) Biocompatibility of clinical implant materials, Vol II. CRC Press, Boca Raton
4. Homsy CA (1973) Implant stabilization-chemical and biomechanical considerations. Orthop Clin North Am 2:295–311
5. Homsy CA, Cain TE, Kessler FB, Anderson MS, King JW (1972) Porous implant systems for prosthesis stabilization. Clin Orthop 89:220–235
6. Kent JN, Lavelle W, Dolan KD (1974) Condylar reconstruction: Treatment and planning. Oral Surg 37:489–497
7. Kent JN, Westfall RL, Carlton DM (1981) Chin and zygomaticomaxillary augmentation with Proplast: long-term followup. J Oral Surg 39:912–919
8. Rhinelander FW (1977) A flexible composite as a coating for metallic implants: Microvascular and histological studies. Int Orthop 1:77–86
9. Rhinelander FW, Stewart CL, Wilson JW, Homsy CA, Previt JM (1982) Growth of tissue into a porous low modulus coating on intramedullary nails. Clin Orthop 164:293–305
10. Griffith MJ, Seidenstein MK, Williams D, Charnley J (1978) Eight year results of Charnley arthroplasties of the hip with special reference to the behaviour of cement. Clin Orthop 137:24–36

The Uncemented Thrust-Plate Hip Prosthesis

A. H. Huggler and H. A. C. Jacob

Introduction

One of the main problems in the implantation of conventional total hip prostheses is the exposure of the host bone to unphysiologic loads. Ideally, an endoprosthesis should be designed in such a way that it distributes loads to the bone in a normal fashion. The physiologic stress pattern in the proximal femur is reflected in the geometry of the trabeculae, which align with prevailing compressive and tensile stresses.

As Scholten et al. (1976) have shown, the dense cancellous bone assumes the main load-transfer function in the area of the femoral head, while at the level of the femoral neck and farther distally, the cortical bone becomes the major load-transfer element. In contrast to the normal situation in the intact femur, the presence of an endoprosthesis with an intramedullary stem sets up circumferential tensile stresses in the femoral cortex. In addition, the rigid stem exerts a "stress shielding" effect which prevents the degree of femoral loading that Wolff's law would require for the maintenance of a mechanically sound bone structure. Experimental stress analyses of the proximal femur, both with and without a cemented intramedullary stem (Jacob et al., 1978, 1980), have demonstrated the biomechanical shortcomings of this type of prosthesis. This problem is also reflected in the variety of designs, sizes, materials and anchoring methods that are currently in use for femoral endoprostheses (Figs. 1 and 2).

Every endoprosthesis is essentially a compromise – especially those that are anchored by an intramedullary stem. It must be borne in mind that sizable transverse forces act between the stem and the lateral femoral cortex, and that the intervening cancellous bone is subjected to large unphysiologic stresses. In addition, stress shielding of the proximal femoral cortex can cause atrophy to develop in that region. Should the endoprosthesis become loose, a particularly unfavorable biomechanical situation will develop, and the high specific loads and relative motion between the bone and implant will accelerate the process of bone resorption, leading to a rapid deterioration of the anchorage.

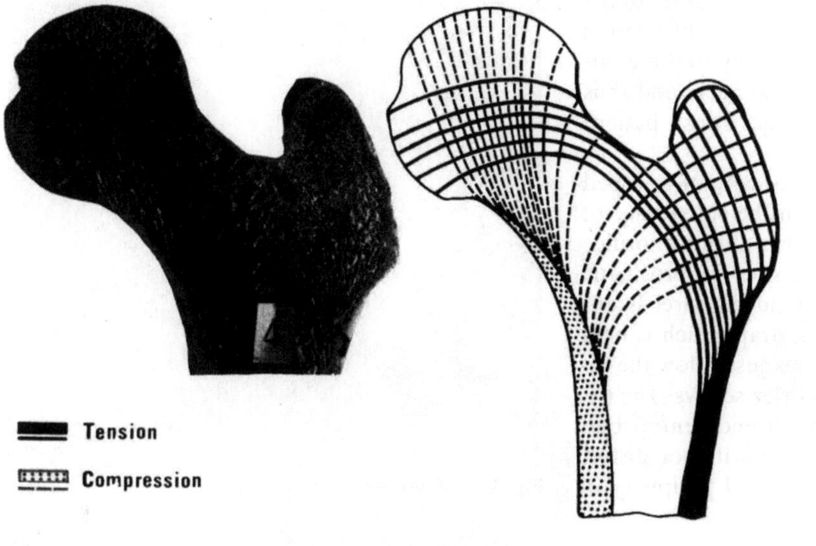

Fig. 1. The trabecular geometry of the proximal femur reflects prevailing lines of tensile and compressive stress

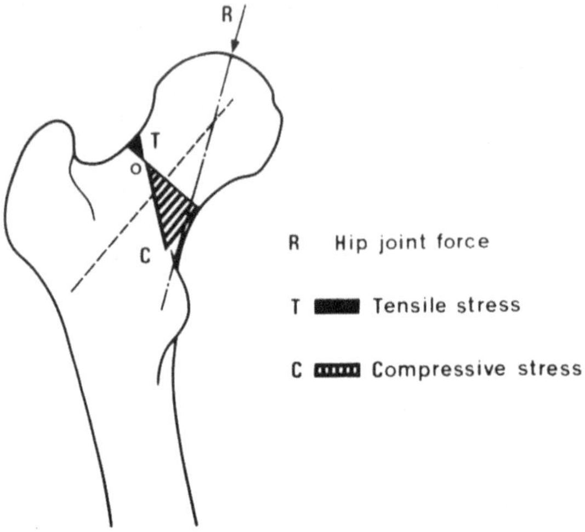

Fig. 2. Stress distribution in the femoral neck

Despite the practical clinical success that has been achieved with both cemented and uncemented femoral endoprostheses, there is no question that long-term results on a scale of 10 years or more are far from satisfactory (Dietschi, 1978). Thus, the intramedullary attachment of a prosthetic stem must generally be regarded as a yet-unsolved biomechanical problem.

Description of the Thrust-Plate Endoprosthesis

A new stemless femoral endoprosthesis, different from conventional types, has been developed in an effort to preserve both the magnitude and direction of physiologic stress transfer in the living bone (Fig. 3). The key feature of the device is the "thrust plate," which enables forces at the hip to be transferred directly to the cortical bone of the resected femoral neck, and thus maintains a largely physiologic stress pattern within the proximal femur.

The prosthesis consists basically of a lipped circular plate that mates with the cut surface of the femoral neck. The plate has a central orifice to accept a mandrel which carries the prosthetic femoral ball. The hollow, rigid mandrel is anchored by a single bolt to a strap which is held onto the lateral femoral cortex just below the innominate tubercle by two cortex screws. The extreme stiffness of the mandrel and central bolt ensures that the femoral neck will not distort under stress and keeps the cranial periphery of the thrust plate seated firmly on the stump of the femoral neck during walking.

To cope with variations in the length of the femoral neck, spherical heads of 32 mm diameter are available in 2 different neck lengths. Studies on the behavior of the bone-plate interface, stress analyses of the different components of the prosthesis, fatigue testing and final sizing were completed in 1978 after 2 years' work (Fig. 4).

A specialized instrument package had to be developed for implantation of the prosthesis: Following resection of the head, a drill guide is used to drill a central hole through the lateral femoral cortex and into the cancellous bone of the femoral neck. This provides a guide for the face milling of the resected neck to create a seat for the thrust plate, and for the reaming of the central channel prior to insertion of the mandrel.

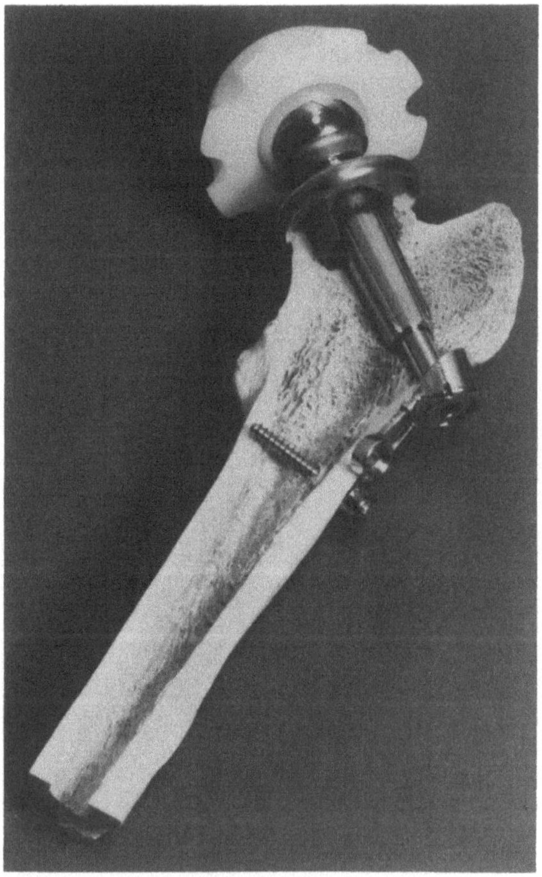

Fig. 3. The thrust-plate prosthesis

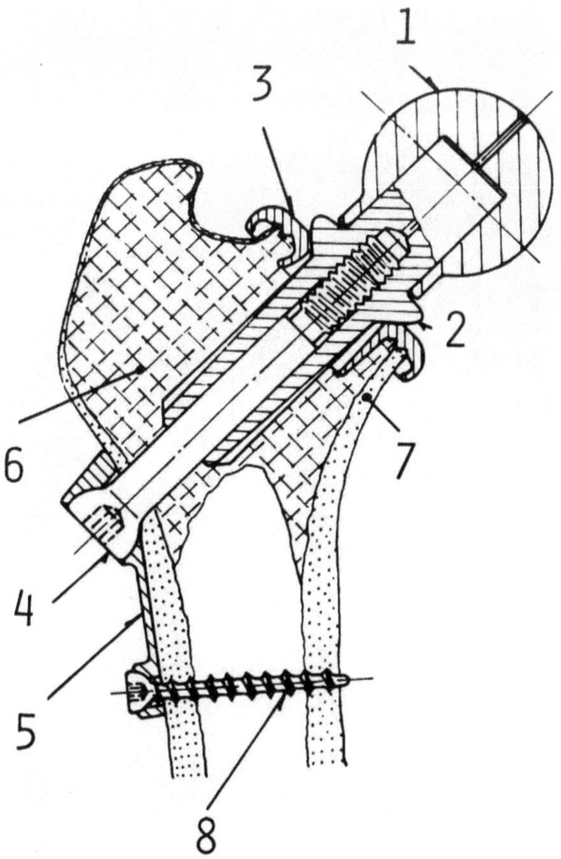

Fig. 4. Components of the thrust-plate prosthesis. *1* – head; *2* – mandrel; *3* – thrust plate; *4* – central bolt; *5* – anchoring strap; *6* – cancellous bone; *7* – calcar; *8* – cortex screw

Surgical Technique

The anterolateral incision of Watson-Jones is recommended. After exposing the hip joint between the gluteus medius and tensor fasciae latae muscles, a Kirschner wire about 15 cm long is placed over the anterior surface of the femoral neck, parallel to its axis. The position of the drill hole in the lateral femoral cortex below the innominate tubercle is marked after the bone has been dissected free. Although a CCD angle of about 125° is the basic objective, it is advantageous to consider the actual CCD angle, without increasing it excessively, since otherwise an undesired increase in leg length could result. The femoral neck is now osteotomized just proximal to its smallest diameter. The femoral head is removed, and a template is pressed onto the cut surface of the femur to mark the center of the cross-section. The leg is then rotated medially, and a drill guide is positioned so that the aiming point on the guide is centered on the template while the drill bit enters the point previously marked on the lateral femoral cortex. A 10-mm hole is drilled through the bone, and then the template and drill guide are removed. The strap is centered over the drill hole and temporarily attached to the lateral femur with two cortex screws. Now the femur is rotated laterally, and the face milling cutter is applied to the cut surface of the femoral neck such that it is centered on the hole in the lateral cortex. The neck is milled until the surface is smooth. As much cancellous bone is removed as is necessary to create a snug seating for the lipped thrust plate.

After the thrust plate has been press-fitted onto the stump, a trial mandrel is inserted through the plate and into the channel that has been reamed to receive it. The trial mandrel is withdrawn, the definitive mandrel is inserted, the femoral ball is attached to the proximal end of the mandrel, and the femur is rotated medially. Now the central bolt is inserted through the strap from the lateral side and tightened. The head of the bolt is secured to the strap with a locking wire.

The acetabular component is inserted just after resection of the femoral neck and before definitive placement of the thrust plate. The posteroinferior rim of the acetabular component (Weber type) should be trimmed to prevent the thrust plate from impinging on the socket when the leg is in full extension and lateral rotation. The acetabular component is protected with a gauze compress until insertion of the femoral component is complete.

Clinical Results

The first two thrust-plate endoprostheses implanted in 1978 have been closely followed. One patient shows an excellent 4-year result, has normal hip function and is free of pain. The second patient had to be reoperated following a fracture of the central bolt due to a flaw in the material supplied by the manufacturer (Figs. 5 and 6).

In close cooperation with the Orthopedic Clinic of the University of Zurich, an extensive field study was started in 1980. The 34 cases reviewed to date show excellent results and will be discussed in a subsequent paper.

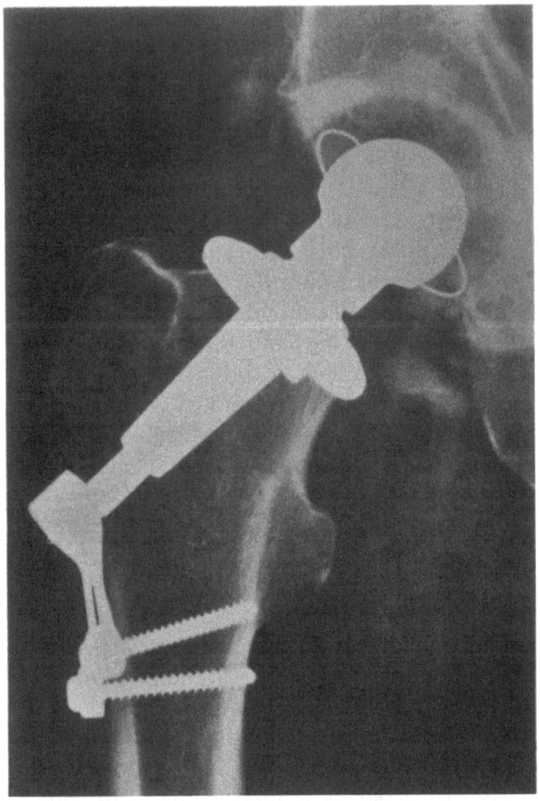

Fig. 5. H.B., 1912, ♂: Three months after implantation of a thrust-plate prosthesis (9-11-78)

The thrust-plate prosthesis (TPP) would be indicated in younger individuals with failed intertrochanteric osteotomies for osteoarthritis, primary and secondary avascular necrosis of the femoral head, and advanced primary osteoarthritis.

It will always be possible to convert the TPP to a conventional stem-type prosthesis should the need for such a revision arise.

Discussion

Based on experimental investigations, including stress analyses, it would appear that cancellous bone is not always able to withstand the mechanical stresses associated with the implantation of endoprostheses (Ritter and Grunert, 1973; Jacob et al., 1976, 1980; Ducheyne et al., 1977; Kolbel et al., 1977). Consequently, a femoral endoprosthesis has been designed which transfers loads directly to the cortical bone, thereby approximating physiologic conditions of stress transfer. This avoids the problems associated with the intramedullary attachment of femoral prostheses with a large amount of bone cement. Another advantage is that the blood supply to the proximal femur is not significantly disrupted owing to a minimum of trauma during implantation. Finally, the TPP is highly amenable to revision, which could be of value in younger individuals.

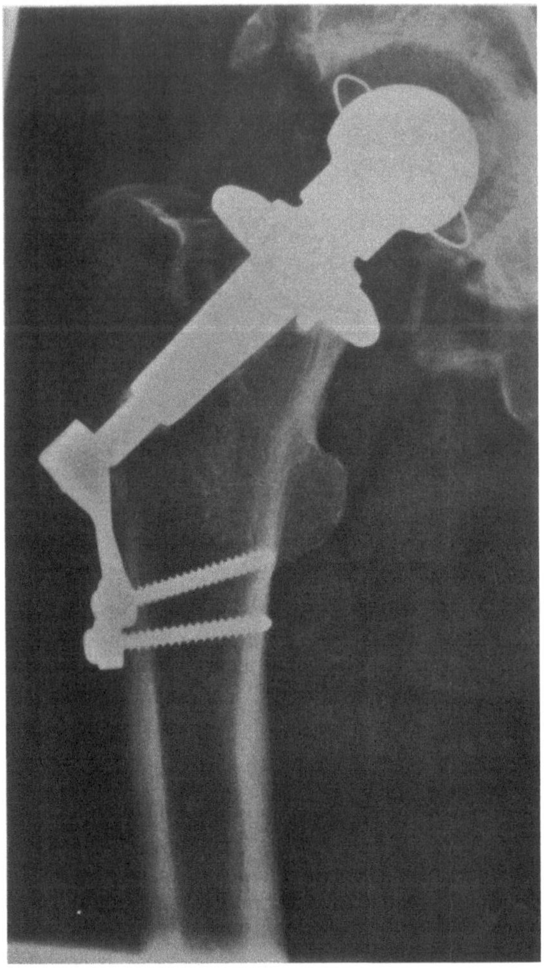

Fig. 6. H.B., 1912, ♂: Four years after implantation of the thrust-plate prosthesis. No bone resorption is evident in the calcar area, which shows a good, dense structure and apparently is providing the necessary support. The functional result is outstanding; the patient is free of pain and has full working capacity (7-21-83)

It is interesting to note that Wiles in 1938 and McKee in 1941 described a very similar femoral implant (McKee, 1967), although that design did not have the essential features of the thrust-plate prosthesis. The prosthesis described here has evolved entirely from recent discoveries in biomechanics and therefore must be considered a fundamentally new concept.

The TPP would provide an excellent substrate for a ceramic or carbon coating; the resulting bone ingrowth would integrate the prosthesis into the bone structure. We are also considering titanium as a material for construction of the thrust plate itself.

We chose to place the axis of the prosthesis in line with the femoral neck axis for two reasons:

1. Because the thrust plate is at right angles to the mandrel and the central bolt, this is the only way to seat the thrust plate on cortical bone of appreciable thickness. If the axis of the prosthesis were positioned more vertically, causing the thrust plate to assume a more horizontal attitude, the medial part of the plate would come to lie above the calcar, where the cortical bone is sparse and offers little support. On the other hand, the trochanteric fossa creates an anatomic constraint which precludes a more horizontal placement of the prosthetic axis.
2. The more vertical the position of the prosthesis, the more it approaches the mechanical situation of an intramedullary stem prosthesis with collar (Jacob et al., 1980). The difference in axial stiffness between the bone and implant would cause the distal end of the central bolt to move within the strap with each load cycle.

To neutralize the transverse forces arising between the thrust plate and the bone, the contact area of the plate was fashioned so as to prevent transverse motion even after the primary tension of the central bolt has subsided.

Stress analyses, loading tests and clinical experience confirm that the thrust-plate prosthesis is entirely capable of withstanding the stresses that are imposed on it. Stress transfer to the femur is far more physiologic than with conventional stem-type endoprostheses. In accordance with Wolff's law, full functional integration with the host bone and improved long-term results may be expected with the new endoprosthetic system.

Summary

A new femoral endoprosthesis of stemless design, different from conventional types, has been developed with the object of preserving the magnitude and direction of stress transfer in the proximal femur. The key feature of the prosthesis is the "thrust plate," which distributes loads on the proximal femur directly to the cortical bone of the resected femoral neck, thereby approximating conditions of physiologic stress transfer. The thrust-plate prosthesis, special instrument package and surgical technique are described. In 1978 two prototypes of the device were implanted in Chur, Switzerland. These initial clinical results are discussed with reference to the encouraging and positive field study launched in 1980 by the Orthopedic Department of the Kanton Hospital in Chur and the Orthopedic Clinic of the University of Zurich.

References

Dietschi C (1978) Problematik des künstlichen Hüftgelenkes: Experimentelle Untersuchungen über die Biomechanik des Hüftgelenkes und Langzeitergebnisse nach Hüfttotalendoprothesen. Habilitationsschrift Dez. 1976. Gentner, Stuttgart

Ducheyne P, Heymans L, Martens M, Aernoudt E, de Meester P, Mulier JC (1977) The mechanical behaviour of intracondylar cancellous bone of the femur at different loading rates. J Biomech 10 (11/12): 747–762

Jacob HAC, Huggler AH (1978) Experimentelle Spannungsanalysen im menschlichen Oberschenkelknochen-Modell mit und ohne Prothese. Forschungsheft, Technische Rundschau, Sulzer, S 73–83

Jacob HAC, Huggler AH (1980) An investigation into biomechanical causes of prosthesis stem loosening within the proximal end of the human femur. J Biomech 13: 159–173

Jacob HAC, Huggler AH, Dietschi C, Schreiber A (1976) The mechanical function of subchondral bone as experimentally determined on the acetabulum of the human pelvis. Biomechan 9: 625–627

Kölbel R, Bergmann G, Rohlmann A, Rauschenbach N (1977) Dynamic implant for application of cyclic loads to bone in vivo. Artif Organs 1/2: 125

McKee GK (1967) Developments in total hip joint replacement. Symposium on lubrication and wear in living and artificial human joints. Institution of Mechanical Engineers, London. Proc 1966/67, vol 181, Part 3 J, Paper 4, 1–5

McKee GK (1970) Development of total prosthetic replacement of the hip. Clin Orthop 72: 85–103

Ritter G, Grünert A (1973) Experimentelle Untersuchungen zu den mechanischen Eigenschaften des Knochens im Hinblick auf die Druckosteosynthesen. Arch Orthop Unfallchir 75: 302–316

Scholten R (1976) Über die Berechnung der mechanischen Beanspruchung in Knochenstrukturen mittels für den Flugzeugbau entwickeltes Rechenverfahren. Med Orthop Techn 6: 130–137

Wiles P (1958) The Surgery of the osteoarthritic hip. Br J Surg 45: 488–497

First Results with the "Thrust Plate" Total Hip Prosthesis

A. Schreiber, H. A. C. Jacob, Y. Suezawa and A. H. Huggler

The concept of the "thrust plate" total hip prosthesis was first presented publically at SICOT in Kyoto by Huggler and Jacob in 1978. This cement-free prosthesis was designed to reproduce a physiologic mode of stress transfer to the proximal femur, thereby avoiding bone resorption and consequent loosening. Another great advantage is that there is no need to open the medullary cavity when the prosthesis is inserted. If revision becomes necessary, all conventional options for revisionary surgery remain open. Having improved certain details of the prosthetic design, and following testing and approval by our Ethical Committee, we implanted a series of 20 thrust-plate prostheses at the Balgrist Orthopedic Hospital in Zurich approximately 2 years ago. Here we shall report on our first clinical results with this system.

At Balgrist and at the Orthopedic Department of the Canton Hospital in Chur, 32 thrust-plate prostheses (TPP) were implanted in 30 patients (22 men and 8 women) between September, 1980, and July, 1981. The length of follow-up is from 1 to 1¾ years, with an average of just over 1½ years. The patients ranged in age from 35 to 79 when the implantation was performed; the average age was 54. Twelve of the patients had necrosis of the femoral head, 28 had idiopathic osteoarthritis, and 9 had undergone prior hip surgery (intertrochanteric osteotomies). No complications arose either intraoperatively or in the immediate postoperative period, and primary wound healing was obtained in all patients.

The clinical results of the operations were rated according to a 3-point scale (0 to 2) with regard to pain, mobility, walking ability and working ability (2 = good, 1 = fair, 0 = poor). These individual scores were then tallied. A total score of 7–8 was rated as "excellent", 5–6 as "good", 3–4 as "fair", and 0–2 as "poor".

The result was rated excellent in 11 patients with 12 prostheses (Fig. 1). Today these patients are entirely free of complaints, and several have regained 100% working capacity (1 farmer, 1 butcher, 3 office workers). The farmer, for example, is able to work all day without discomfort 1 year after surgery. Fifteen patients with 15 TPPs have mild, transitory complaints. They are able to walk for 2 hours, on the average, and have only minimal restriction of hip mobility. The overall result for this group is rated "good". About one-third of all patients complained of pain in the area of the greater trochanter in the immediate postoperative period, but this abated spontaneously within 6–8 months. Results were rated "fair" in 2 patients and "poor" in 3 [sic] patients. One of the patients with a "fair" result has a consolidated arthrodesis in the contralateral hip. The sub-optimum improvement of mobility with the TPP obviously has a negative effect on the subjective result rating by the patient. In the 2 patients with a poor clinical result, the prosthesis had to be removed and a further replacement performed due to clinical and radiographic loosening:

- In one patient with bilateral necrosis of the femoral head, a TPP was inserted in the right hip in October, 1980. So far the result for this prosthesis is excellent. Seven weeks after the first operation a second TPP was implanted in the left hip, but complaints due to loosening arose within a week. Reexposing the hip and retightening the central anchoring bolt 6 months postoperatively relieved complaints for a while, but within 6 months the TPP had to be removed because of renewed loosening and associated complaints, at which time it was replaced with an uncemented titanium prosthesis. The poor results of the revision are probably due to the insidious infection that was detected on histologic examination.
- The second patient, a 52-year-old man, had femoral head necrosis of the left hip that was treated in 1980 with a TPP 3 years after an

unsuccessful intertrochanteric osteotomy. One week postoperatively, lumboischialgia developed on the left side in association with a herniated disk at L5/S1; this was treated operatively after radiologic confirmation. 3–4 weeks later the patient again complained of pain in the buttock and groin radiating to the anterior thigh. At 6 months postoperatively the hip was reexposed, the greater trochanter was revised, and the iliotibial tract was split longitudinally. Two months later, however, it became necessary to remove the TPP due to loosening and associated complaints and replace it with an uncemented titanium pros-

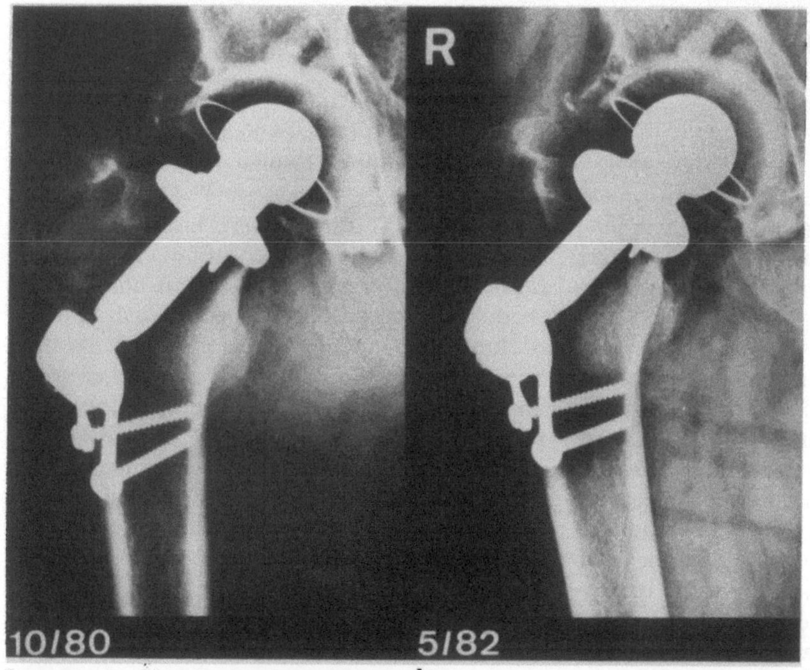

a b

Fig. 1 a, b. H.F., ♂, 1928, Pt. No. 274829. More than 1½ years after surgery the patient is entirely free of complaints and is able to work without disability. The x-rays show no evidence of loosening

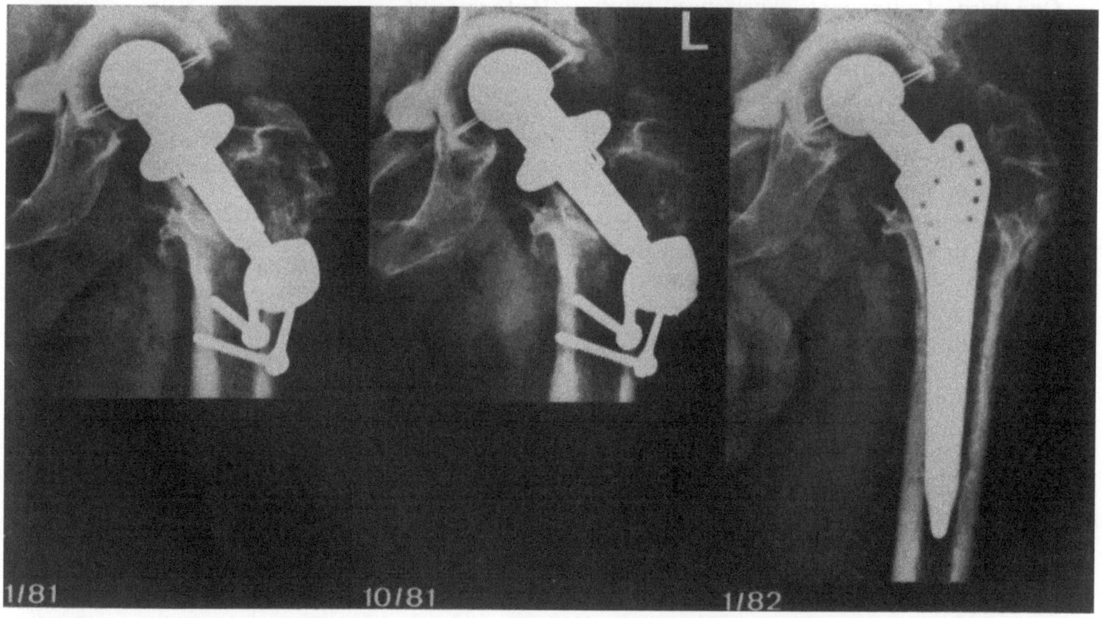

Fig. 2. F.S., ♂, 1928, Pt. No. 263490. There is loosening of the thrust-plate prosthesis, probably due to chronic infection. The TPP was replaced with an uncemented titanium-stem prosthesis of the Zweymueller type

thesis. Histologic examination disclosed a chronic plasmacytic infection. The result of the revision has not been satisfactory (Fig. 2).

The projecting portion of the TPP distal to the greater trochanter caused local pain and bursa formation in about one-third of all patients. However, these complaints abated spontaneously in almost all cases. On the whole, the first clinical results of the new thrust-plate prosthesis may be rated as highly encouraging.

Discussion

An improved model of the original thrust-plate prosthesis (Huggler and Jacob, 1980) was produced by improving the material of the central bolt and by reshaping the area of the thrust plate that comes in contact with the bone. Then, after testing by our Ethical Committee, 20 prostheses of this type were implanted without cement in 19 patients at the Balgrist Orthopedic Hospital in Zurich. A review of the Balgrist cases as well as cases from the Canton Hospital in Chur shows that the clinical results in general have been very good: No clinical or radiologic signs of loosening was apparent in 28 out of 30 patients. In the 2 cases where loosening did occur, it was presumably due to the presence of a chronic infection that was demonstrated histologically.

One-third of all patients experienced transitory pain and bursa formation in the area of the greater trochanter, apparently due to irritation from the projecting head of the anchoring bolt. These complaints disappeared within 6–8 months postoperatively in almost all patients. In the present series of 32 THRs, we used the traditional, cemented polyethylene acetabular component in all cases to avoid introducing an additional variable into the field study. The uncemented screw-type socket of Endler, which we have used in the past, is not easily combined with the thrust-plate prosthesis, because the minimal femoral neck resection hinders insertion of the very large thread-cutting instrument. A new cement-free acetabular component of our own design that could be combined more easily with the thrust-plate prosthesis is currently undergoing clinical testing.

Summary

The first clinical results of a field study conducted at the Balgrist Orthopedic Hospital in Zurich and at the Canton Hospital in Chur with the new, uncemented "thrust-plate" hip prosthesis are reported. (This prosthesis is inserted into the stump of the femoral neck without cement and is anchored by means of a central bolt which produces compression between the cut surface of the femur and the thrust plate.) A conventional polyethylene acetabular component was implanted in the usual fashion with bone cement. Since September of 1980, a total of 32 thrust-plate prostheses have been implanted in 30 patients. The clinical result was rated fair to excellent in 28 of the patients (29 prostheses). In the 2 patients whose result was poor, chronic infection was considered the probable cause of failure.

References

Huggler AH, Jacob HAC (1980) A new approach towards hip-prosthesis design. Arch Orthop Traumatol Surg 97: 141–144

Jacob HAC (1981) Die Druckscheiben-Hüftendoprothese: ein neues Hüftprothesenkonzept. Swiss Med 3/9:55–56

Schreiber A, Huggler AH, Jacob HAC (1981) The thrust plate hip prosthesis, a new approach towards hip-prosthesis design. In: XV World Congress in Rio de Janeiro, August 30–September 4, 1981: abstract. Sponsored by SICOT. S.I.s.n., 1981, pp 258–259

Uncemented, Ceramic-Coated, Electrically-Nonconductive Implants With Physiologic Stress Transfer

A. Engelhardt

An analysis of the biomechanical and chemical factors involved in skeletal implantation has led to a new concept for attaching an implant to the bone.

Our first use of endoprostheses was for the bridging of bony defects left by tumor resections. We observed the formation of a supporting bony pedestal at the distal end of the implant about 3–4 months postoperatively, and the first calcifications were visible on x-ray around the proximal part of the cone between the 3rd and 5th postoperative month (Fig. 1). After 1½ to 2 years, x-rays revealed a sheath of calcified material surrounding the endoprosthesis for 70–80% of its length. We interpret these findings as evidence of a process aimed at incorporating the implant actively into the skeletal system. We have taken these processes into account in designing our total hip replacement system.

The most critical areas in the hip prosthesis appear to be located in the plane of the resection (Fig. 2). There we have observed bone resorption that in some cases amounted to several angular degrees, analogous to the demineralized zone in bone fractures. We have also identified three developmental stages that are visible in postoperative x-rays:

1. By the 2nd–3rd postoperative month, appositional growth appears on the medial femoral neck and is oriented according to prevailing load lines. This growth was not visible preoperatively and appears as deposits on the cortical bone.
2. By the 3rd–6th month the femoral neck appears to broaden, and the bone appears to grow around the anterior edge of the implant and gradually acquire a lateral orientation on the cranial surface of the prosthetic collar. After ¾ to 1 year, calcium shadows can be seen medial to the greater trochanter in a thin layer on the upper edge of the implant.

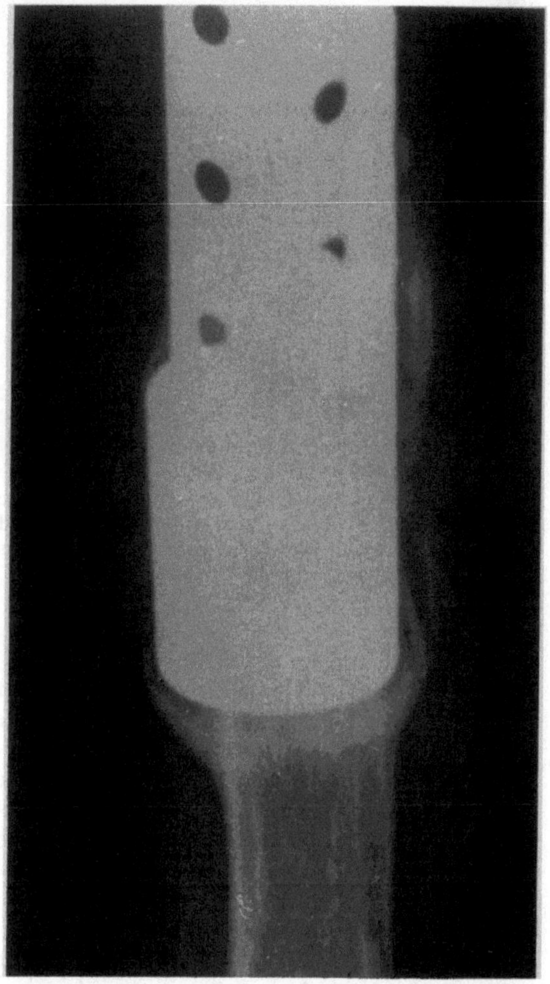

Fig. 1. Status 4 months after insertion of implant. A bony pedestal has formed distally, and bone is starting to grow around the implant. The implant was inserted to bridge a ¾-length resection of the proximal humerus for a giant-cell tumor (cementless fixation)

In addition, there is an apparent ingrowth of osteons into the apron region, which may enhance the rotational stability of the implant.

In a similar fashion, new radiodense structures appear about the roof of the acetabulum

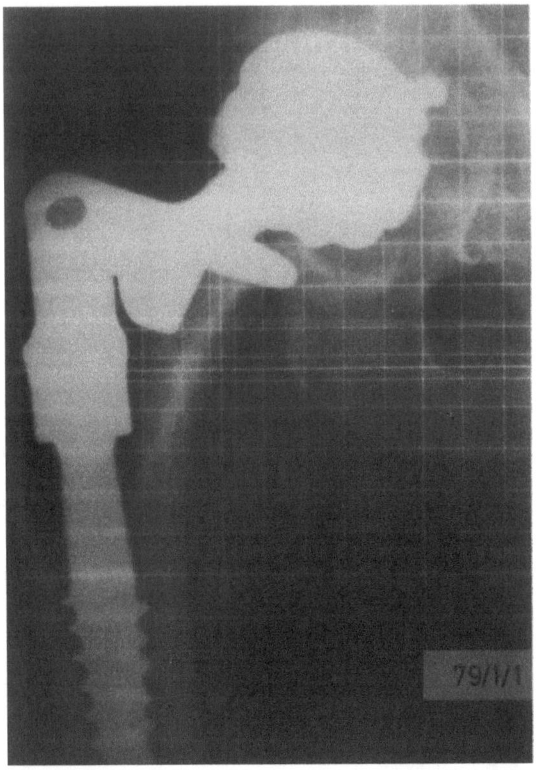

Fig. 2. Uncemented total hip prosthesis with ceramic coating and physiologic stress transfer (42-year-old man who had arthroplasty for femoral head necrosis and extensive damage of the hip joint)

in response to implantation of an acetabular prosthesis, and the closure of cysts cranial to the natural acetabulum becomes evident. Our observations in the acetabular region must be viewed somewhat more critically, however, because, unlike the femur, it was not possible to position the pelvis reproducibly for every x-ray.

These observations, which are identical to those made with tumor endoprostheses that were implanted more than 8 years ago, provide unmistakable evidence of an active incorporation of the implant into its bony environment.

It would appear, then, that by promoting these processes through refinements of prosthetic design and surgical technique, it would be possible to encourage a gradual bony investment of the proximal part of the implant that will enhance the biological anchorage of the prosthesis.

What must be done to achieve this? At present this question can be answered only by radiologic and other noninvasive clinical studies. Histologic results are not yet available in human patients. Thus, today we are able to obtain only a partial confirmation of our implant concept and therapeutic approach.

The guiding principle of our developmental work was the theory of "causal histogenesis," which we have modified or expanded on the basis of new discoveries. Basically, this theory states that bone becomes oriented structurally along prevailing lines of force, and that shear forces stimulate the formation of connective tissue. Moreover, it is known that collagen fibers provide the structural framework for bone, and that these fibers, as a crystalline material, are capable of generating bioelectrical impulses. The potentials that are produced under mechanical loads, together with direct mechanical effects, are believed to exert a "trigger" function through which genetically predetermined biochemical processes are set into motion. They thus play a key role in the formation and maturation of osseous tissue.

Recognizing the importance of these processes, we may state the following requirements for endoprosthetic components:

1. The implant must be inserted in such a way that
   a) it causes minimal interruption of the bony structure in the area of contact;
   b) physiologic stress transfer is not disturbed under either static or dynamic loads, and unphysiologic shear forces are eliminated.
2. Processes of development and maturation in the defect-bridging bone tissue must not be disturbed by excessive mechanical stresses during the healing period.
3. Negative physical and physicochemical influences should be minimized. This means eliminating the effects of bone cement (heat, monomers), corrosion products, and temperature elevations during cutting and reaming of the bone.

Remarks on 1a: In the acetabulum, this is achieved by adopting a socket design that will spare as much cortical bone stock as possible. Only three 5-mm drill holes are made around the resultant load line F_R (Fig. 3). The knobbed anchoring pegs (the two cranial pegs are eccentrically placed) are press-fitted into the drill holes, utilizing elastic deformation of the bone as an anchoring mechanism. The pegs abut on the posterior surface of the cortical bone. This fixation method avoids gross disruption of the presumed bioelectrical impulse pattern while preventing undesired stress concentrations and unphysiologic edge stresses that could lead to bone resorption.

In the area of the distal anchoring screw, only a portion of the thread engages the bone. As time passes, stress competence will be increased by appositional bone growth in a mathematically predictable fashion (Fig. 4).

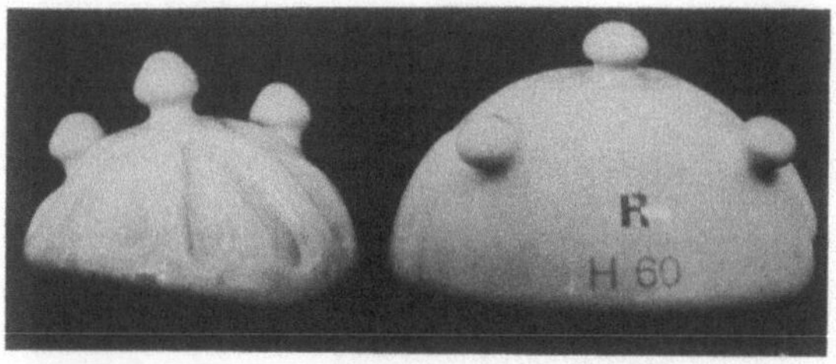

Fig. 3. Acetabular component designed for cementless fixation: *right* cranial view; *left* caudal view

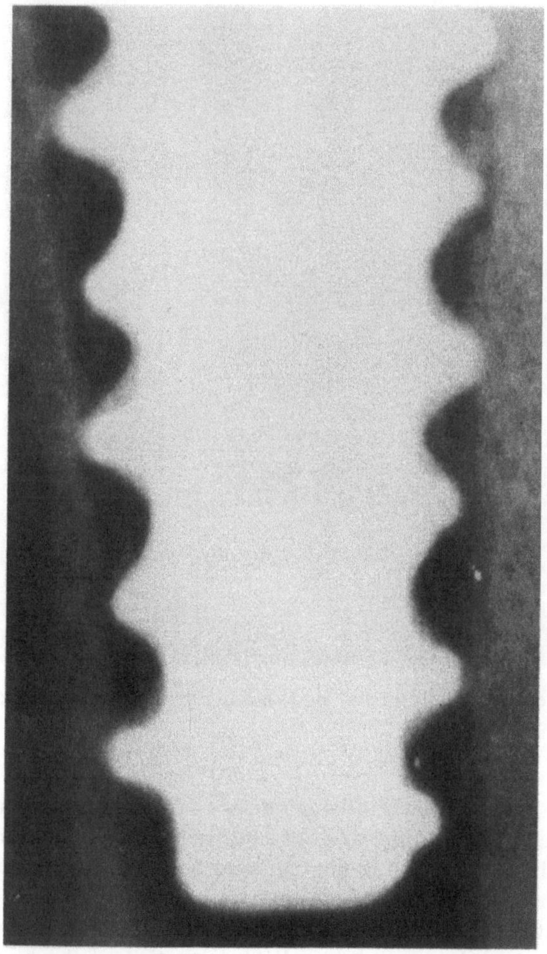

Fig. 4. Appositional bone growth around the intramedullary anchoring screw (4–6 months postoperatively)

Bone resorption at interfacial zones in this area was so slight that it could not be demonstrated by x-ray. This does not mean that no resorption occurred, but that the resorbed areas were too small to be detected by ordinary methods. Solid primary contact between the bone and anchoring screw may be assumed.

In performing the femoral neck resection, the principle of "minimal injury" must be adhered to, for the bearing surface of the implant on the cut surface of the femur must be set at right angles to the resultant of the osteon axis at the calcar to ensure that only perpendicular loads will be transferred to the bone and that large, unphysiologic shear loads will be minimized.

In contrast to other anchoring regions, this requirement necessarily involves a radical interruption of the bony architecture.

Remarks on 1b: Angular relationships in the proximal part of the implant are adjusted to ensure a physiologic load transfer to the bone (Fig. 5a, b). Angles are measured from two plane x-rays made with a special radiographic technique. In addition, the surgical instrumentation is designed so that both 2- and 3-dimensional orientation can be maintained during the operation. Finally, a joint is provided so that the "stress shielding" effect known from internal fixation techniques can be avoided.

Remarks on 2: A carefully supervised program of graduated weight-bearing, measured by the normal component of ground forces transmitted to the hip, is started postoperatively to avoid excessive stresses. As more is learned about bone properties and their measurement, it may become possible to individualize the exercise regimen on that basis.

Remarks on 3: By the use of a ceramic, inert, electrically neutral coating, cementless fixation, and friction reduction through proper matching of the articulating surfaces, corrosion and other chemical effects can be avoided, and wear reduced to a point that is not harmful to host tissues.

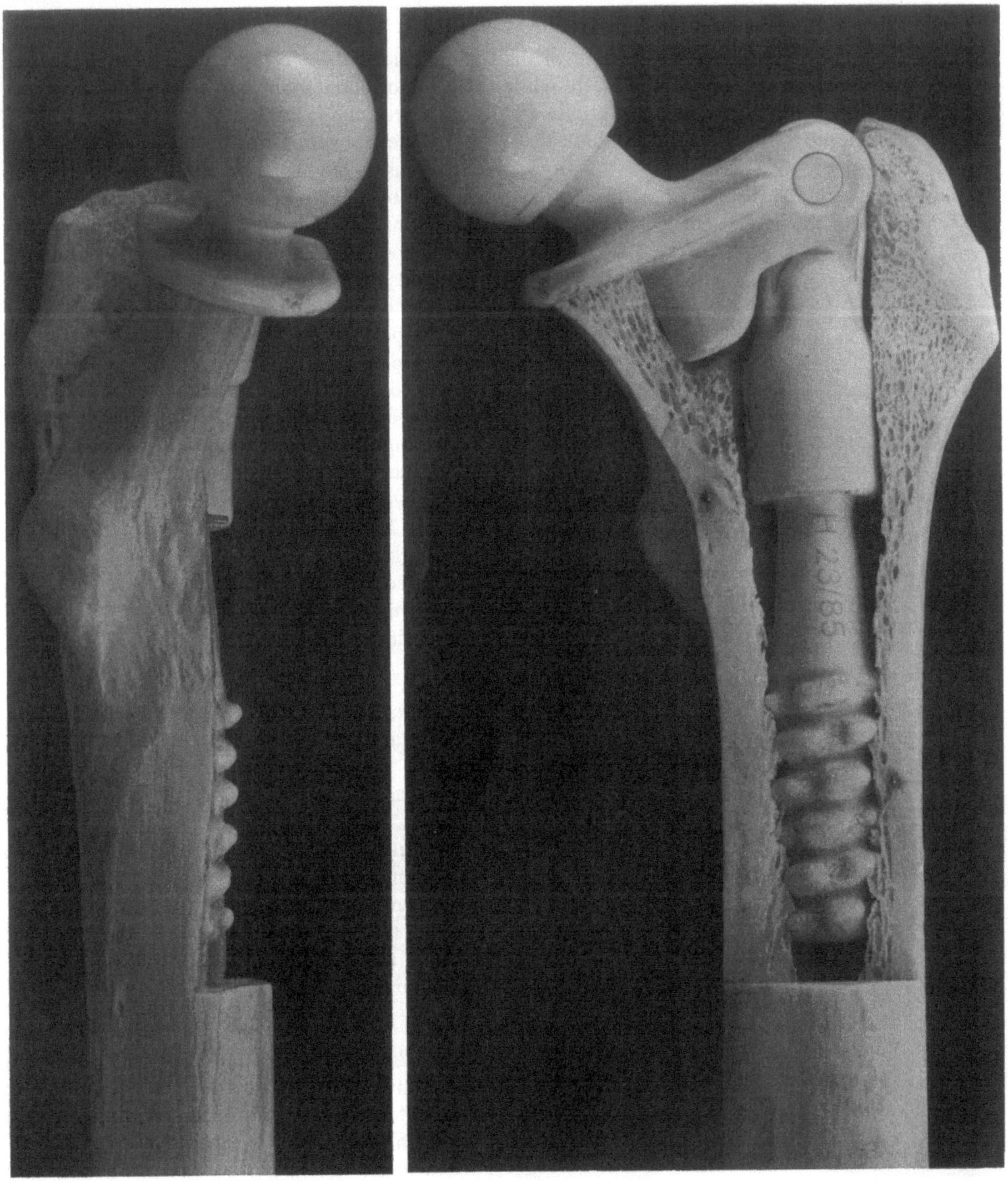

a b

Fig. 5 a, b. Cut-away preparation showing the inserted implant. **a** Medial view; **b** anterior view. Note the anterior inclination of the cut surface of the femur, perpendicular to the osteon axis

Results

The system places rigorous demands on both therapy and patient. The results depend upon strict adherence to specified procedures, taking note of the following points:

The anchoring of the acetabular and femoral components proceeds according to a specific program, and large stresses can be borne within a short time without causing component malposition. The biologic tissues behave in a predictable, calculable fashion.

We believe that the femoral neck resection and consequent radical disruption of the bony architecture may cause relatively high resorption rates in that area. These rates vary in accordance with individual parameters that are not yet fully understood. The resorptive processes are essentially the same as those occurring in fracture therapy. Hence, we have started placing the plane of resection at a 95° to the osteon axis, rather than the usual 90°. This extra 5° appears to be useful in reducing the degree of resorption.

Instrument-monitored walking exercises are started during the first postoperative days, with allowance made for wound conditions and circulatory status.

The loads placed upon the operated hip are graduated in 20% increments, based upon the normal component of ground forces and body weight. Generally these increments are made at intervals of one month. In some cases it is prudent to start with a 4–6 week period in which floor contact is allowed but no weight is borne (rolling the foot from heel to toe).

Active mobility in the hip joint is gained as muscular atrophy regresses. Full hip mobility is achieved from 6 to 9 months postoperatively, on the average. The range of mobility will depend upon the extent to which preexisting contractures have been relieved, and on how well the muscles respond to rehabilitation.

We found that most patients experienced muscular pain each time the load was graduated, but that the pain seldom persisted more than 14 days.

At 6–9 months after surgery, the great majority of patients required no walking aids, and a very few required one cane.

At 1 year after surgery, younger patients reported that they were able to walk distances of 20 km without crutches or other aids.

To date, the endoprostheses have been implanted in 10 patients ranging in age from 30 to 58.

So far no revisions have become necessary due to system failure. However, strict adherence to the specified procedures is imperative, for excessive stresses of the femoral neck area during the healing period can seriously interfere with bone repair processes. Alterations in biomechanical relationships can have a negative cumulative effect. The reparative processes may require a year or more before they are complete, especially if pharmacologic therapy is necessitated by intercurrent disease. No data are yet available on the connection between the primary status of the bone and bone repair, although it is reasonable to assume that such a connection exists. Experiments are currently being done to resolve this question.

Due to the varying number of parameters and the limited number of operations, we are not yet able to make a meaningful statistical analysis of our results. This will require a broader investigative approach, particularly with regard to primary bone data.

Beginning this year, all patients will undergo a preoperative gait examination with goniometry, and an EMG will be obtained for selected muscles. The tests will be repeated postoperatively as soon as 100% weight-bearing has been instituted. Then clinical and radiologic examinations will be conducted after 3 months, 6 months, and then at yearly intervals.

Results to date justify the hope that, with further improvements in the biological anchorage, our endoprosthetic system will be of value even in younger patients. We base this prognosis both on 9 years' experience with tumor implants and on the results of the hip operations begun in 1979.

The primary diseases of the patients that had undergone previous surgery were distributed fairly evenly among idiopathic necrosis, degenerative arthritis associated with dysplasia or dislocation, femoral head necrosis secondary to hepatic disease, and one case of necrosis following cortisone therapy.

Full, normal mobility of the hip joint was achieved in all cases.

In all cases x-ray showed calcifications at the apex of the greater trochanter, in the area of attachment of the gluteus medius muscle. These shadows were of operative origin and did not hamper mobility.

One of the patients, who had been treated abroad, has applied for a pension at the age of 59. He is a farmer by trade.

Summary

The principle of causal histogenesis appears to be of definite value in the development of skeletal endoprostheses and the planning of therapy, provided the differences with respect to conventional fracture therapy are recognized, as they are here. Good agreement is found between calculated and test results. Discoveries to date indicate that further improvements are possible, especially with regard to individual prognosis; a significant shortening of the primary fixation time is a particularly interesting prospect. The use of suitable inert surfaces in zones of bone-implant contact and of appropriate material combinations in articulating areas rounds out the concept. The technique is more costly and time-consuming than other therapies and is more susceptible to error. It may be practiced only in centers that are equipped to meet the rigorous therapeutic and operative demands, and by physicians that are able to manage their patients in a consistent fashion. Patient compliance is also an important factor, for the insertion of an implant that is "quasi-active" in physiologic terms can easily lead to failure if the biologic tissue is unduly stressed during the primary healing and fixation period.

References

1. Engelhardt A (1980) Probleme der zementfreien Prothesenverankerung. Med Orthop Techn Heft 1/80
2. Engelhardt A, Grell H, Komitowski D et al. (1976) Trends in the development of permanent ceramic implants. In: Schaldach M, Hohmann D (eds) Engineering in medicine, vol 2. Advances in artificial hip and knee joint technology, pp 475–492. Springer, Berlin Heidelberg New York
3. Engelhardt A, Scholten R, Burkhard KH, Sollbach B (1977) Kraftflußberechnungen zu zementfrei implantierbare Hüftgelenksprothese mit physiologischer Krafteinleitung. Ber. BMFT
4. Engelhardt A, Sencar M, Scharbach H, Komitowski D, Andreef I (1978) Results after implantation of ceramic-coated humerus endoprostheses. Sicot Konf. 14
5. Engelhardt A, Sencar M, Heipertz W, Kooke D et al. (1979) Implantate zur Defektüberbrückung nach Tumorresektionen. Acta Facult. Med. Univ. Brunensis, S 64
6. Engelhardt A, Sencar M, Scharbach H, Grell H, Andreef I (1981) Erfahrungen mit zementlós verankerten Implantaten. Z Orthop 119/6:789–791
7. Grell H (1976) Ursachen der Lockerung von Hüftendoprothesen und konstruktive Abhilfemaßnahmen bei Verwendung biokompatibler Werkstoffe. Dissertation, Universität Stuttgart
8. Kummer B (1978) Mechanische Beanspruchung und funktionelle Anpassung des Knochens. Verh Anat Ges 72:21–45
9. Pauwels F (1965) Gesammelte Abhandlungen zur funktionellen Anatomie des Bewegungsapparates. Springer, Berlin Heidelberg New York
10. Scholten R, Röhrle H (1977) Kraftflußberechnungen in Knochenstrukturen und Prothesen – Phase II. Ber. BMFT

Experience with the Lord Prosthesis

G. Rupp

We have been using the cement-free Lord total hip system in our department for four years. Our confidence in this system is based upon the very high strength that is achieved when the components are implanted correctly. This strength derives not only from the interlock produced by bony ingrowth into the madreporic surface of the prosthesis but also from the manner in which the femoral component is seated within the medullary cavity and upon the greater trochanter. To achieve the strongest possible bond between the components and surrounding bone, Lord provided his components with a "madreporic" surface, i.e., a surface that is roughened by the deposition of numerous tiny beads, each having the shape of a ¾ sphere. This enlarges the surface area by a factor of 3 while providing a framework for bone ingrowth. Animal studies have shown that this form of surface enlargement is superior to "negative" forms in which pores or recesses are used to increase surface area. With the madreporic surface, the tiny bone structures that invade the spaces between the spherules are not as susceptible to fracture as the bone ingrowth into porous surfaces. Animal implantations have also demonstrated how firmly the bone encloses and "grips" the madreporic implant, creating a highly accurate prosthesis-to-bone fit.

A variety of stem sizes are available, and the acetabular component comes in various sizes and shapes. The regular stem diameters are 13 mm, 15 mm and 18 mm, and a "miniature" femoral component with a stem diameter of 11 mm is available for dysplasic hips. The stem lengths range from 15 to 20 cm. The stems also come in several neck lengths – short, medium and long. The heads are interchangeable and have three different depths of the neck socket. This makes it possible to vary the head-neck length over a total range of 2 cm. The head diameter is 32 mm. The regular acetabular components, which are externally threaded, come in diameters of 50 mm, 54 mm, 58 mm and 62 mm. Diameters of 42 mm and 46 mm are available for patients with dysplasia. Each socket comes with a polyethylene insert which, like the head, is interchangeable. Thus, if wear becomes excessive and the stem and acetabular ring are still firmly seated, it is necessary only to replace the head and the socket insert. It is also possible to use a snap-in socket with the femoral component, thus combining the Lord and Moor systems. In this case the correct socket size is chosen, the socket is mounted on the Lord stem, to which is attached the appropriate head, and the system is simply inserted into the acetabulum with no further preparation of the acetabular area. The best candidates for this system are elderly patients with femoral neck fractures, in whom other treatment methods probably could not prevent avascular necrosis of the femoral head.

For the operation itself, the patient is placed in lateral recumbency. I use a longitudinal incision that curves slightly distally and posteriorly over the greater trochanter. The fascia lata is incised in the same direction (a notch may be made in the posterior edge of the incision if additional exposure is needed). Then the external rotators are snared near their attachment in the trochanteric area and divided in their tendinous portion. Now part of the posterior capsule is excised, the cranial part of the capsule is notched following retraction of the gluteal muscles that insert there, and the hip is dislocated by careful medial rotation of the femur. During this process the assistant holding the leg flexes the knee to about 80° while carefully rotating the thigh medially, until the lower leg is approximately vertical. The dislocation can be further assisted by inserting broad-blade elevators into the joint. The femoral head having been dislocated, the assistant rotates the limb about 10° farther medially so that the lower leg passes the vertical and is inclined toward the front of the patient. In this position the surgeon can resect the femoral neck with an oscillating saw, using two cuts. The first cut starts at the junction of the greater trochanter with the femoral neck and runs parallel to the long axis of the femur. The second cut is made horizontally, starting about 1 cm proximal to the lesser trochanter and forming an angle of about 85° with the first cut. The plane of the bearing surface forms a 90° angle with the long axis of the femoral shaft. Next the medullary cavity of the femur is rasped for insertion of the prosthetic stem. The rasp for the 13-mm stem is the first to be used. If a good fit cannot be obtained in this way, the next larger rasp size is tried. The preoperative x-rays are a useful guide in this respect, as well as in determining the necessary size of the prosthetic components. It is important that the rasp fit snugly within the femoral shaft. If difficulties are encountered during rasping due to a distal constriction of the medullary cavity, and much force would be needed to drive the rasp through the constricted area, it is imperative that an intramedullary reamer be used to widen the cavity. The cavity should be reamed to within 0.5 mm of the desired stem diameter. Thus, for a stem diameter of 15 mm, the medullary cavity is reamed to an inside diameter of 14.5 mm. Following preparation of the medullary cavity, the acetabulum is prepared to receive the threaded socket. Suitable acetabular reamers are used to increase the diameter of the bony acetabulum. In addition, the acetabulum should be deepened so that the threaded socket is surrounded on all sides by a firm, stable bony ring. When this has been done, the thread for the screw-in socket is precut in the acetabulum. At this time it will become apparent whether a firm seating can be achieved for the threaded acetabular ring. If the thread-cutting instrument does not gain sufficient purchase in the acetabular bone, it will be necessary either to deepen the acetabulum or go to the next larger socket diameter, depending on local bone conditions. When the seat for the acetabular ring has been adequately prepared, I recommend sealing the bony wound with a mixture of fibrin and autologous cancellous bone taken from the resected femoral head and neck. For this purpose the cancellous bone is ground into a fine powder and mixed with the adhesive components fibrinogen and thrombin. While still pasty, the mixture is packed into the bony wound and spread over the surface of the bone bed. At this point the threaded acetabular ring is screwed into the acetabulum. This provides a very strong and accurate seating for the component while encouraging bone growth around the prosthetic ring. Next the acetabular ring, which is positioned at a 45° angle to the horizontal plane and in 15–20° anteversion, is provided with the matching polyethylene insert. After the bone wound in the femoral shaft has been sealed as described above for the acetabulum, the proper stem is driven into the cavity, and the appropriate head is attached. (Alternatively, one may first insert a smooth-stemmed trial prosthesis that is compatible with various head sizes to check the selected head–stem combination for accuracy of length.) Insertion of the stem should be done with an instrument that allows the stem to be securely held and guided as it is driven into the femoral shaft. Once the stem has been driven into place, it generally is no longer possible to extract it; this indicates that a firm primary seating has been achieved. The sequence in which the acetabular and femoral components are inserted is largely a matter of individual preference and may be reserved if desired. After both components have been inserted, the hip is reduced by traction and lateral rotation of the femoral shaft. If now the leg is extended and rotated medially by 10°, and longitudinal traction is applied to the limb, the femoral head should emerge from the acetabular cup by about ½ to ¾ of the head diameter. This is a sign that the correct system has been selected.

About 2 years ago I did a follow-up and evaluation of the first 100 patients to receive the Lord prosthesis. At that time the prostheses had been in place for periods ranging from 1½ to 2½ years. The patients consisted of 30 men and 70 women. The youngest patients were in their 30's and the oldest in their 80's at the time of operation; most were in their 60's. In 36 cases the arthroplasty was performed for conditions secondary to trauma. In 62 cases the conditions were due to non-traumatic causes, and in 2 cases no cause could be ascertained. The longest period of hospitalization was 102 days, the shortest 12. The average hospitalization was 20–30 days, including preparation time and primary postoperative care.

The length of observation postoperatively was 3 months in 82% of the patients and up to 6 months in 18%. Complications consisted of 5 trochanteric fractures, 7 cases of postoperative phlebitis, and 10 cases of periarticular ossification (7 mild, 3 severe). These ossifications had to be excised in 2 patients. In 9 patients a plaster dressing was applied to immobilize the hip. Two patients had a previous Voss "hanging hip" operation, 6 had post-traumatic necrosis of the femoral head, and 5 had failed cemented arthroplasties. Weight-bearing on the operated limb was started between the 2nd and 5th postoperative day, with crutches used to restrict the load to about one-half the body weight. Full weight-bearing was allowed between 3 and 6 weeks postoperatively, and the majority of patients were able to walk without crutches at that time. Exceptions were cases in which the implantation could not be performed with the desired degree of precision at reoperation. These hips were put in plaster for 3–4 weeks postoperatively, and weight-bearing was deferred for 3–6 months.

It would be useful at this point to examine several cases that illustrate the kind of problems that can arise in this type of operation. One case involved a juvenile patient who, at age 16, suffered a severe central hip dislocation that precipitated a very painful and disabling degenerative arthritis. At 22 the patient underwent a THR in which a ceramic femoral head was used. About 1½ years later the head became fractured during a jump from a wall. In a revisionary operation the head and polyethylene insert of the acetabular cup were replaced. The operation went smoothly, and 4 weeks later the hip was fully sound and could bear weight without discomfort. The patient was able to return to work.

Another problem concerns fractures of the trochanter. If the seat of the femoral prosthesis on the greater trochanter is incorrectly prepared, i.e., if too much of the trochanter is left by the resection, there is a danger that the trochanter will break off when the stem is driven into the femur. If this occurs, the trochanter can be replaced and reattached with a cancellous bone screw. Alternatively, the wound may be closed and the limb immobilized in plaster for 3–4 weeks, during which time weight-bearing is allowed. After about 6 weeks the greater trochanter should be stable enough that the fracture will cause no significant complaints and will go on to bony union with no impairment of function. It is best, of course, to avoid trochanteric fractures through accurate preparation of the bone. If the rasp makes too deep a groove in the greater trochanter during rasping of the femur, this is a sign that additional resection of the trochanter is needed. Insertion of the rasp should make no more than a very shallow track in the greater trochanter. When the trochanteric resection is correctly done, there should be no danger of fracture during prosthetic insertion. This danger is greatest in cases where the Lord prosthesis is inserted to replace a cemented prosthesis, for cemented prostheses invariably lead to embrittlement of the bone.

The first follow-up of 2½ years ago encompassed 100 patients. Over the past 4 years, I have implanted a total of 547 Lord prostheses. In that time there has been one case of acetabular loosening and one case of stem loosening. Both failures were due to primary errors of technique. The acetabular component had not been anchored securely enough in the bony acetabulum. The acetabular ring diameter (54 mm) was too small, and the next larger size (58 mm) should have been used. This error was corrected at revision, whereupon the acetabular component was stable. The stem loosening was the result of a similar error. The 13-mm stem diameter did not match the canal well, and this allowed the stem to wobble and loosen. At revision the stem was removed and replaced with an 18-mm stem. The patient reported slight discomfort immediately after surgery which increased somewhat over the next 1½ years, but no signs of infection were apparent.

Another case illustrates that a deep-seated acetabular component that protrudes into the lesser pelvis is very well tolerated. A cemented component had to be removed, thus leaving a very wide and deep acetabulum. The floor of the acetabulum was packed with cancellous bone and fibrin before inserting the revisional prosthesis. Only 4 months later the x-rays showed excellent appositional bone growth that completely filled the original gaps. For 2½ years the patient has been entirely free of complaints.

Yet another case demonstrates the load-bearing capabilities of the Lord prosthesis. It involved a young woman who, at age 18, suffered a severe central hip dislocation during an auto accident. Walking was extremely painful, and a progressive adduction contracture developed over a period of about 4 years. Transposition of the adductor muscles was of only transitory benefit. Three and one-half years ago the patient was treated with a Lord prosthesis. This enabled her to walk without discomfort. About 1½ years after the operation the patient was involved in another traffic accident, at which time she sustained a severe comminuted fracture of the ipsilateral femur with involvement of the distal end. The peripheral half of the right femur was affected. The implant itself withstood the trauma without irritation. The peripheral fracture was operatively reduced and stabilized with a plate and screws. The fracture healed completely, and following removal of the internal fixation material the patient was able to walk as before the accident.

Another patient, a women just over 60, suffered a traumatic dislocation about 1½ years after implantation of the total hip. The dislocation was reduced under general anesthesia, and the limb was immobilized in plaster for 3 weeks. A short time after removal of the fixation (about 4 weeks) the dislocation recurred during normal movement, the hip was again put in plaster for 6 weeks, and again it dislocated a few weeks later. At reoperation it was found that the lateral rotators, which had been detached from the femur and then reattached during the primary operation, had been torn from the bone by the trauma, and that the capsule was badly stretched in its posterior portion. The lateral rotators were resutured, the stretched capsule was resected and the defect closed, and the operated hip was immobilized in plaster for 3 weeks. Since that time (more than 6 months) the dislocation has not recurred, and the patient has remained free of complaints. In this case the intercurrent trauma of the hip dislocation was sufficient to rupture the lateral rotators and stretch the posterior capsule, allowing recurrent dislocations of the joint.

Finally, I would like to relate my experience with a failed arthroplasty, which, like most failures, is highly instructive. The patient, a women over 60, was transferred to my unit with a fistulous wound of the thigh following prior surgery for a femoral neck fracture. The fracture had been stabilized with a 3-layered pin, and an infection had developed. As the fistulous drainage indicated, the path of infection led into the pin, through the femoral head into the joint. The pin was extracted, the head resected, the joint drained, and the limb immobilized. The operative wound healed well, and the fistulous tract closed. Six months after closure of the fistula, a Lord prosthesis was inserted. Initially it appeared that the prosthesis would be tolerated without complications. But after 4 weeks the fistula reappeared and this time persisted despite suction irrigation, gentamycin, immobilization in plaster, etc. It became necessary to remove the prosthetic components. At this time it was found that the acetabular component was very firmly seated but could be easily screwed out of the bone with the wrench. This was not the case with the stem, which was so firmly impacted in the femoral shaft that, during extraction, a portion of the femoral shaft came away with the stem. This fragment, a cylindrical segment about 12 cm long, had to be split before it could be removed from the prosthesis. Because of the large defect in the femur, an attempt was made simply to replace the bone fragment in the shaft and then immobilize the leg in a hip spica, maintaining suction irrigation of the wound. The wound healed well, and the fistula closed a second time – this time permanently. Remarkably, postoperative films demonstrated a complete revitalization of the reimplanted bone segment, and the hip has functioned satisfactorily as a Girdlestone.

Finally, the data presented below represent an overall evaluation of the results of the first 100-case review. Essentially the same results have been obtained in subsequent patients, and so the data are basically valid for the 547 operations that have been performed to date.

The patients were classified into four groups as follows:

Group 1: patients who have a mobility of at least ⅔ the normal range and are able to walk without discomfort and with an apparently normal gait.

Group 2: patients who have from ½ to ⅔ the normal range of motion and have mild, intermittent complaints related to weather conditions or overexertion.

Group 3: patients who have from ⅓ to ½ the normal range of motion and must use a cane when walking.

Group 4: patients who have less than ⅓ the normal range of motion, have hip pain and must use 2 crutches or canes when walking.

The percentage breakdown of the patients by group is as follows:

Group 1: 70%, including 3 patients with a bilateral Lord prosthesis.

Group 2: 23%, including 2 patients with a bilateral Lord prosthesis.
Group 3: 5%.
Group 4: 2%.

When reporting on a prosthesis that is expected to provide many years of problem-free service, but for which only 4 years of follow-up are available, one should avoid being overly optimistic. This period simply is not long enough for a definitive evaluation to be made. However, it may be sufficient to enable certain conclusions to be drawn, and provides some basis for reporting on our experience with the system. Results to date and parallels with other cases give us reason to hope that this prosthesis will fulfill the expectations placed upon it in terms of longevity and long-term compatibility in the human body.

Experience with the Lord Total Hip Replacement: Biomechanics and Clinical Results

H. Seidel

Introduction

Even today, satisfactory long-term results in total hip replacement arthroplasty often remain an elusive goal. The changeover of prosthetic systems that has been taking place in all large hip centers is evidence of the disappointing results obtained with the old-generation prostheses. The surgeon who must decide what type of hip prosthesis to use often finds himself overtaxed or in a conflict of conscience, owing to the widely diverging implant philosophies in many large hip centers.

This is illustrated by the problem of the prosthetic collar, which is viewed quite differently by Mueller, for example, than by Buchholz, Harris or Lord. While Buchholz uses cemented prostheses exclusively, Lord has completely rejected this fixation concept.

We believe that the best information in this area is provided by a critical analysis of operative results.

Review of Total Hip Replacements

In reviewing 187 revision total hip arthroplasties, the author has observed the following:

1. Wear of the cement mantle around the prosthetic stem as a result of alternating bending loads on the prosthesis.
2. Prosthetic fracture as a consequence of cement wear.
3. Prosthetic fracture associated with deficient medial support of the prosthesis.
4. Ceramic wear in the socket and head due to too much verticality of the acetabular component.
5. Subsidence of the femoral prosthesis due to a deficient area of proximal support.

Isolated loosening of the stem was found in 70% of the patients (mean implantation time 5 years).

Biomechanical Studies

To clarify the importance of prosthetic stem support, I performed biomechanical tests using fresh human femurs into which various total endoprostheses had been cemented. Loads were applied to the specimens using a tension-compression apparatus of the type described by Frank. The forces were applied at an angle of 16° to the center of the femoral head. The condyles were rigidly cemented to the base, and the greater trochanter was supported externally.

Prostheses with a broad area of collar support and a short stem, which had additionally been implanted with a restrictor plug (Seidel), were the most stably anchored.

Collarless prostheses sank into the femoral shaft under loading, fracturing the cement mantle or the femur itself.

A Lord total hip prosthesis taken from a patient who had died 8 months postoperatively from pulmonary embolism was tested 2 days postmortem in the same fashion. When the static load was increased, the prostheses sank into the femur. Under a cyclic load of 2000 N, the femur displayed a spring action that was like that of a normal femur without a prosthesis. Under a cyclic load of 3000 N, the femur fractured obliquely at the tip of the prosthesis.

A second femur with a Lord prosthesis was subjected to the same test. Under a cyclic load of 2000 N, the relatively loose basal support remained unchanged. At a load of 4000 N, the prosthesis sank into the shaft until the collar was in flat contact with the femur. After 10 cycles at 10,000 N the bone fractured, again at the tip of the prosthesis.

These experiments indicate that the primary stability of the Lord prosthesis is based upon a "wedging" of the prosthesis within the S-shaped femoral shaft. This primary stability is on the order of 2000–3000 N.

The madreporic surface of the prosthesis does not contribute to primary stability.

Stability increases markedly following the ingrowth of cancellous bone into the prosthesis. The elastic behavior of the femur is hampered, however, by the long, rigid stem of the Lord prosthesis, which creates a site of predilection for fractures at the distal tip of the device.

Clinical Results

I have had clinical experience with 100 Lord total hip prostheses, 85 of which I inserted personally.

The straight Lord stem causes problems during implantation of the prosthesis and during the postoperative period.

The straight stem must be inserted carefully into the medullary cavity. Particular care must be taken to avoid undue stresses between the femoral cortex and prosthesis, since a shaft fracture could result. The trochanteric resection must be relatively deep, and it is important that the posterior femoral neck cortex be adequately resected.

Among our patients, complete or partial fractures of the femur have occurred intraoperatively in two instances.

This can be avoided if an accurate seating for the prosthesis is fashioned during the resection, so that the trochanteric bearing surface is parallel and contiguous to the femoral rasp.

From March, 1979, to December, 1981, I implanted Lord total hip prosthesis in 85 patients. The indications were osteoarthritis, femoral neck fractures, degenerative arthritis secondary to pelvic fractures, migrated endoprostheses, and loose total prostheses.

The average age of the patients was 56. The youngest patient was 18.

In 68 cases I implanted a Lord socket and Lord stem. In the remaining patients the Lord socket or stem was combined with other models.

The excellent biocompatibility of the material was my principal motive for using the Lord prosthesis, which I implanted even in a few selected young patients. Based on the experience of Lord and my own observations, the bone tends to grow around the prosthesis, which contrasts with cemented prostheses in which a broad interfacial layer forms between the cement and bone. I feel that the greatest advantage of cementless fixation is the gain in bone stock compared to cemented prostheses, which invariably lead to some loss of bone substance.

Aside from five failures, all of which were due to massive periarticular ossification, I observed no poor results.

Summary

Biomechanical tests show that the prosthetic collar has an important bearing on the primary stability of the prosthesis. The Lord prosthesis satisfies the requirement of a broad proximal seating through its contact with the cut surface of both the femoral neck and the trochanter. The madreporic surface of the prosthesis enhances secondary stability as a result of cancellous bone ingrowth. Postmortem studies have demonstrated excellent biocompatibility of the metal and madreporic surface with the bone.

The straight stem of the Lord prosthesis alters the elastic behavior of the femur, however, and under heavy loading the femoral bone at the tip of the prosthesis is predisposed to fracture, as clinical and experimental observations confirm.

This disadvantage of the straight stem is offset by the "anti-swing" stem with a madreporic-like surface of the author's own design.

Early Results of Judet Total Hip Replacement Arthroplasty

D. Schöllner and K. H. Elsner

The general interest in the prevention of problems associated with the use of bone cement in total hip replacements, together with the relatively high incidence of loosening of uncemented prostheses, directed our attention toward the uncemented THR of Judet. This shift of attention does not mean that we have entirely abandoned conventional cemented prostheses. We continue to favor cemented THRs for patients over the age of 60. At our hospital, then, the Judet THR is not considered a routine procedure, but is reserved for special indications. We felt that the design of the prosthesis, with its rough surface that creates a mechanical interlock with the bone, was excellently suited for long-term stability and maximum longevity, perhaps for the lifetime of the patient. This remains to be determined. The prime candidates for the Judet THR at our hospital are patients under 60 years of age in whom a hip replacement either is mandatory or is the most attractive of several alternatives. Arthrodesis has never been considered a viable option. We have also used the Judet system in patients over 60 years of age in whom the single or repeated loosening of a cemented prosthesis appeared to contraindicate the further use of cemented components.

In the present paper we shall review the early results of 50 Judet operations performed at our hospital. Follow-ups are available for only 40 of these patients, because 4 failed to keep their follow-up appointments, and 6 others had not yet had their prostheses for 3 months at the time of the review.

The *indications* for the arthroplasties are listed in Table 1. The relatively high prevalence of osteoarthritis secondary to dysplasia and of femoral head necrosis, accounting for nearly ⅓ of all cases, is due to the fact that these conditions occur at a relatively young age and thus fall within the domain of the uncemented Judet THR.

As shown by the *age distribution* in Table 2, only 6 of the patients in the present series were over 60 years of age.

Intraoperative complications arose in a relatively high percentage of cases (Table 3). In the 8 cases of femoral shaft penetration, it is noteworthy that the penetration did not significantly impair the outcome and did not necessitate removal of the endoprosthesis. In all cases adequate stability could be obtained by applying Judet clamps to the shaft and by other adjunctive measures. Poor seating of the collar is actually more of an asthetic problem, because a firm collar seating is not critical for obtaining a firm seating of the endoprosthesis. In one case

Table 1. Indications (n = 50)

Osteoarthritis	22
Osteoarthritis secondary to dysplasia	10
Femoral head necrosis	6
Failed primary arthroplasty	7
Rheumatoid arthritis	2
Fracture or pseudarthrosis	2
Osteoarthritis secondary to protrusio	1

Table 2. Age at operation (n = 50)

21 – 30	2
31 – 40	4
41 – 50	20
51 – 60	18
61 – 70	5
71 – 80	1

Table 3. Intraoperative Complications (n = 50)

Femoral shaft penetration		8
Poor anchorage of acetabular component		6
→ packing with cancellous bone	2	
→ threaded socket	4	
Poor collar seating		4
Dislocation		3
Trochanter avulsion (screw fixation)		2

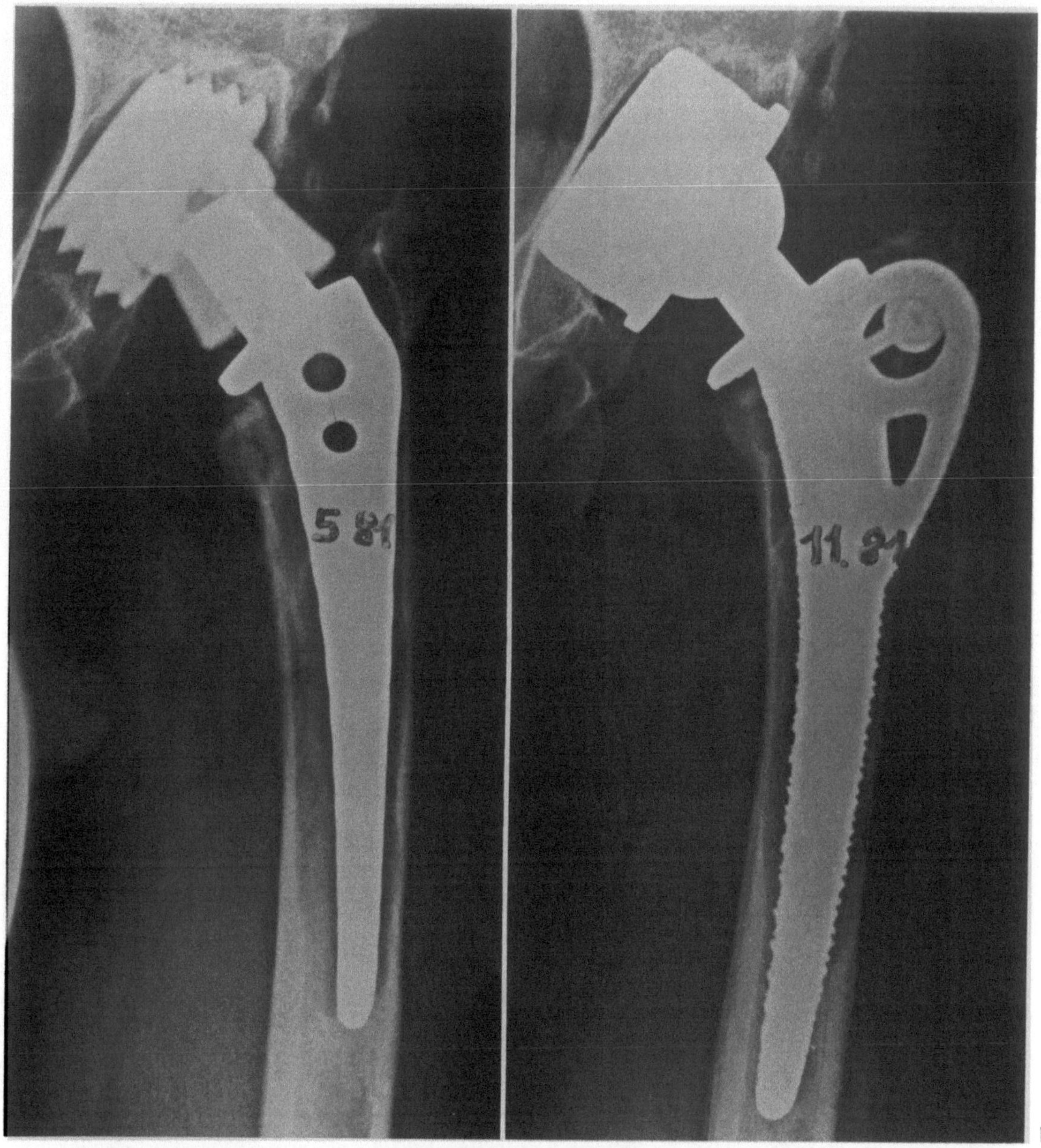

a b

Fig. 1. **a** 21-year-old man with loose, uncemented ceramic endoprosthesis (Autophor stem) in the left hip. **b** After insertion of the Judet THR the hip is free of pain and can bear weight normally

the prosthesis was already impacted so tightly in the femoral shaft when the collar was applied that further insertion of the stem was impossible. Intraoperative dislocation of the prosthetic joint was episodic in character, and the joint showed no tendency to dislocate following wound closure.

The *postoperative complications* included in the present series (Table 4) were those arising between the completion of the operation and the patient's discharge from the hospital. The high incidence of peroneal nerve paresis is undoubtedly due to our preference for the "southern approach," which can easily lead to stretching or contusion of the sciatic nerve. In one case a towel clip for the leg drape was inadvertently clamped to the common peroneal nerve at the head of the fibula.

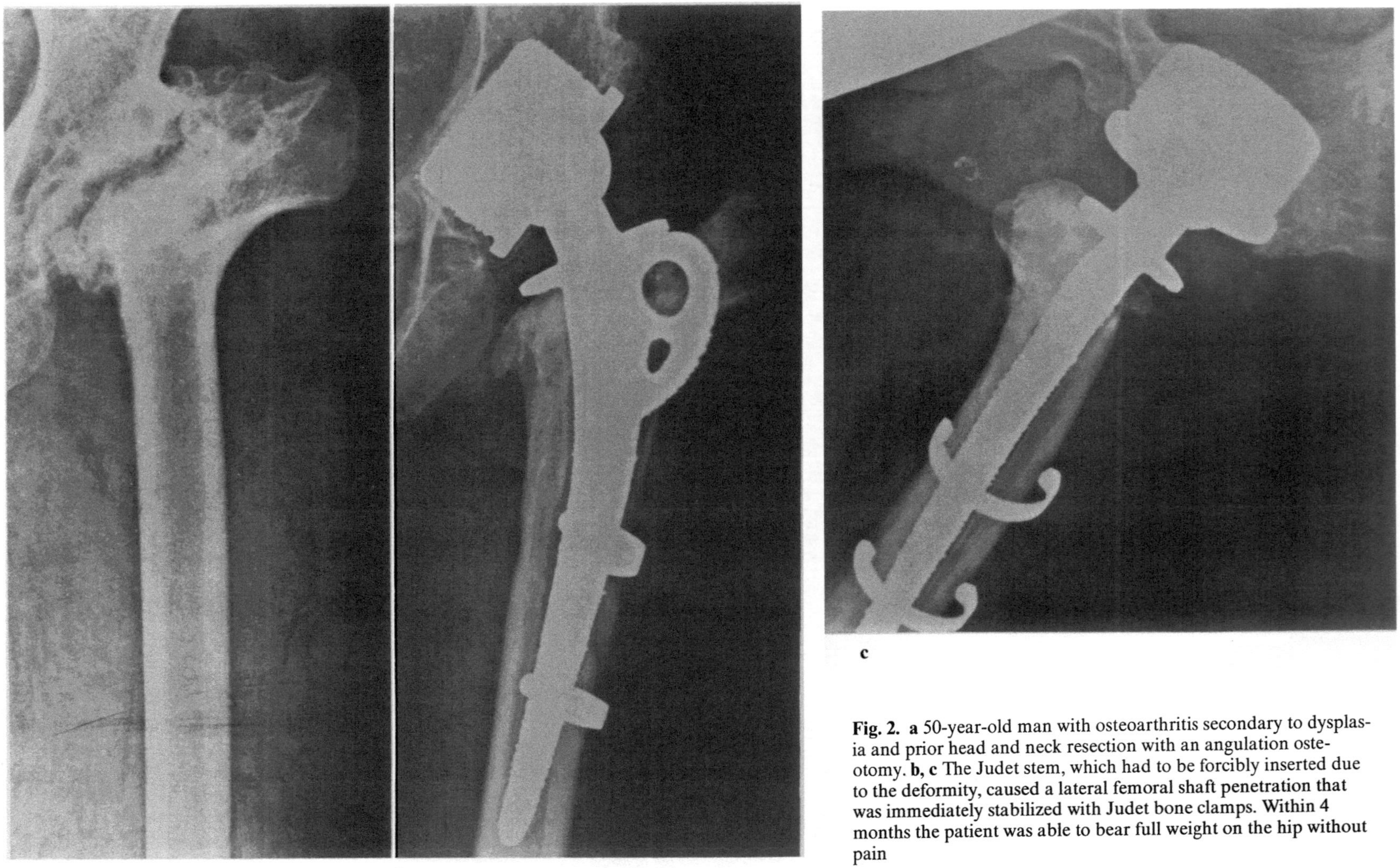

a b c

Fig. 2. **a** 50-year-old man with osteoarthritis secondary to dysplasia and prior head and neck resection with an angulation osteotomy. **b, c** The Judet stem, which had to be forcibly inserted due to the deformity, caused a lateral femoral shaft penetration that was immediately stabilized with Judet bone clamps. Within 4 months the patient was able to bear full weight on the hip without pain

Table 4. Postoperative Complications (n = 50)

Peroneal nerve paresis	4
Fistula following hematoma evacuation	1
Infection → removal	2
Infection, removal and replacement	1
Delayed wound healing	2
Thrombosis (suspected)	2

Table 5. Surgical Approaches (n = 50)

"Southern approach" in lateral recumbency	48
Lateral approach (Watson-Jones) in supine position	2

Table 6. Primary vs. Secondary Operations (n = 50)

Primary operations	36
Secondary operations	14

Table 7. Three-Month Results of Judet THR (n = 40)

Leg lengths:	equal	34
	1/2 cm longer	4
	1/2 cm shorter	2
Mobility:	better	27
	unchanged	7
	worse	6

Table 8. Ratings of Results

Subjective rating by patient:	
excellent	16
good or fair	21
poor	3
Objective rating by physician:	
excellent	19
good or fair	18
poor	3

Our marked preference for the southern approach (Table 5) is based upon the shape of the Judet THR. The ring-shaped trochanteric protrusion on the femoral prosthesis is a formidable obstacle to the conventional Watson-Jones approach without trochanteric osteotomy and is likely to cause trauma to the gluteus medius muscle. Moreover, a solid anchorage in the trochanter is not possible if this structure has been previously detached. Hence, we have followed the recommendation of Hopf that the "southern approach" be used for this type of endoprosthesis.

The high percentage of *secondary operations* (Table 6) is explained by the special range of indications.

The first follow-up were done at 3 months postoperatively. Results are presented only for the 40 cases that were available for follow-up, as stated earlier (Tables 7 and 8). *Leg length* adjustments may be somewhat more difficult with the Judet prosthesis than with cemented prostheses, because occasionally the stem becomes solidly impacted in the femoral shaft before it has been inserted all the way. This accounts for the four cases of leg lengthening. On the other hand, the *reduction of mobility* postoperatively in 6 patients is not specific for the Judet endoprosthesis, but is based upon the peculiar range of indications. Generally, it was our impression that hip mobility following the Judet arthroplasty was very good and painless.

Three cases were given a "poor" rating by both patient and physician. These included the two cases in which the endoprosthesis finally had to be removed, and one refractory case of peroneal nerve paralysis (Table 8).

In summary, we may draw the following conclusions from our early results:

By and large, the Judet THR has met with expectations. The design of the prosthesis makes the implantation technique somewhat more difficult than with other prostheses. This usually means a somewhat longer operating time, although the absence of bone cement saves time in other areas. Postoperative mobility is relatively good. The incidence of intraoperative complications is relatively high at present but presumably will decline as experience is gained and instrumentation is improved.

First Clinical Experience with an Uncemented Modular Femoral Prosthesis System with a Wrought Ti-6Al-4V Stem and an Al_2O_3 Ceramic Head

K. Zweymüller

Introduction

The experience gained with uncemented implants at the Orthopedic Clinic of the University of Vienna dates back to 1972, when ceramic materials were primarily used to bridge bone defects and to replace joints following tumor resections (Salzer 1975, 1976). In the region of the hip joint, a ceramic socket was implanted without the use of acrylic bone cement, and ceramic sockets were also used at that time for arthroplasties in osteoarthritic hips (metal/ceramic composite prostheses) performed partially without bone cement (Zweymüller 1977, 1978). Gradually it became clear that the conventional method of attaching the femoral component by means of bone cement would also have to be replaced eventually by a cementless method. Following the short-term and limited use of a type of femoral prosthesis developed at another institute (Chiari 1977), we decided to initiate the development of a new cementless prosthesis system based on evaluations of our own experience. In the present paper we shall describe the concept of the new femoral prosthesis (Zweymüller, Semlitsch 1981), which has been in clinical use in its original form since October, 1979, and present the clinical results and experience acquired thus far.

Concept of the Modular System and Fixation Principle

The hot-forged femoral straight-stem prosthesis is constructed of a tianium alloy (Ti-6Al-4V Protasul®-64 WF). The conical middle and distal portion of the stem has a three degree taper. The distal portion ends in a rounded tip, while the proximal stem flares in the frontal plane (Fig. 1). The flared proximal portion and the cross-sectional shape of the stem in the middle and distal portion help to absorb torsional forces and thus enhance the primary fixation.

Fixation of the stem is achieved through contact of the prosthesis with the diaphyseal cortex. Given the anatomic features of the proximal femur in the sagittal plane, i.e., the S-shaped curvature resulting from anteversion-anteflexion and antecurvation, all four corners of the stem cross-section can have contact with the cortical bone only in ideal circumstances. As shown in Fig. 2, this cortical contact can be broad at several points, approaching the ideal case and thus ensuring implant stability.

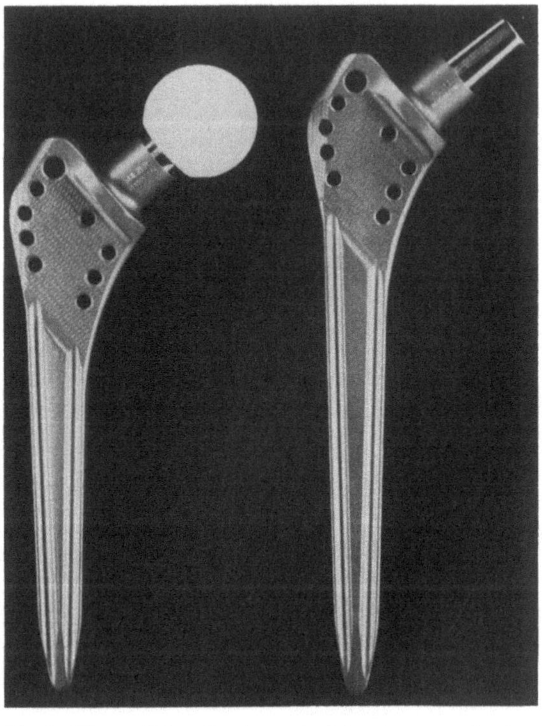

Fig. 1. View of the titanium straight-stem prosthesis from the anterior side with and without the slip-on ceramic head. The small collar is for marking and not for support. Consequently the implant has no contact with the cut surface in the intertrochanteric region

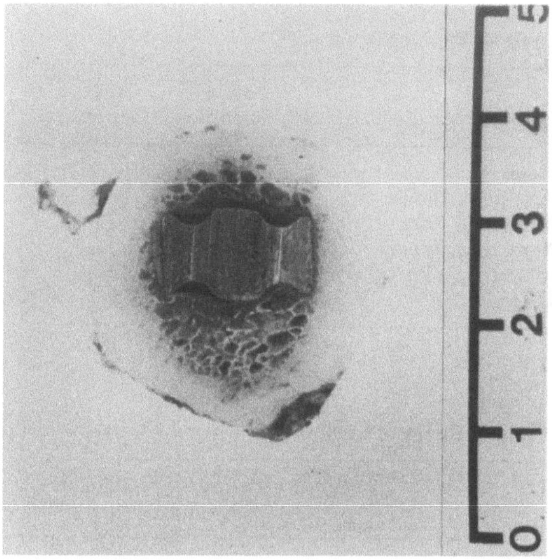

Fig. 2. Sagittal section of the stemmed prosthesis implanted in patient A.A. (cf. Fig. 3). The sides of the implant are in close apposition with the adjacent cortical bone

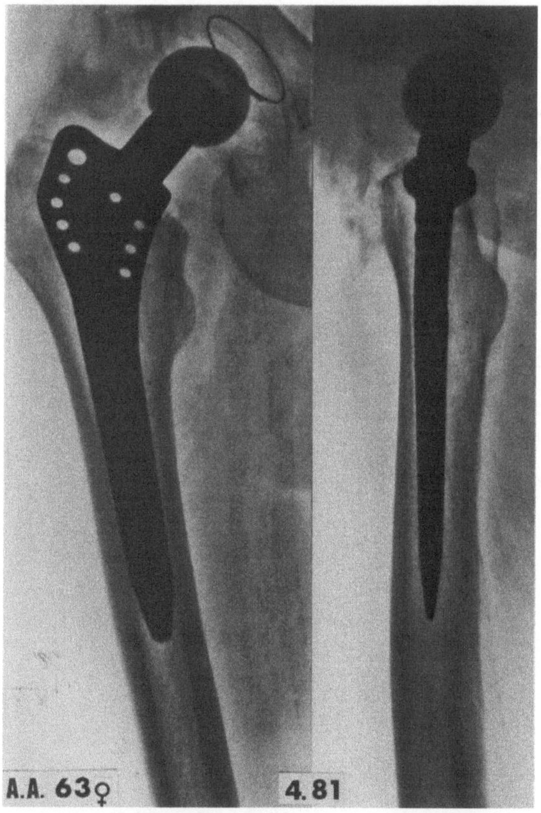

Fig. 3. Radiograph taken three months after operation. The patient A.A. (female), who was able to walk without the aid of a crutch, died of renal failure four months after the operation. The axial radiograph shows the narrow aspect of the prosthesis in relation to the two proximal curvatures of the femur

The shape of the prosthetic stem is dictated by the S-shaped curvature of the femur, for a straight body can be inserted into an S-shaped channel only if it is narrow (Fig. 3).

The prosthetic stem is available in seven different sizes. Experience to date has shown that it is suitable for implantation into femurs of all shapes. For each prosthesis size there is a special surgical rasp for preparing the osseous bed to receive the implant. Three ceramic heads (Al_2O_3 sintered ceramic Biolox) with three different neck sizes are also available. Thus, while the modular prosthesis system consists of only 10 components, 21 variations are possible.

During the operation, the surgeon first implants the acetabular socket and then the stem. He then determines the necessary neck length, selects the appropriate ceramic head and press-fits it onto the conical post atop the femoral stem. The polyethylene, externally-threaded socket designed by Endler (Endler 1982, 1982) has been successfully used for more than two years in conjunction with the ceramic head.

Clinical Experience

291 femoral prostheses of this cementless modular system were implanted from October, 1979, to June, 1982. During this period not a single arthroplasty had to be revised due to loosening, though there was one case of infection requiring removal of the prosthesis. Presented below is an analysis of clinical findings only in those patients who underwent total hip arthroplasty two or more years ago.

Seventeen male and 20 female patients were operated in this series. One of the female patients required a total arthroplasty in both hips. The patients ranged in age from 32 to 70 years, the average age being 54.5 years. The length of follow-up was from 19 to 31 months after surgery, with an average of 24.4 months.

In one case pulmonary embolism occurred in the sixth postoperative week, and the patient died (Table 1). One prosthesis had to be removed because of deep staphylococcal infection. In this case the hip was left as a Girdlestone. The only intraoperative complications were two femoral shaft fractures at the distal tip of the prosthesis. These were attributable to deficiencies of instrumentation. After optimum in-

Table 1. Uncemented Femoral Prostheses (October 1979 – June 1980)

Number of hips: 43	Number of patients: 42
Deaths in the postoperative period:	1
Deaths later:	2
Number of removed prostheses:	1
Follow-up not possible:	1
	38 hips/37 patients

Table 2. Diagnosis

Idiopathic osteoarthritis	20
Femoral head necrosis:	9
Dysplasia:	5
Rheumatoid arthritis:	2
Post-traumatic state:	1
Slipped femoral epiphysis:	1
	38 hips/37 patients

Table 3. Complaints

	Before operation	After operation
None	0	29
Sensitivity to weather conditions, scar pain	/	8
Slight pain on weight-bearing	2	/
Slight, constant pain	/	/
Severe pain on weight-bearing	5	1
Severe, constant pain	31	/

Table 4. Walking Ability

	Before operation	After operation
None	/	/
Around the house	10	/
More than 100 m	10	2
More than 500 m	9	2
More than 1 km	9	12
Unlimited	0	22

Table 5. Range of Motion

	Before operation	After operation
Flexion	73	94
Abduction	7	27
Adduction	8	23
Lateral rotation	10	27
Medial rotation	3	9

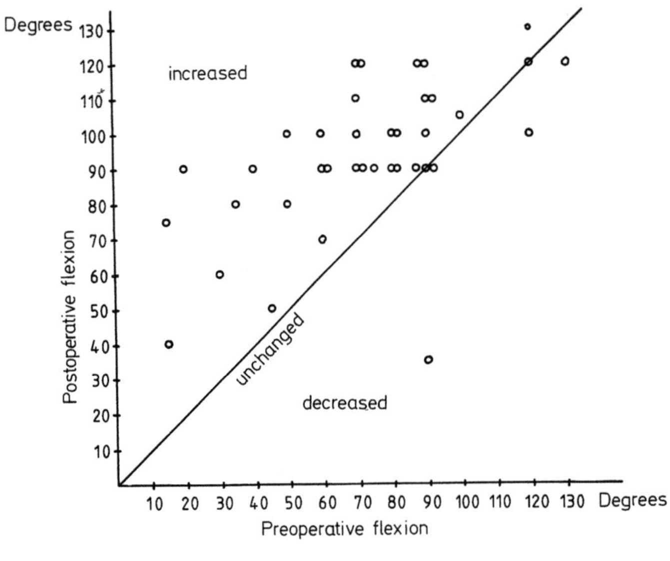

Fig. 4. Preoperative vs. postoperative flexion of the hip joint. Points falling on the 45° diagonal indicate no change. Points plotted above the diagonal indicate an increase in the range of flexion; points below indicate a decrease

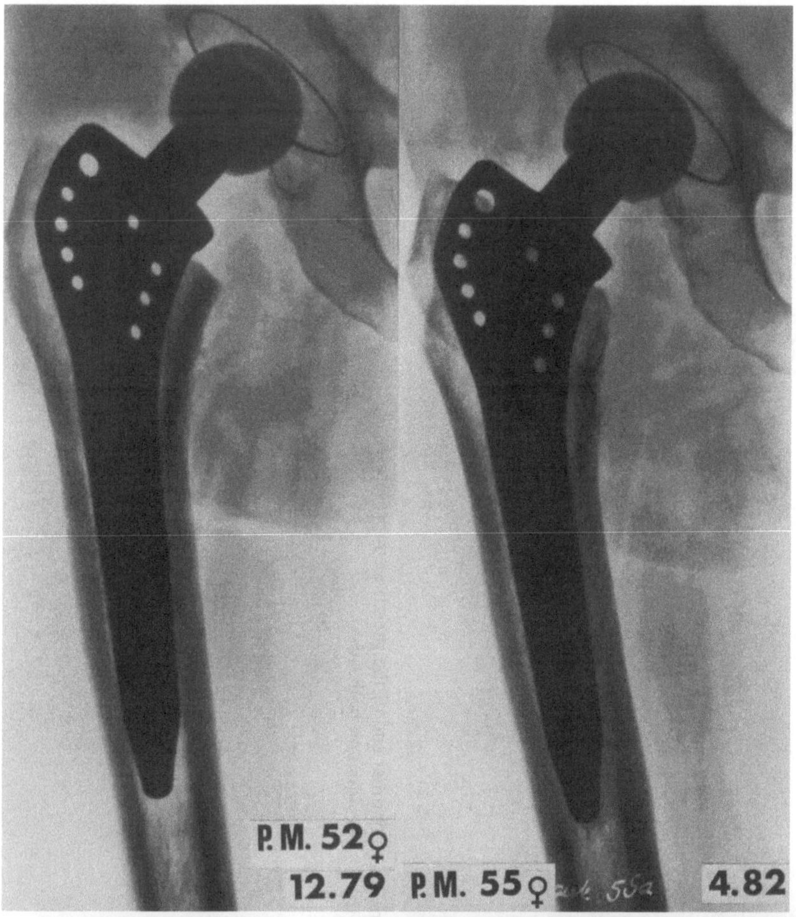

Fig. 5. X-ray follow-up over 2½-year period. There has been slight atrophy and consolidation of the calcar, and there is close apposition between the bone and prosthesis

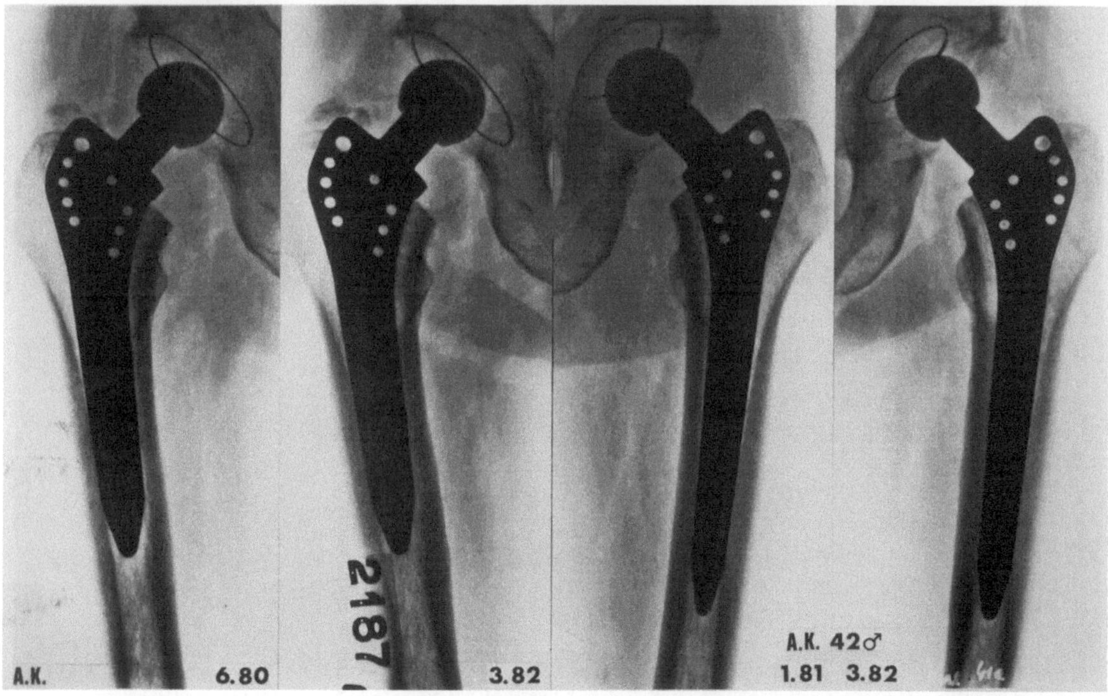

Fig. 6. Two-year result (right hip) in a patient who underwent a bilateral arthroplasty. Cortical thickening above and below the end of the prosthesis is apparent in the right femur

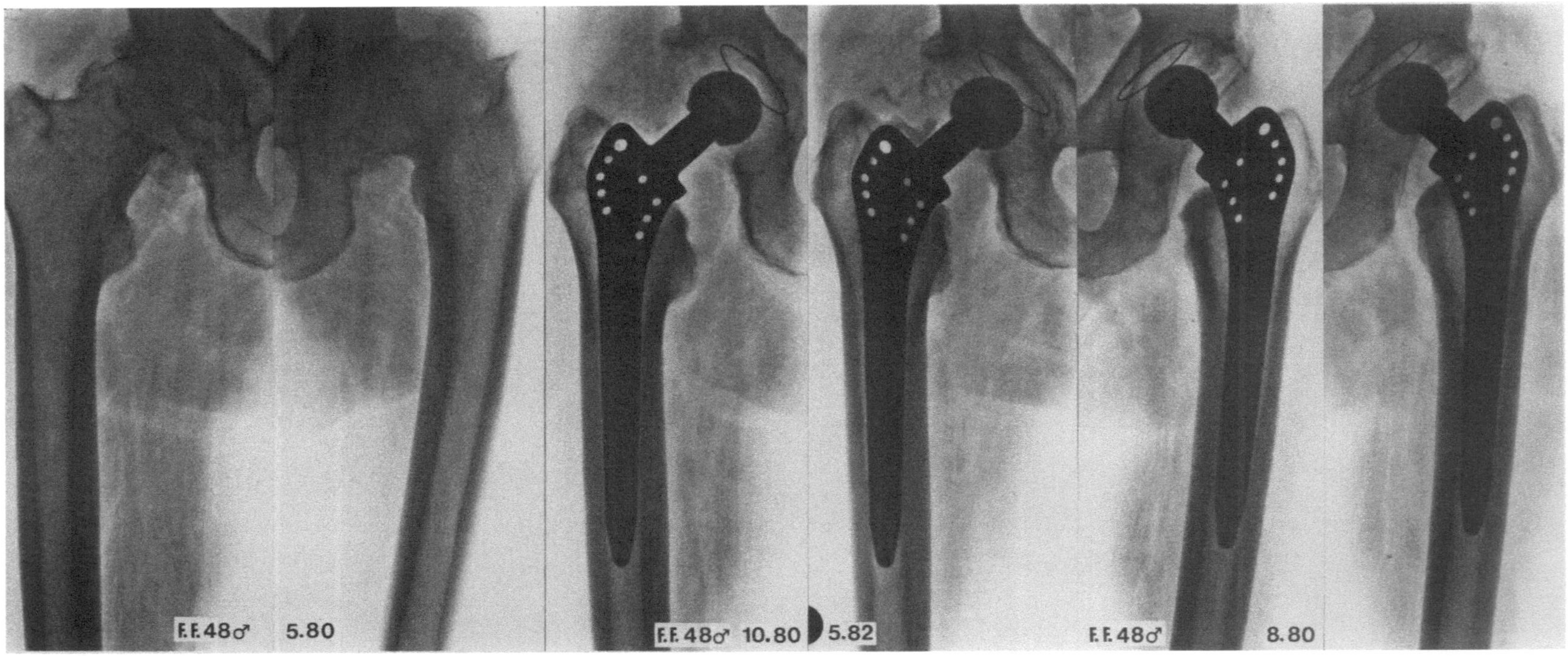

Fig. 7. Two-year result (left) of bilateral arthroplasty for degenerative arthritis secondarly to epiphysiolysis. Slight femur varum. The fine double contours at the proximal end of the prosthesis represent cancellous scars. Adaptation of the calcar is evident on both sides

struments had been developed, no case of shaft fracture occurred during the following 250 operations. The two patients affected were placed in a short Whiteman's plaster for three weeks, and both recovered fully.

The patients' complaints are listed in Table 3. In eight cases there was sensitivity to weather conditions or scar sensitivity. This was attributed to a trochanteric bursitis. One patient complained of severe pain in the operated leg on weight-bearing after a pain-free period of 1½ years. In this case the patient proved to be a malingerer who feigned severe continuous pain in order to fraudulently obtain a welfare allowance (and who subsequently admitted to the deception).

Because of the diaphyseal stem anchorage, most radiographs showed a slight atrophy of the calcar, which became consolidated after about six months. It appears that the cortical bone in proximity to the plane of resection adapts itself to the altered mechanical situation (Fig. 5). In other cases a moderate hypertrophy of the cortical bone may be observed adjacent to the middle and distal portions of the prosthetic stem (Fig. 6). The double contours which are frequently seen adjacent to the proximal part of the stem may be attributed to healing processes within the cancellous bone (Fig. 7). If they were resorption lines, they would be observed over the entire length of the stem.

Summary

This paper deals with a series of 38 uncemented titanium prosthetic stems which were implanted from 2 to 2½ years ago. It presents clinical experience gained with the modular femoral endoprosthesis and explains the principle of the stem fixation method.

References

Chiari K, Zweymüller K, Paltrinieri M et al. (1977) Eine keramische Hüfttotalendoprothese zur zementfreien Implantation. Vorläufige Mitteilung. Arch Orthop Unfallchir 89:305–313

Endler M (1982) Theoretisch-experimentelle Grundlagen und erste klinische Erfahrungen mit einer neuen zementfreien Polyäthylenschraubpfanne beim Hüftgelenkersatz. Acta Chirurgica Austriaca, suppl. 45:1–20

Endler M, Endler F (1982) Erste Erfahrungen mit einer zementfreien Polyäthylenschraubpfanne beim Hüftgelenkersatz. Orthop Prax 18/4:319–323

Salzer M, Locke H, Engelhardt H, Zweymüller K (1975) Keramische Endoprothesen der oberen Extremität. Z Orthop 113:458–468

Salzer M, Zweymüller K, et al. (1976) Further experimental and clinical experience with aluminium oxide endoprostheses. J Biomed Mater Res 10:847–856

Zweymüller K (1978) Knochen- und Gelenkersatz mit biokeramischen Endoprothesen. Facultas, Wien

Zweymüller K, Semlitsch M (1982) Concept and material properties of a cementless hip prosthesis system with Al_2O_3 ceramic balls heads and wrought Ti-6Al-4V stems. Arch Orthop Trauma Surg 100:229–236

Zweymüller K, Zhuber K, Locke H (1977) Eine Metall-Keramik-Verbundprothese für den Hüftgelenkersatz. Wien Klin Wochenschr 89:548–551

Cementless Implantation of a Modified Mueller Straight-Stem Prosthesis

D. Parpan and R. Ganz

The history of hip endoprosthetics began with cementless fixation and later experienced a "golden age" of cement fixation. Today, increasing efforts are being made to dispense with the use of methacrylate and return to the age of the uncemented arthroplasty. These efforts are chiefly motivated by reports of high loosening rates, whose morphologic picture at revision is one of a more or less pronounced resorption of the bone bed.

In recent years a large number of cementless prosthetic systems have been introduced, all claiming to ensure permanent fixation without the use of cement [1–8]. This has prompted us to perform trial implantations of the Mueller straight-stem prosthesis, which is impacted into the medullary cavity without cement. We modified the stem slightly by providing first 4 and later 2 longitudinal slots in its proximal portion. These enable bony bridges to grow across the implant, stabilizing it against rotation. If removal becomes necessary, the bridging bone can be easily drilled out owing to a longitudinal groove that runs along the line of the slots.

Since 1978 we have implanted a total of 45 such prostheses for primary and secondary osteoarthritis of the hip. All the prostheses were implanted without cement, and none of the patients had had prior arthroplasties. The patients were selected on the basis of radiographic criteria, which included a conical taper of the proximal medullary cavity and/or a good fit between the cortex and the stem template. A definitive decision for cementless fixation was made intraoperatively if, after rasping of the canal, an adequately snug fit was obtained on insertion of the selected trial prosthesis.

Of the 20 cases that had been operated more than 1 year previously, 13 could be followed up (Table 1). Of the remaining 7, 1 patient had died, 1 patient had to have his prosthesis removed due to infection, and 5 foreign patients were unavailable for follow-up.

Three patients were free of all subjective symptoms 1, 2 and 4 years after surgery. One patient reported a feeling of instability in the operated hip. Mild, load-dependent pain associated with subjective instability was found in a total of 7 patients after 1, 2, 3 and 4 years. Pain on vibration and rotation was reported by 2 patients after 1 and 2 years (Table 2).

Three signs of prosthetic movement could be seen radiologically (Table 3). A slight subsidence of the stem was witnessed in all patients. Except for 2 cases in which the stem size apparently was too small, allowing a progressive subsidence throughout the observation period, no further distal movement of the prosthesis was noted after the first year of observation.

A bony "pedestal" was seen to form below the tip of the prosthesis in cases where stem subsidence was 2 mm or more, though in one case this was observed 1 year postoperatively after a subsidence of only 1 mm. Pedestal formation was always associated with the 3rd sign – the formation of a discrete radiolucent seam around the proximal third of the stem, visible in lateral films. Only 3 patients showed no evidence of pedestal or seam formation 1–4 years after surgery. All patients with pedestal formation experienced mild complaints. Two patients complained of pain on vibration and rotation (Figs. 1 and 2).

Hip mobility at follow-up was good to nearly normal. It is noteworthy that rehabilitation of the abductor muscles was more difficult and time-consuming than usual.

An analysis of these decidedly preliminary results yields several insights, tendencies and questions. The self-locking fixation of the prosthesis within the medullary cavity is an excellent means of neutralizing bending forces over a long period of time, though only a few, selected patients make good candidates for a cementless arthroplasty with the modified straight-stem prosthesis. The problem of proximal stabili-

Table 1. Prostheses Implanted and Followed up

Years after operation	Number	Followed up	Women/Men
1	7	4	3/4
2	5	4	3/2
3	4	3	2/2
4	4	2	1/3
	20	13	9/11

Absent for follow-up:	5
Girdlestone:	1
Deaths:	1
Average ages:	women, 62 years men, 57½ years

Table 2. Clinical Findings

	1 year	2 years	3 years	4 years
No complaints	1	1	–	1
Feeling of instability	–	–	1	–
Feeling of instability plus pain				
mild	2	2	2	1
severe	–	–	–	–
Pain on vibration and rotation	1	1	–	–

Table 3. Roentgenologic Findings

	1 year (n=4)	2 years (n=4)	3 years (n=3)	4 years (n=2)
Subsidence:				
1 mm	3	1	–	–
2 mm	–	2	–	1
3 mm	–	1	2	1
>3 mm	1	–	1	–
Prox. marginal seam:	2	3	3	2
Pedestal formation:	2	2	3	2
Loosening:	–	–	1	–

zation against rotation is considerably more critical. Anchoring the prosthesis in the cancellous bone does not appear favorable from a biomechanical standpoint, even if, as in younger patients, the quality of the bone is good (Staner and Eulenberger, 1982, personal communication). If loosening occurs, uncemented prostheses lead to less osteolysis than would be the case with cemented devices.

For broader applications, a self-locking straight-stem prosthesis would require additional modifications of the stem, especially in its proximal portion. Further studies are needed to define the place of the cementless fixation of femoral prosthesis and to clarify the advantages and disadvantages of stress transfer across a "rigid interlock" as compared to a "softer" mode of attachment.

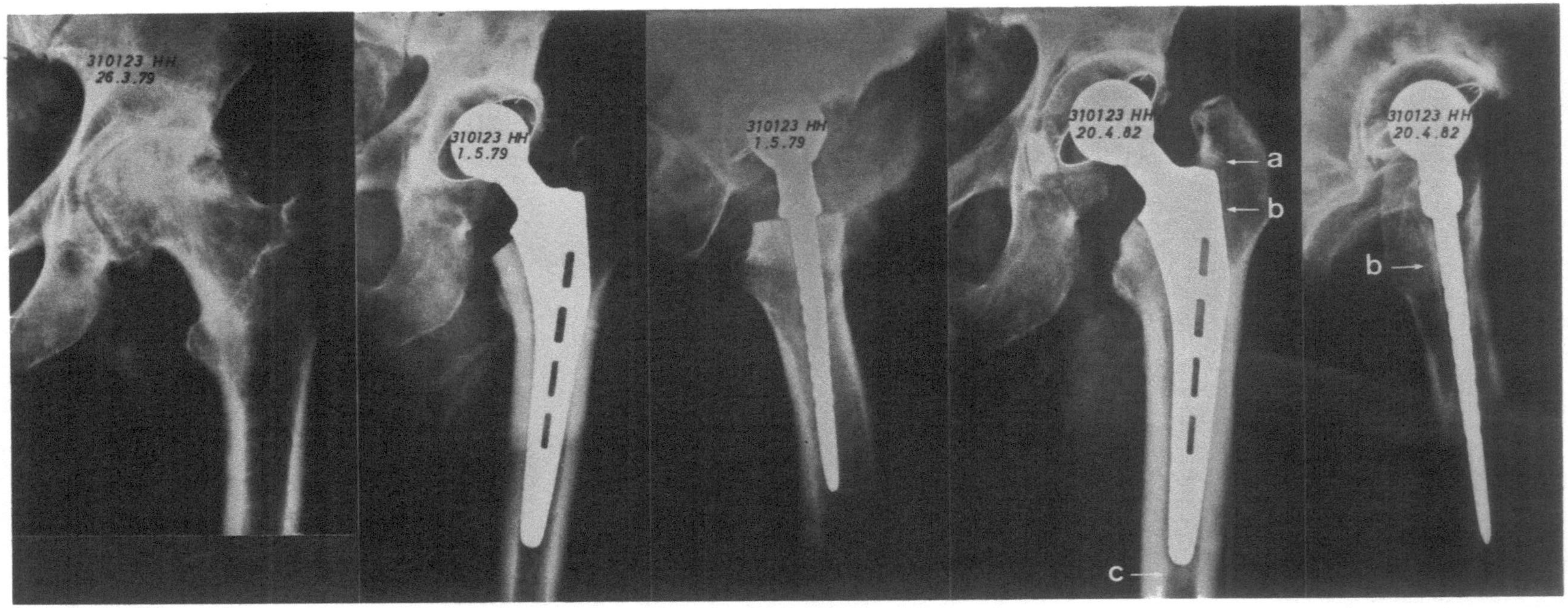

Fig. 1a–e. **a** 59-year-old man (H.H.) with femoral head necrosis of the left hip. **b, c** Total hip replacement inserted on 5-1-79, femoral component not cemented. **d, e** 3 years later the femoral component shows a 5-mm subsidence (1), marked peripheral seam formation is evident in the apical and axial views (2), and distal pedestal formation is pronounced (3)

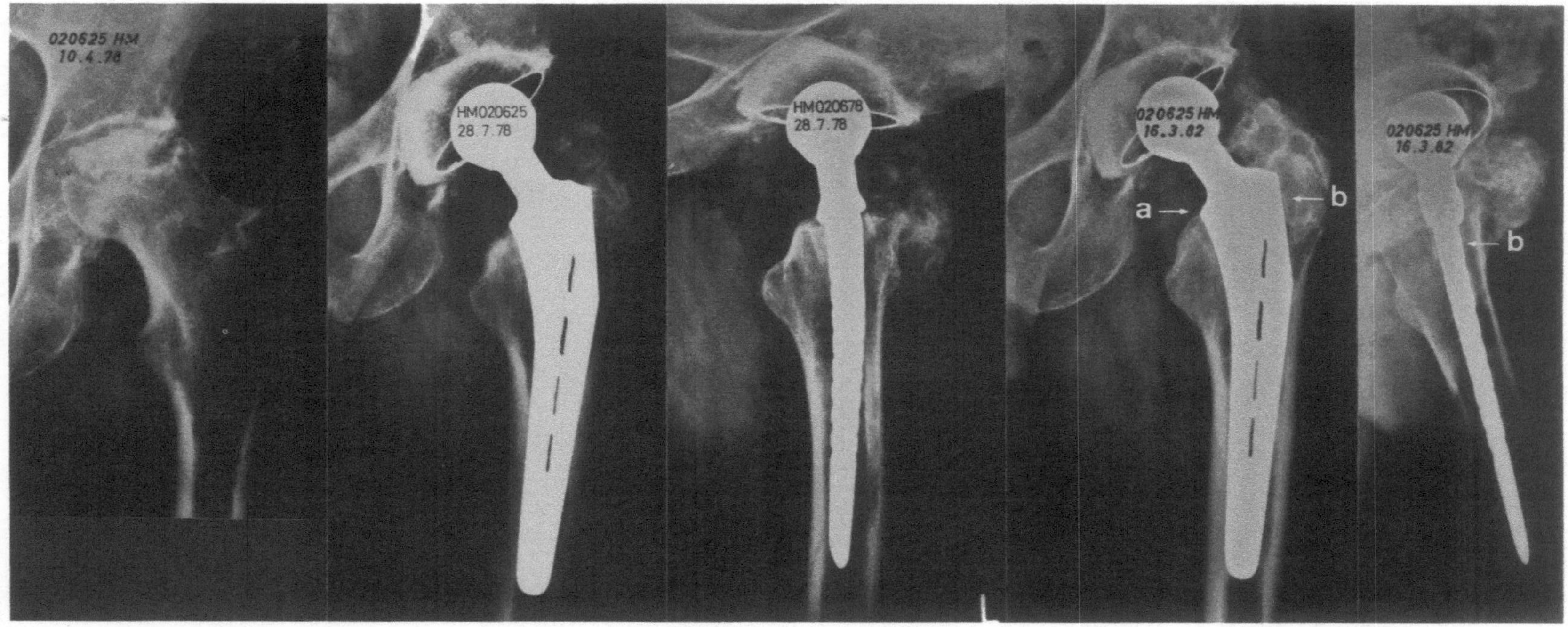

a b c d e

Fig. 2a–e. **a** 57-year-old man (H.M.) with femoral head necrosis of the left hip secondary to psoriasis. **b, c** Total hip replacement inserted on 4-11-78, femoral component not cemented; anterior periarticular calcification is apparent after 3½ months. **d, e** 4 years postoperatively the femoral component shows a subsidence of 2 mm (*a*), and a proximal marginal seam is visible in the a.p. and axial films (*b*)

References

1. Jentschura G (1979) 4jährige klinische Erfahrung mit teilweise zementfrei implantierten Keramik-Endoprothesen. Z Orthop 117:482–484
2. Judet R (1979) Derzeitiger Stand der zementfreien Verankerung. Zementfreie Verankerung von Hüftendoprothesen. Z Orthop 117:476–477
3. Lord GA, Hardy JR, Kummer FJ (1979) An uncemented total hip replacement. Experimental study and review of 300 madreporique arthroplasties. Clin Orthop 141:2–16
4. Mittelmeier H (1979) Keramik-Tragrippen-Prothesen ohne Zement. Langenbecks Arch Chir 349:315–319
5. Morscher E, Bombelli R, Mathys R (1981) The treatment of femoral neck fractures with an isoelastic endoprosthesis implanted without bone cement. Arch Orthop Traumatol Surg 98:93–100
6. Motta A, Callea C, Roncaglia L (1979) Sulle arthroprotesi senza cemento nella coxarthrosi. Giorn Ital Orthop 5:71–78
7. Ring PA (1978) Five to fourteen year interim results of uncemented total hip arthroplasty. Clin Orthop 137:87–95
8. Zweymüller K, Semlitsch M (1981) Konzept und Materialeigenschaften einer zementfreien Hüftendoprothese mit Al_2O_3-Keramikkugel und Ti-6 Al-4V Schmiedeschaft.

Radiologic and Clinical Follow-Ups of Uncemented Femoral Endoprostheses with and without Collars

M. Salzer, K. Knahr and P. Frank

Among the unsolved problems of hip replacement arthroplasty is the question of how to anchor a prosthetic stem permanently in the femoral shaft. Because the traditional fixation of endoprostheses with bone cement is associated with a high incidence of loosening [2, 6, 7], increased attention has been focused on means of anchoring femoral endoprostheses permanently without the use of cement [3, 4, 5, 8, 9]. In the present paper we shall describe our own attempts to develop a new design for an uncemented stem endoprosthesis.

Material (Table 1)

The Weller Long-Stem Prosthesis (Fig. 1 a)

At the General Orthopedic Department in Vienna-Gersthof, the use of uncemented total hip prostheses was begun in 1976. Because the prosthetic stems designed specifically for cement-free implantation were still in the early testing stage at that time, the first model to be implanted without cement was the traditional Weller long-stem prosthesis. The candidates were patients in whom a mechanically-stable primary fixation could be achieved, the principal criterion being a narrow medullary cavity. A total of 57 such prostheses were inserted without cement. Since then, 10 of the patients have died, and the remaining 47 have been closely followed. These consisted of 33 women and 14 men ranging in age from 52 to 80. The average age at operation was 68.6 years.

Modified Stem Prosthesis with a Collar (Fig. 1 b)

Stems with larger diameters were introduced so that uncemented arthroplasties could also be done in patients with wide medullary cavities. Initially only the stem diameter was increased, but shortly thereafter a lateral wing was added to enhance rotational stability. Eighty-seven prosthetic stems of both variants were implanted. Since that time four patients have died, and one patient with bilateral arthroplasties traveled abroad shortly after the operation. Thus, a total of 81 hip joints were available for follow-up. The patients consisted of 59 women and 22 men between 31 and 77 years of age; average age at operation was 59.3.

Table 1. Femoral Endoprostheses Implanted Without Cement (n = 193) (Gen. Orth. Dept. Vienna-Gersthof, June 1976–September 1980)

Type of prosthesis	Operations	Deaths	Lost to follow-up	Followed	Age	Female	Male
Weller	57	10	0	47	68.6 (52 – 80)	33	14
Modified stem with collar	87	4	2	81	59.3 (31 – 77)	59	22
Modified stem without collar	49	2	0	47	59.6 (33 – 75)	28	19
Total	193	15	2	175	61.9 (31 – 80)	120	55

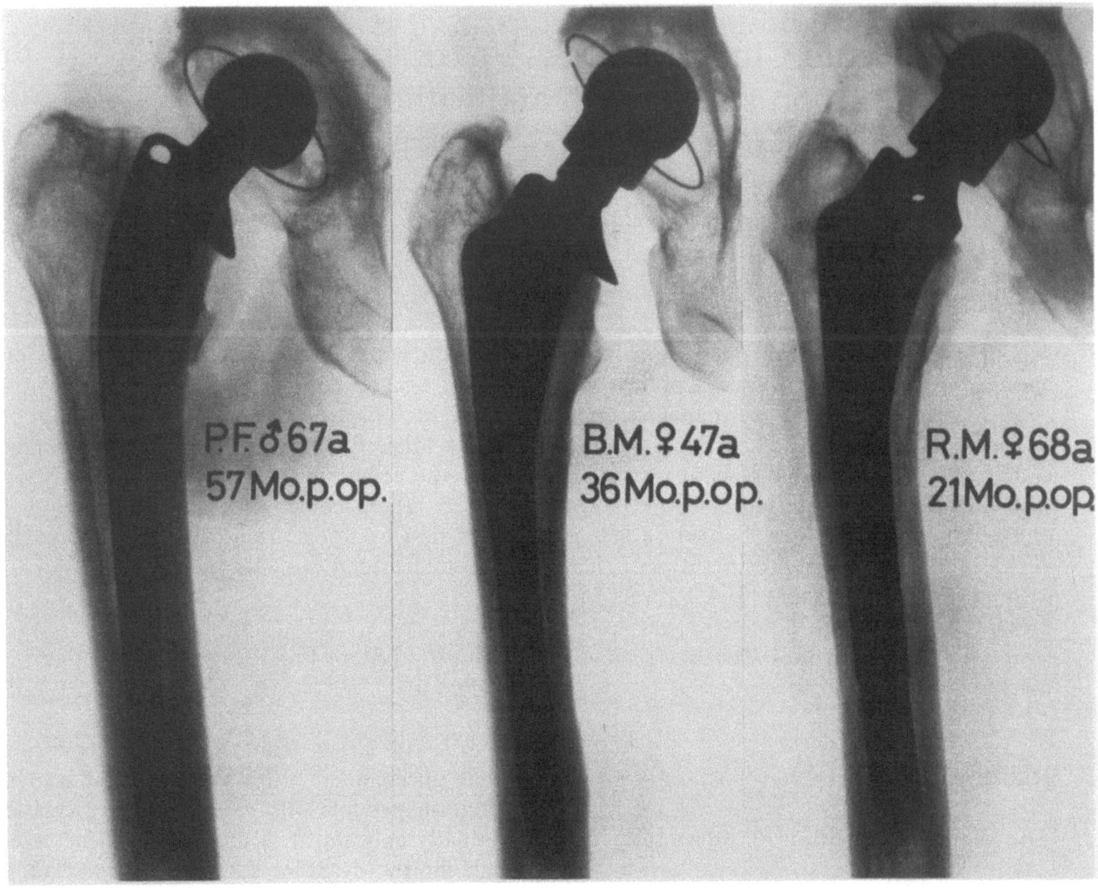

a **b** **c**

Fig. 1. a Uncemented Weller long-stem prosthesis. **b** Modified stem prosthesis with collar. **c** Modified stem prosthesis without collar

Modified Stem Prosthesis without a Collar (Fig. 1c)

The third type of stem is distinguished by the absence of a collar. Omission of the collar was prompted by radiologic follow-ups which showed that collars often prevented the implant from settling into the femoral canal and becoming stably impacted there. Forty-nine of these collarless prostheses, which consist of a stem and removable head with a variable neck length, had been implanted by September of 1980. Since then 2 patients have died, and the remaining 47 (28 women, 19 men) have been closely followed. The age at operation was between 33 and 75 (average 59.8).

The present review covers a total of 175 uncemented stem endoprostheses. The patients, consisting of 120 women and 55 men, were followed for a minimum of 18 months. The age at operation ranged from 31 to 80, with an average of 61.9.

Results (Table 2)

The clinical results were evaluated using the Harris 100-point scale, with a score of 100 representing an optimum result [1].

For the 47 Weller endoprostheses, the average length of follow-up was 58 months. The results were rated excellent (higher than 90 points) to good (80–89 points) in 62% of the patients, fair (70–79 points) in 17%, and poor (less than 70 points) in 21%.

For the 81 patients with a modified stem with collar, average follow-up was 36.9 months.

The result was excellent to good in 61%, fair in 16% and poor in 23%.

Average follow-up for the 47 collarless stems was 22.0 months and showed an excellent to good result in 64% of cases, a fair result in 17%, and a poor result in 19%.

Complications

The most frequent intraoperative complication associated with the prosthesis itself was fracture of the femoral shaft. The incidence of this complication was relatively low with the Weller prostheses (3.5%) but quite high with the modified stems with collars (17.2%). In these cases the attempt to achieve a snug fit between bone and stem led to a fissure fracture of the shaft. Most of these fractures were invisible on radiographs, and all could be easily stabilized with cerclage wires. Extensive shaft fractures occurred in only three patients. There were three instances of postoperative dislocation, and all could be stably and permanently reduced. Two cases of peroneal nerve paresis have improved somewhat with passage of time, and one case of femoral nerve paralysis proved refractory to treatment. A fatal pulmonary embolism developed in one patient (Table 3).

A complication having considerable bearing on the functional outcome is periarticular ossification. Using the scheme of Arcq, this complication was classified into three degrees of severity. Third-degree ossification, which causes

Table. 2. Clinical Results (Harris Evaluation) of Uncemented Femoral Endoprostheses (Min. Length of Follow-Up 18 Months)

Type of prosthesis	Number	Average length of follow-up in months	Excellent or good (in %)	Fair (in %)	Poor (in %)
Weller	47	58.0 (48 – 68)	62	17	21
Modified stem with collar	81	36.9 (26 – 50)	61	16	23
Modified stem without collar	47	22.0 (18 – 26)	64	17	19
Total	175	38.5 (18 – 68)	62	17	21

Table 3. Complications of Uncemented Femoral Endoprostheses (n = 193)

Type of prosthesis	Intraoperative	Postoperative		
	Femoral shaft fracture	Dislocation	Paresis	Pulmonary embolism
Weller	2 (3.5%)	0	2	1 (fatal)
Modified stem with collar	15 (17.2%)	3	1	3
Modified stem without collar	4 (8.1%)	0	0	2
Total	21 (10.8%)	3	3	6

Table 4. Periarticular Ossification with Uncemented Femoral Endoprostheses (n = 175)

Type	1st degree (in %)	2nd degree (in %)	3rd degree (in %)
Weller	17.0	2.1	0
Modified stem with collar	13.6	8.6	6.1
Modified stem without collar	38.2	8.5	4.2
Total	21.1	6.8	4.0

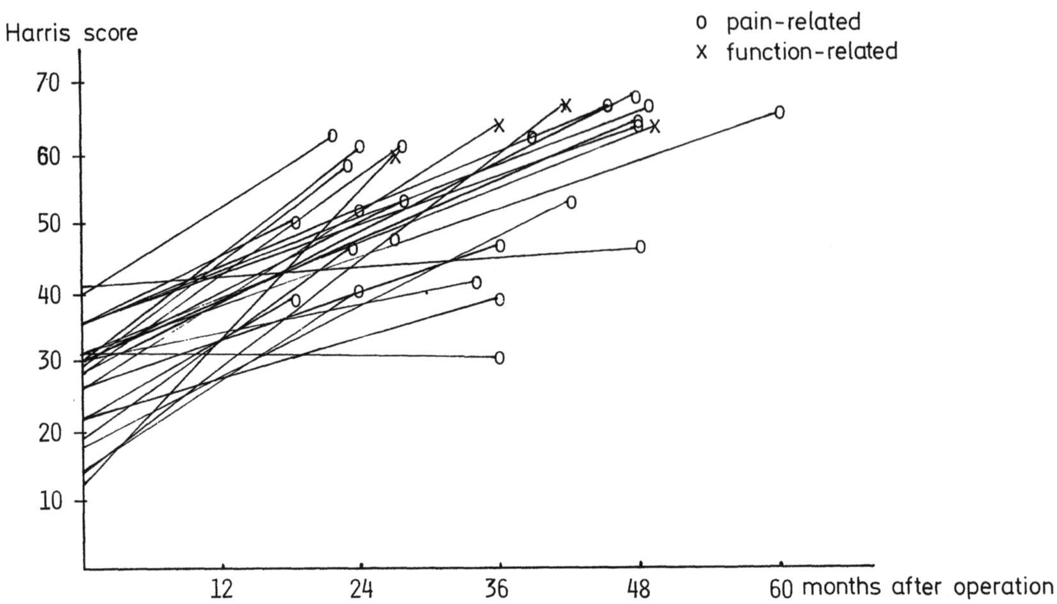

Fig. 2. Clinical analysis of poor results according to the Harris scale. Change in point score relative to preoperative values: O = pain-related, X = function-related

gross restriction of motion, occurred in 4% of cases. This corresponds roughly to the incidence reported in the literature (Table 4).

Analysis of the Poor Clinical Results

According to the Harris evaluation scale, a clinical result is poor if given a score below 70 points. In 24 patients the cause of the poor rating was pain in the operated hip. In 4 patients it was restriction of hip motion. In 10 patients it was loosening that necessitated reoperation (Table 5). However, comparing the clinical result in the "poor" cases with the preoperative status of the hips, we find that nearly all of the patients were better off after surgery than before (Fig. 2). This was not the case, of course, in the patients that required reoperation.

In all 10 reoperated hips, clinical evidence of loosening appeared within a year after the primary operation. Even at the first routine follow-up 3 months postoperatively, the patients complained of discomfort. A typical clinical symptom of loosening appears to be pain on weight-bearing as well as pain on medial rotation of the limb.

Radiologic Follow-Up

Follow-up radiographs were taken in order to document position changes in the form of varus or valgus angulation, subsidence of the stem in

Table 5. Analysis of Poor Clinical Results (< 70 Harris Points)

Type of prosthesis	Number	Poor result due to pain	Poor result due to restr. motion	Revision
Weller	10	5	1	4
Modified stem with collar	19	11	3	5
Modified stem without collar	9	8	0	1
Total	38	24	4	10

the femoral shaft, the cortical reaction to the distal end of the prosthesis ("pedestal" formation within the medullary cavity), and the remodeling of the cortex around the stem (Fig. 2).

Varus angulation was seen most frequently in the prostheses with collars. This was especially common with the Weller prostheses (85%), but the modified, thicker stem also showed a marked tendency toward varus angulation in 26% of cases. Varus angulation was rare with the collarless prostheses, but 24% of the stems showed some degree of valgus deviation. Both forms of deviation are a mechanism for achieving a definitive, stable position of the prosthesis within the femoral shaft (Table 6).

Subsidence of the prosthetic stem was apparent in about ¼ of the Weller prostheses. This occurred when the medullary cavity was too wide relative to the stem, allowing the prosthesis to settle despite the presence of a collar. Half of the collarless stem prostheses showed a subsidence of up to 5 mm – a process that is entirely desirable. Subsidence in excess of 5 mm was seen in only 2 of the operated hips. When subsidence occurred, it became apparent a short time after the operation and seldom progressed further with passage of time. The greatest amount of subsidence was 1 cm (Table 7).

Another typical radiologic change in the femoral shaft is an appositional growth of the cortex about the distal part of the prosthesis in response to increased varus or valgus loading. Like subsidence of the stem, this reaction showed little if any progression with time. Bone-forming processes of this type may well account for the femoral pain that was frequently reported by the patients.

With all types of prosthesis, the appearance of a bony pedestal at the distal end of the prostheses was a very common finding. While this pedestal does assist in supporting the prosthesis, it is not essential to a stable anchorage.

Another phenomenon, seen mainly in the modified stem prostheses with collars, was a porosity increase in the cortical bone of the femoral shaft. This was interpreted as a disuse atro-

Table 6. Radiologic Follow-Up of Uncemented Femoral Endoprostheses

Type of prosthesis	Varus angulation		Valgus angulation	
	Slight	Marked	Slight	Marked
Weller	50	35	0	0
Modified stem with collar	20	6	5	1
Modified stem without collar	4	0	20	4

Table 7. Subsidence of Prosthetic Stems

Type of prosthesis	≦5 mm (in %)	>5 mm (in %)
Weller	24	2
Modified stem with collar	6	0
Modified stem without collar	50	4

Table 8. Radiologic Follow-Up of Uncemented Femoral Endoprostheses

Type of prosthesis	Cortical reaction		"Pedestal" formation		Increase of bone porosity (in %)
	Slight (in %)	Marked (in %)	Slight (in %)	Marked (in %)	
Weller	22	17	26	70	46
Modified stem with collar	21	8	40	51	64
Modified stem without collar	13	7	37	48	46

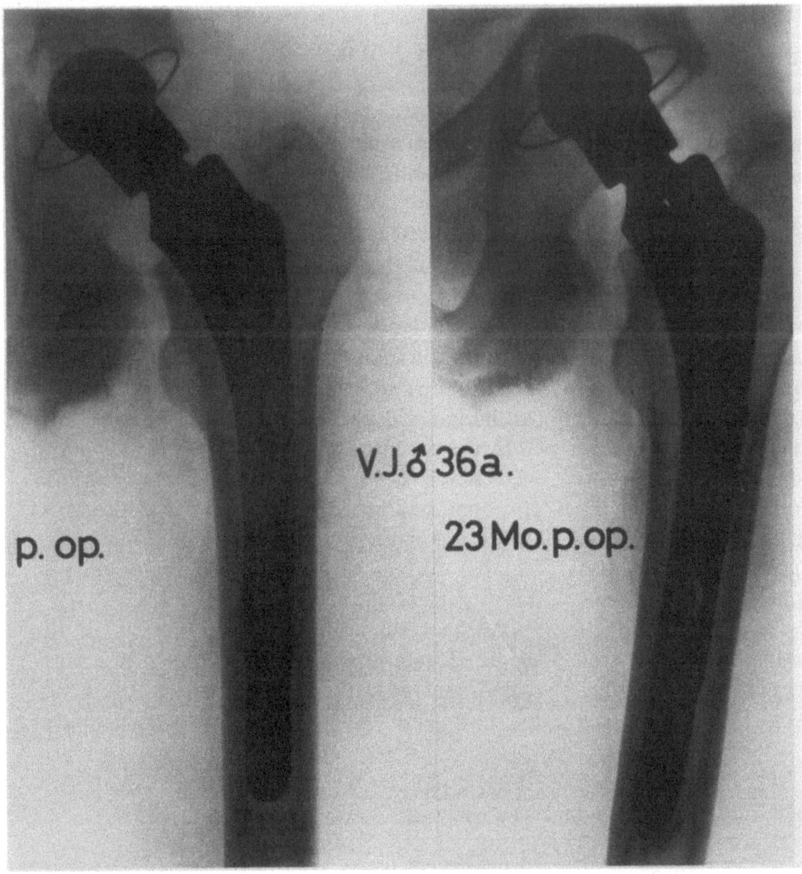

a b

Fig. 3a, b. 36-year-old man with total left-hip replacement for Bekhterev's disease. The 23-month film shows settling of the stem with valgus deviation, an increase in cortical bone porosity, and distal pedestal formation in medullary cavity

phy resulting from the restriction of stress transfer to the calcar area and the tip of the prosthesis (Table 8).

Discussion

In contrast to cemented endoprostheses, our uncemented stems have shown a relatively high incidence of early loosening. This appears to be a function of design, however, for the collarless prostheses were less apt to loosen than the Weller prostheses. This demonstrates the great importance of design improvement in the development of stable stem implants.

While revisional operations for loose cemented endoprostheses usually show extensive destruction of the bone bed caused by wear debris from the bone cement, uncemented endoprostheses are usually found to be separated from the bone by a connective-tissue buffer that has no injurious effects on the surrounding bone. Hence, the cementless technique would appear to be more favorable from a biologic standpoint, and it would be reasonable to assume that the high incidence of late loosening of cemented prostheses could be reduced by cement-free implantation. However, because it would take 10–15 years to prove such an assertion scientifically, one should still be extremely cautious when weighing the indications for a total hip replacement in younger individuals.

References

1. Harris WH (1969) Traumatic arthritis of the hip after dislocation and acetabular fractures: Treatment by mold arthroplasty. J Bone Joint Surg [Am] 51:737–755
2. Huggler AH, Schreiber A (1978) Alloarthroplastik des Hüftgelenkes. Thieme, Stuttgart
3. Judet R, Siguier M, Brumpt B, Judet T (1978) A noncemented total hip prosthesis. Clin Orthop 137:76–84

4. Knahr K, Salzer M (1980) Zweijahresresultate bei zementfrei implantierten Hüftendoprothesen. Med Orthop Techn 100:44–48
5. Lord GA, Hardy JR, Kummer FD (1979) An uncemented total hip replacement: Experimental study and review of 300 madreporique arthroplasties. Clin Orthop 141:2–16
6. Maier S, Griss P, Rahmfeld T, Dinkelacker T (1977) Nachuntersuchungsergebnisse der totalen Alloarthroplastik der Hüfte unter besonderer Berücksichtigung der Spätkomplikationen 4 bis 7 Jahre post operationem. Z Orthop 115:274–283
7. McBeath AA, Foltz NR (1979) Femoral component loosening after total hip arthroplasty. Clin Orthop 141:66–70
8. Mittelmeier H, Harms J (1979) Derzeitiger Stand der zementfreien Verankerung von Keramik-Metall-Verbundprothesen. Z Orthop 117:478–481
9. Morscher E, Bombelli R, Schenk R, Mathys R (1981) The treatment of femoral neck fractures with an isoelastic endoprosthesis implanted without bone cement. Arch Orthop Trauma Surg 98:93–100

Fiber Titanium: Animal Studies and Clinical Trials

A. Gächter and J. Galante

Introduction

Since 1968, Galante and Rostoker have been using a meshwork of sintered titanium fibers for bone replacement and for the cementless attachment of implants to bone. The material has undergone a lengthy series of mechanical and biomechanical tests. Animal studies have been conducted in rabbits, dogs and baboons, and 10-year implants are currently being evaluated in the baboons. "Fiber titanium" has also been in use since 1976 for bone replacement in tumor patients. Following thorough evaluation of the experimental results, a total hip prosthesis was developed which featured a fiber titanium coating. At this writing, uncemented total hip and knee prostheses have been used in human patients for more than 15 months. The first clinical results are now available.

For production of the fiber titanium, the titanium, wires are first kinked, cut into short lengths, and then pressed into the desired shape. The pressed wires are sintered together in a vacuum annealing furnace at over 1000 °C. This produces a stable meshwork with an interconnecting pore size of 200–300 μ that is not unlike the trabecular structure of bone. The elasticity of the sintered body can be controlled by varying the sintering temperature. Fiber titanium is intended as a surface coating for uncemented implants, providing a network of interconnecting pores that are receptive to bone ingrowth. Titanium is well known for its excellent compatibility with tissues. Because the surface area available for bone contact is very large in porous bodies (about 5 times larger than in smooth bodies), it is essential that the material used be as nontoxic as possible. The excellent biocompatibility of titanium makes it decidedly superior to vitallium, for example, which contains relatively toxic substances such as cobalt, chromium and molybdenum.

The compatibility studies, in which the release of various substances (including titanium) into the tissues was investigated, were followed by various experiments to determine the optimum pore size. It was found that the rate of bone ingrowth was best with a pore size of 200–300 μ. Segmental bone replacement operations with fiber titanium implants were performed in more than 150 long bones of adult baboons. As a supplement to many previous publications [1–9], we shall present a yet-unpublished series of experiments designed to explore the possibilities of fiber titanium bone replacement.

Method

At operation, a segment was excised from the femur, tibia or humerus of the baboon and replaced with a fiber titanium cylinder (see Fig. 1). The replacement segment was stabilized by means of a central intramedullary rod. Fixation was provided by two flanges at each end of the replacement segment, which were fitted into corresponding notches in the proximal and distal cortices of the remaining bone. To achieve optimum stability, a semitubular titanium plate was then attached to both cortices, using the compression device of the ASIF (Association for the Study of Internal Fixation). This enabled postoperative care to be administered without the need for plaster or other external fixation. The animals were placed in large cages so that they could ambulate with little restriction.

A total of 22 segmental bone replacements were performed in 10 femora, 8 tibiae and 4 humeri. One baboon received 3 different implants, and the others received 1 implant each. The length of the replacement segment was 5 cm for the humerus, 6.3 cm for the tibia, and 7.6 cm for the femur. The segments for the tibia

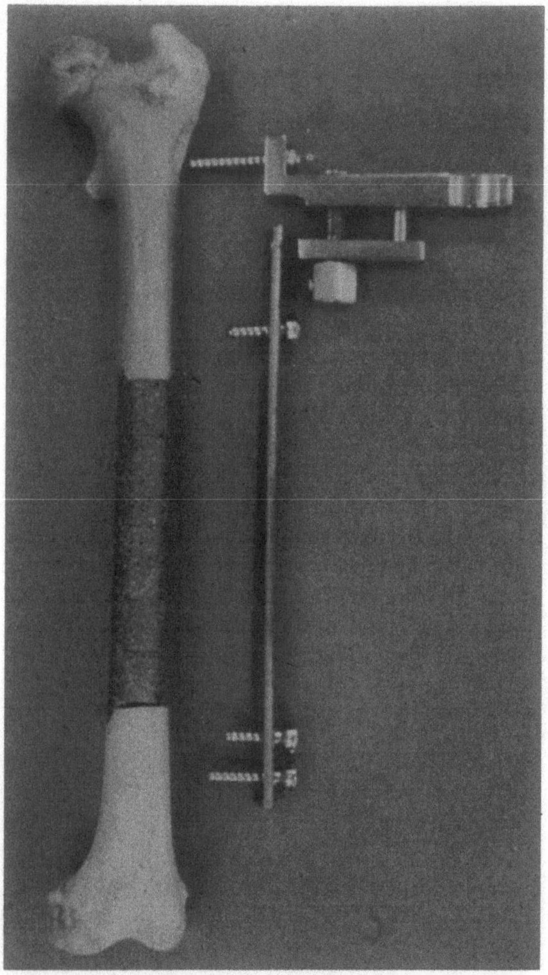

Fig. 1. Arrangement for segmental bone replacement with fiber titanium. The implant is stabilized by a titanium plate applied under compression (using ASIF instruments)

and femur had a circular cross-section, while the humeral segments had a triangular cross-section. Each segment consisted of a Ti6% Al4% V cylinder onto which the fiber titanium was sintered. To improve rotational stability, two flanges were placed on each end of the cylinder to be fitted into the remaining cortices. An intramedullary rod, also with a fiber titanium coating, was inserted for additional stability. Temporary fixation was provided by a semitubular plate attached with four steel screws from the small-fragment set of the ASIF. The bone segment was resected subperiosteally (s.p.) in 6 femora and extraperiosteally (e.p.) in 4 femora, 8 tibiae and 4 humeri. In 7 of the e.p. resections, no bone grafts were used. In the remaining 9, autologous grafts from the resected bone segment were applied. The grafts were grouped around the prosthetic segment and were also placed at the junction between the segment and bone. The compression instruments of the ASIF were additionally used in 6 cases. Standard sterile technique and antibiotic prophylaxis were employed for the implantation. The femoral segments were implanted through a lateral approach, and the tibial and humeral segments through an anterior approach. No external fixation was used, and the baboons were free to move about in their relatively large cages. The animals were killed between 4 and 32 months following implantation. The implants were tested manually for stability. The entire bone and surrounding soft tissues, as well as all internal organs, were removed for histologic study. In addition, a contact radiograph was made of each implant. The specimens were embedded in PMMA and sectioned (< 50 microns). Besides the 5–10 horizontal sections, one vertical section was obtained through the interfacial zone between the titanium, cylinder and bone. The following point system was used:

0 = pseudarthrosis,
1 = less than 0.5 cm bone ingrowth into implant,
2 = bone ingrowth of 0.5 cm or more.

Bone ingrowth into the coated intramedullary rods was evaluated separately:

0 = no ingrowth,
1 = ingrowth limited to a few layers,
2 = ingrowth permeates coating and reaches central core.

Results of Segmental Replacement

Macroscopic evaluation showed no gross evidence of intraoperative infection. The animals with a s.p. resection showed extensive bone formation around the implant, except for the area below the plate. In the e.p. resections without bone grafting, a thin, adherent layer of connective tissue formed around the shaft. Some of these implants showed rotational instability. Two of the unstable specimens showed black discolorations between the plate and cylinder that were interpreted as corrosion or wear. In one humerus there was a fracture of the intramedullary rod, and one of the distal screws

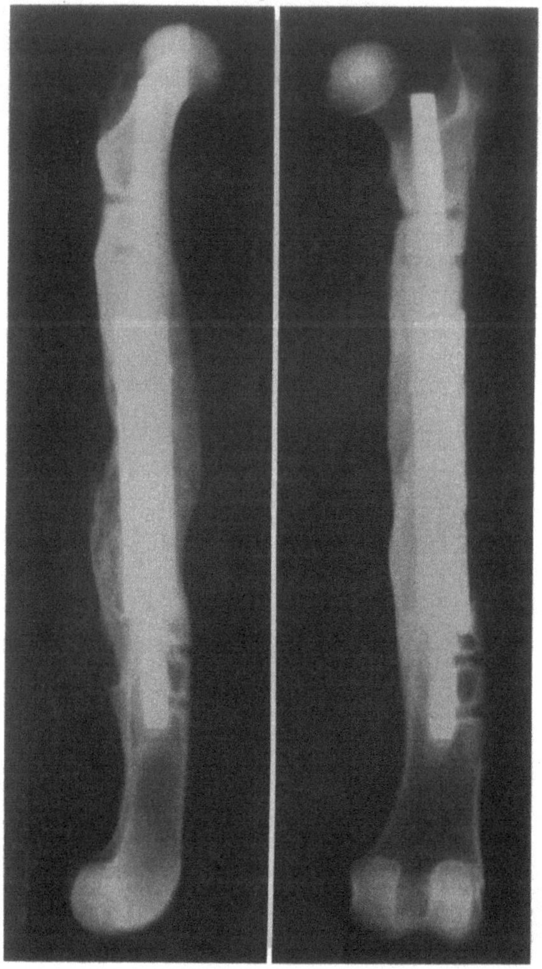

Fig. 2. Radiographic views of a baboon femur 5 years after implantation of a porous fiber titanium segment. Except for the area under the compression plate, the cylinder is entirely covered by a thick layer of bone. No loosening of the cylinder or intramedullary rod is apparent

was also fractured. In all these segments, bone was found covering the fiber metal cylinder. In addition, a solid bridge had formed from the proximal bone fragment across the intramedullary rod to the distal fragment.

Radiologic evaluation revealed a pseudarthrosis in two of the s.p. resected femurs, in two of the e.p. resected bones that had not been grafted or compressed, and in one e.p. resected tibia without grafting or compression. All e.p. resections in which compression and grafting had been used showed satisfactory radiologic conditions at the bone-implant interface. No radiolucent zones were found around either the cylinder or the intramedullary rod. A bony sheath was found around the fiber metal cylinder in 83% of the s.p. resections and in 78% of the grafted resections (Fig. 2).

Histology

Only 2 of the s.p. segments showed bone ingrowth at the proximal and distal interfaces. Bone ingrowth was apparent histologically in 6 of the 12 interfacial zones. In the e.p., non-grafted group (7 implants), only one segment showed bone infiltration at its proximal and distal ends. Out of 14 interfaces, only 4 (in 3 animals) were solidly fused by ingrowing bone. In the e.p. group with grafting and without compression, only 1 out of 3 segments showed bone ingrowth at both interfaces. The resections with both grafting and compression showed both proximal and distal bone ingrowth in 5 of the 6 segments examined. In addition, a complete

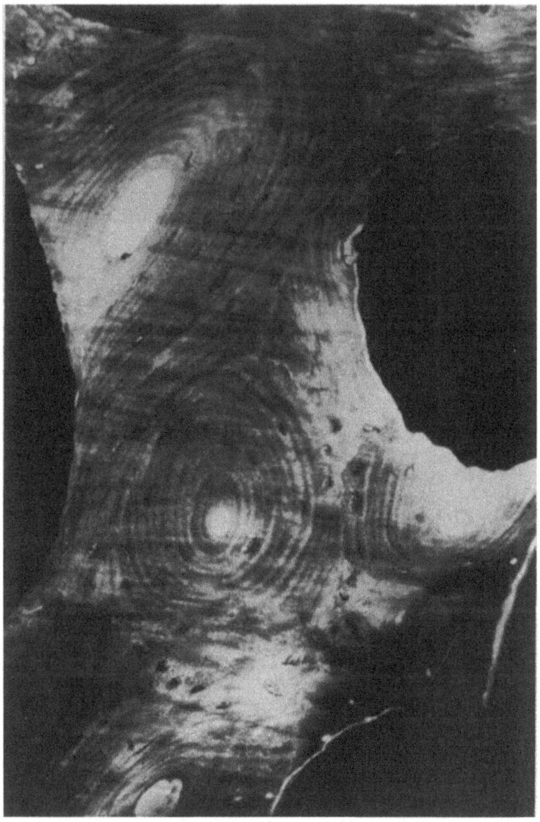

Fig. 3. Microscopic examination of thin sections reveals viable osteons in immediate contact with the titanium mesh (×100, 3 years post-implantation)

bony mantle was found around the titanium cylinder. In the regions with ingrowing bone, contact between the bone and fiber titanium was direct, with no intervening connective tissue (Fig. 3). No osteoclastic activity could be demonstrated in the stable implants. In about 50% of the implants the bony mantle showed circumferential ingrowth into the fiber metal. Bone ingrowth from the endosteum into the intramedullary rod was apparent in 95% of the cross-sections from all 22 implants (Fig. 4).

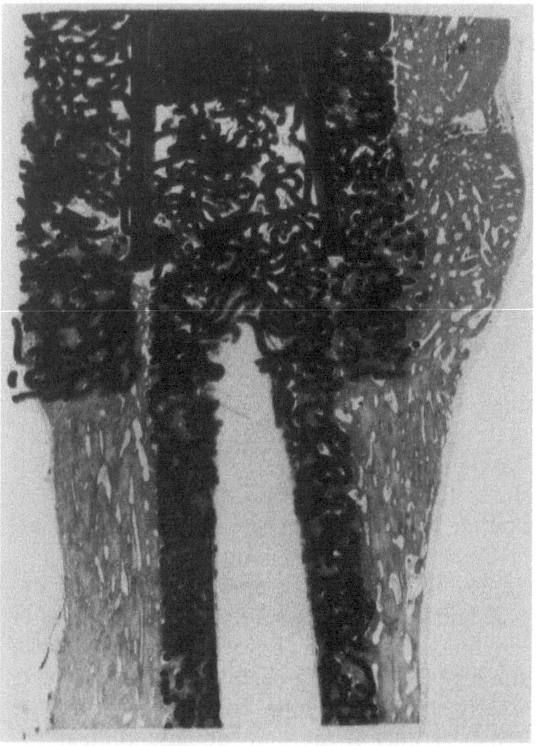

Fig. 4. Longitudinal section through the junction of the titanium cylinder and the bone. No signs of instability are visible, and there is deep bone ingrowth down to the metal core of the intramedullary rod (removed)

The timing of the bone ingrowth was determined by means of tetracycline labeling. This revealed the presence of immature bone among the fibers as early as 6 weeks after implantation. After 3 months the bone was fully mature.

Implantations in Human Patients

Since 1976, fiber titanium implants have been used at the Rush Medical Center in Chicago and at the Mayo Clinic for bone replacement in patients with malignant and semimalignant tumors. The fiber titanium cylinders have an intramedullary flange attached rigidly at each end. The implant are additionally secured by means of a titanium plate applied under compression, and by bone grafting. So far about 50 of these implants have been inserted. The biocompatibility of the titanium has proved excellent in this series, and a problem-free bone ingrowth has been witnessed when conditions are stable.

Initially there was doubt as to whether the fiber titanium would be suitable for the coating of endoprostheses. It was reasoned that the massive ingrowth of bone into the interconnecting pores would make removal of the prostheses

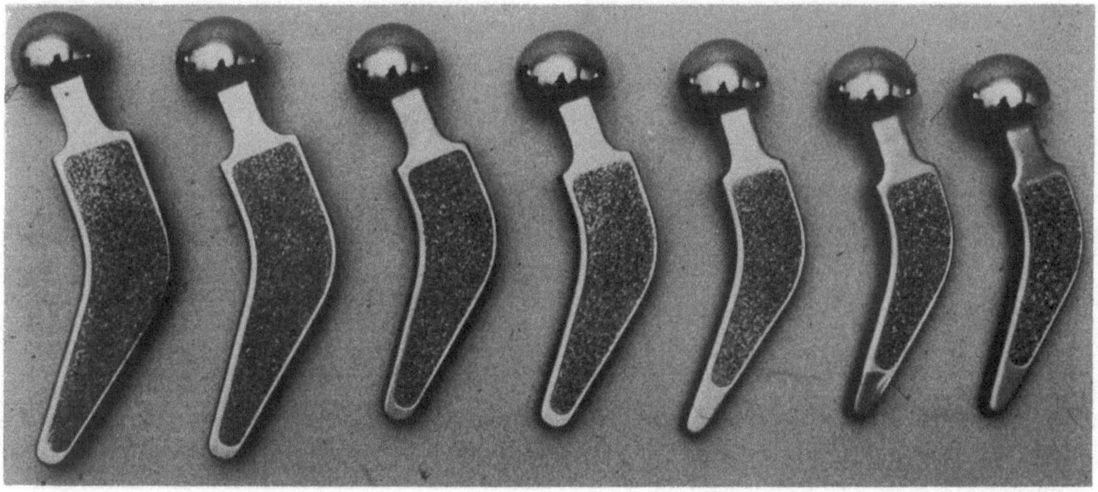

Fig. 5. The femoral endoprosthesis has a porous, fiber titanium coating on its anterior and posterior surfaces. The range of stem diameters enable a secure press-fit to be achieved in all patients

extremely difficult. One of the first rules of endoprosthetics is that every implant should be removable. This is particularly important in the case of hip prostheses. Using the technique of finite element analysis, a computer-assisted design for a new type of femoral endoprosthesis was produced. The prosthesis, shown in Fig. 5, features a collarless intramedullary stem with an unusual degree of angulation. It consists of a Ti-Al-V core with a fiber titanium coating on its anterior and posterior surfaces. The stems are available in 7 different widths for an optimum stem-to-canal match. In all cases, full weight-bearing has been started no later than 3 months postoperatively. The clinical and radiologic results to date are highly encouraging. An illustrative x-ray is shown in Fig. 6. In knee prostheses, fiber titanium has also been used to coat the artificial tibial plateau.

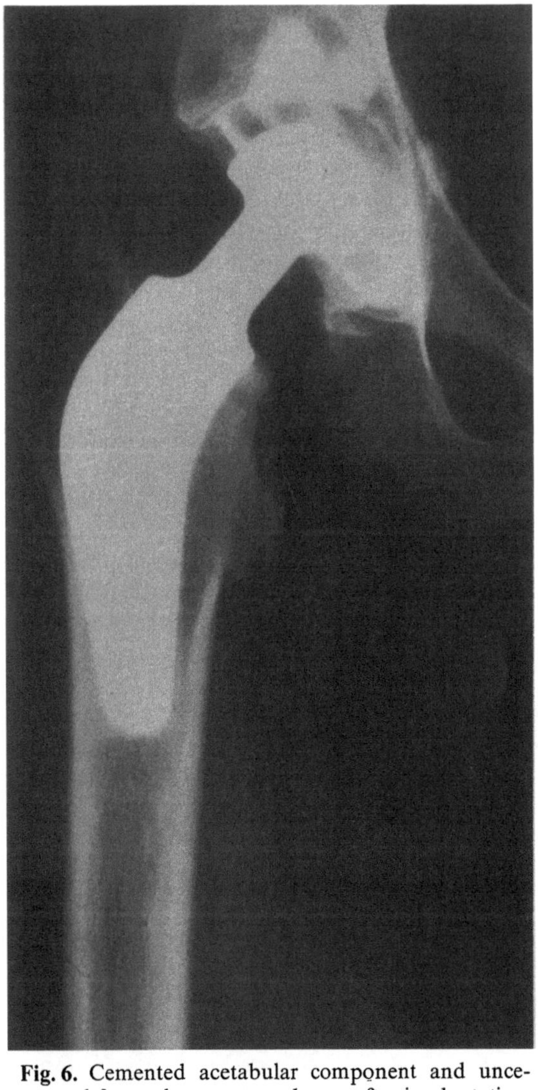

Fig. 6. Cemented acetabular component and uncemented femoral component 1 year after implantation. The patient has borne full weight on the hip since the 9th postoperative week and is free of complaints. Note the areas of increased bone density in the calcar area and at the distal tip of the stem

Discussion

Various porous materials are used to coat imlants and improve their attachment to the bone. Fiber titanium is well tolerated and has an excellent affinity for bone. The elasticity of the sintered material can be closely matched to that of the bone. In addition, the material contains an extensive interconnecting pore system that can provide a strong mechanical interlock through bone ingrowth. Histologic studies often show direct contact between the bone and titanium, provided a very stable primary attachment was achieved at operation.

The fiber titanium is deformable to some degree and so can adapt somewhat to the shape of the bony canal during insertion. Comparative studies of skeletal segmental replacements have clearly shown that good bone ingrowth can be achieved only if there is intimate contact between the implant and bone, with no relative motion between them. The additional application of cancellous bone grafts is of value in improving and accelerating bone ingrowth.

The meshwork of multiply sintered wires is invulnerable to stress fractures and cannot fail by the propagation of cracks. The fiber titanium has undergone extensive testing, both mechanically and in animal studies. Histologic evaluations of 10-year implants in animals are contributing significantly to the advance of implant research.

With all uncemented implants, deep bone ingrowth is possible during the non-weight-bearing period. During subsequent weight-bearing, however, the implant may loosen secondarily if its elasticity is too different from that of the surrounding bone. In the case of fiber titanium, the elastic modulus can be matched to that of the bone by selecting the proper sintering temperature. The deformation properties of the fiber metal are very similar to those of the surrounding trabecular bone. Fiber titanium satisfies the following basic requirements for bone ingrowth into a porous implant:

1. intimate contact between implant and bone,
2. good primary stability,
3. large area of stress transfer to the implant so that bone remodeling can occur.

Stress transfer to the implant is of particularly great importance in the hip region and is a key factor in the prevention of secondary osteolysis. Bone ingrowth in the proximal third of the stem is essential. This requirement can be met either by applying the porous coating only to the proximal part of the implant, or by using a very short, collarless prosthesis that will concentrate stresses in the proximal femur. Fiber titanium is distinguished from other porous materials by its excellent biocompatibility and corrosion resistance. The material can be sintered into any shape desired. It possesses an interconnecting pore system that is conducive to bone ingrowth. The elasticity of the implant can be matched to that of the bone.

Fiber titanium has also demonstrated outstanding longevity in extended animal studies (10 years). In human patients, it has been used for several years as a replacement for resected bone in tumor operations, and for 1½ years it has served as a coating for hip and knee prostheses. Results are encouraging, but it is still too early for definitive conclusions to be drawn.

References

1. Andersson GJ, Gächter A, Galante JO, Rostoker W (1978) Segmental replacement of long bones in baboons using a fiber titanium implant. J Bone Joint Surg [Am] 60:31–40
2. Escalas F, Galante JO, Rostoker W, Coogan P (1976) Biocompatibility of materials for total joint replacement. J Biomed Mater Res 10:175–195
3. Galante JO, Rostoker W (1972) The use of fiber metal composites as a method of fixation of skeletal prostheses. Rush-Presbyterian-St. Luke's Med Bull 11:143–150
4. Galante JO, Rostoker W (1973) Fiber metal composites in the fixation of skeletal prostheses. J Biomed Mater Res 7:43–61
5. Galante J, Rostoker W, Ray RD (1970) Physical properties of trabecular bone. Calcif Tissue Res 5:236–246
6. Galante JO, Rostoker W, Lueck R, Ray RD (1971) Sintered fiber metal composites as a basis for attachment of implants to bone. J Bone Joint Surg [Am] 53:101–114
7. Lembert E, Galante JO, Rostoker W (1972) Fixation of skeletal replacement by fiber metal composites. Clin Orthop 87:303–310
8. Lueck RA, Galante JO, Rostoker W, Ray RD (1969) Development of an open pore metallic implant to permit attachment of bone. Proc Am Coll Surg 20:456–457
9. Rostoker W, Galante JO, Shen G (1974) Some mechanical properties of sintered fiber metal composites. J Test Eval 2:107–112

The Current Status of Uncemented Tantalum and Niobium Femoral Endoprostheses*

H. Plenk Jr., G. Pflüger, S. Schider, N. Böhler and F. Grundschober

Summary

Ingrowth-type femoral endoprostheses constructed of cold-worked tantalum and niobium were implanted without cement in beagle dogs for unilateral total hip replacement. Twenty-one tantalum stems and 6 out of 13 niobium stems were evaluated after observation periods up to 14 months. Four loose tantalum stems and 3 loose niobium stems were discovered. The remaining stable implants were shown to be solidly anchored to the bone by the histologic examination of thin sections. The patterns of attachment were characteristic of uncemented femoral endoprostheses.

By employing suitable powder metallurgical techniques, dispersion hardening and cold-working, it is possible to greatly enhance the strength properties of tantalum and especially of niobium. This, together with the corrosion resistance and biocompatibility of these materials, make them excellent candidates for the manufacture of heavy-duty, cement-free endoprostheses for human use.

The high-melting metals tantalum and niobium, with their excellent corrosion resistance and biocompatibility, have already proven their value as diagnostic aids and as light-duty surgical implants (Mears, 1979). Through advances in powder metallurgy, it has become possible to increase the mechanical strength of these metals to a point where their application in heavy-duty situations also appears feasible (Schider and Bildstein, 1982).

In the present article we shall summarize the results of animal implantations of uncemented tantalum and niobium femoral endoprostheses with ingrowth surface finishes, and we shall examine progress that has been made in the development of heavy-duty tantalum and niobium implants.

In the annealed condition, both tantalum and niobium are very soft and workable, and their mechanical strength can be improved substantially by cold working in this condition, though this necessarily reduces the workability of the materials. However, by using dispersion hardening, which is equivalent to mild alloying, it is possible to increase ultimate tensile strength significantly without sacrificing workability (Fig. 1). Because good cyclic-load endurance is an even more important criterion for heavy-duty implants, preliminary studies were done in which tantalum and niobium materials worked in various ways were tested for this property using the ultrasound resonance technique. Cold-worked tantalum, of the kind used for the femoral endoprostheses in the present animal experiments, shows a relatively low tensile strength but exhibits a cyclic-load endurance for

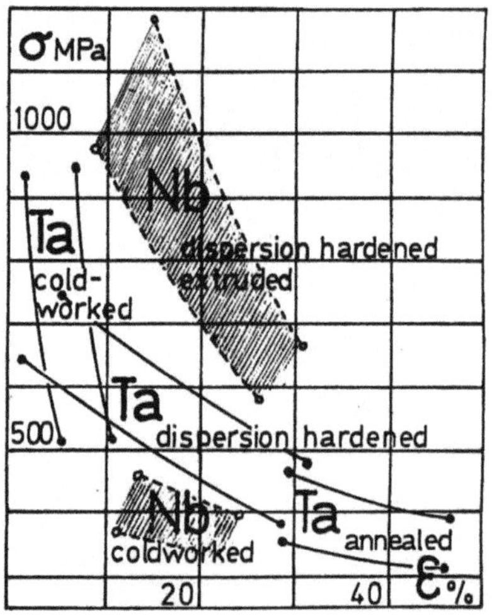

Fig. 1. Ranges of tensile strength (in MPa) and strain (ε%) of tantalum and niobium wires (0.8–1.5 mm diam.) in the annealed, cold-worked and dispersion-hardened condition

* These studies were supported by Metallwerke Plansee A.G., Reutte, Austria, and by the Research Promotion Fund of the Gewerbliche Wirtschaft of Austria, Project No. 3/1851-I/P

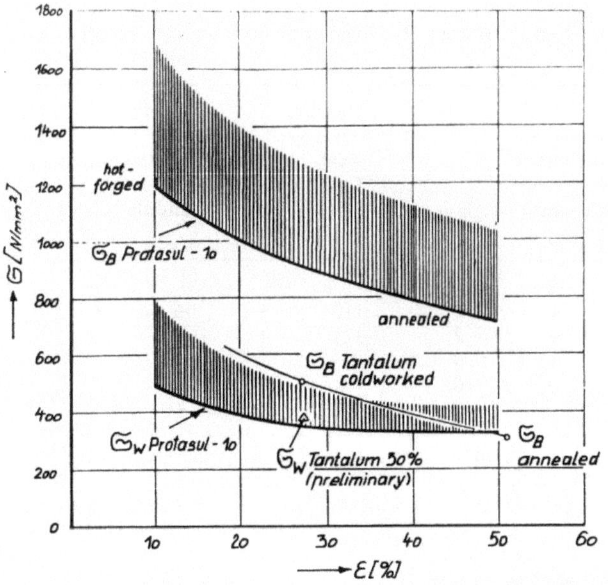

Fig. 2. Ultimate tensile strength (σ_B) of cold-worked tantalum and corresponding cyclic-load endurance (σ_W) for a given strain (ε%) compared to the strength ranges reported for Protasul 10 (*shaded* areas, in N/mm²)

a given strain (Fig. 2) that is comparable to that reported for the prosthetic material Protasul-10 (Sulzer Bros., Winterthur, Switzerland). Moreover, the cyclic-load endurance of tantalum and niobium is practically unaffected by a corrosive environment, which, together with the low susceptibility to notch cracking of both metals, enables the production of implants with an ingrowth surface relief for direct skeletal attachment without cement.

The stems of the femoral endoprostheses were constructed of cold-worked tantalum and niobium and were provided with small, conical surface pits 900 μm in diameter (Fig. 3a, b). The tantalum stems were combined with tantalum heads and necks (Fig. 3a), and the niobium stems with aluminium oxide heads and tantalum necks (Fig. 3b). The heads and necks were interchangeably attached to the stems by means of a screw connection or self-locking cone. Cementable polyethylene acetabular prostheses completed the system, which was implanted unilaterally in beagle dogs (tantalum stems in 21 dogs, niobium stems in 13). The implants were removed for histologic study after observation periods of 6 weeks to 14 months, using polyfluorochrome sequential labeling and microradiography in undecalcified thin sections. In addition, tissue specimens taken from the regenerated capsule and from local and central lymph organs were examined by light and electron microscopy.

The studies on the tantalum stems (Pflüger et al., 1982) have been completed following a maximum observation period of 14 months. Of the 21 stems studied, 4 showed clinical or histologic evidence of loosening. The results are summarized in Table 1. With most of the stable implants, points or areas of dense bony contact

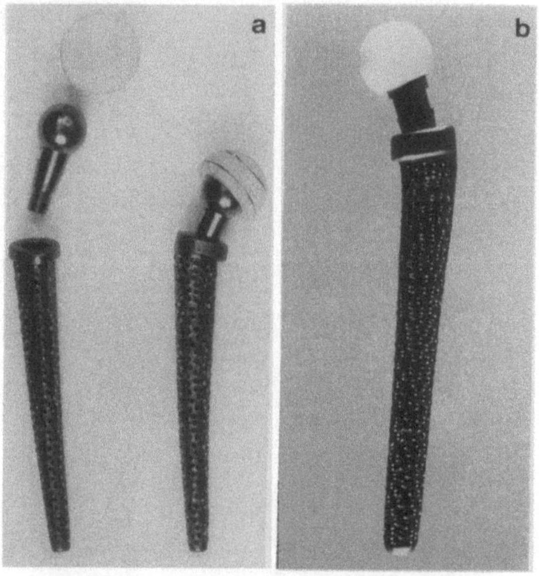

Fig. 3a, b. Femoral endoprostheses with ingrowth surfaces used for dog implantations. **a** Tantalum stem with interchangeable tantalum head and neck. **b** Niobium stem with aluminum oxide head and tantalum neck. Both models were used with cementable polyethylene acetabular prostheses

Table 1. Results of Experimental Studies on Tantalum Stem Prostheses (21 Dogs) and Niobium Stem Prostheses (13 Dogs, 6 Evaluated to Date)

Implantation time	no.	Tantalum				no.	Niobum			
		stem firm loose	Solid bony attachment				stem firm loose	Solid bony attachment		
			proximal	middle	distal			proximal	middle	distal
6 weeks	1	1/0	+	+	+	0				
up to 3 months	3	2/1	+	+	+	1	1/0	+	+	+
up to 6 months	3	2/1	+/−	+	+	2	1/1	+	+	+
up to 9 months	4	4/0	+/−	+	+	0				
up to 12 months	7	5/2	+/−	+	+	0				
up to 14 months	3	3/0	+/−	+	+	3	1/2	+	+	+

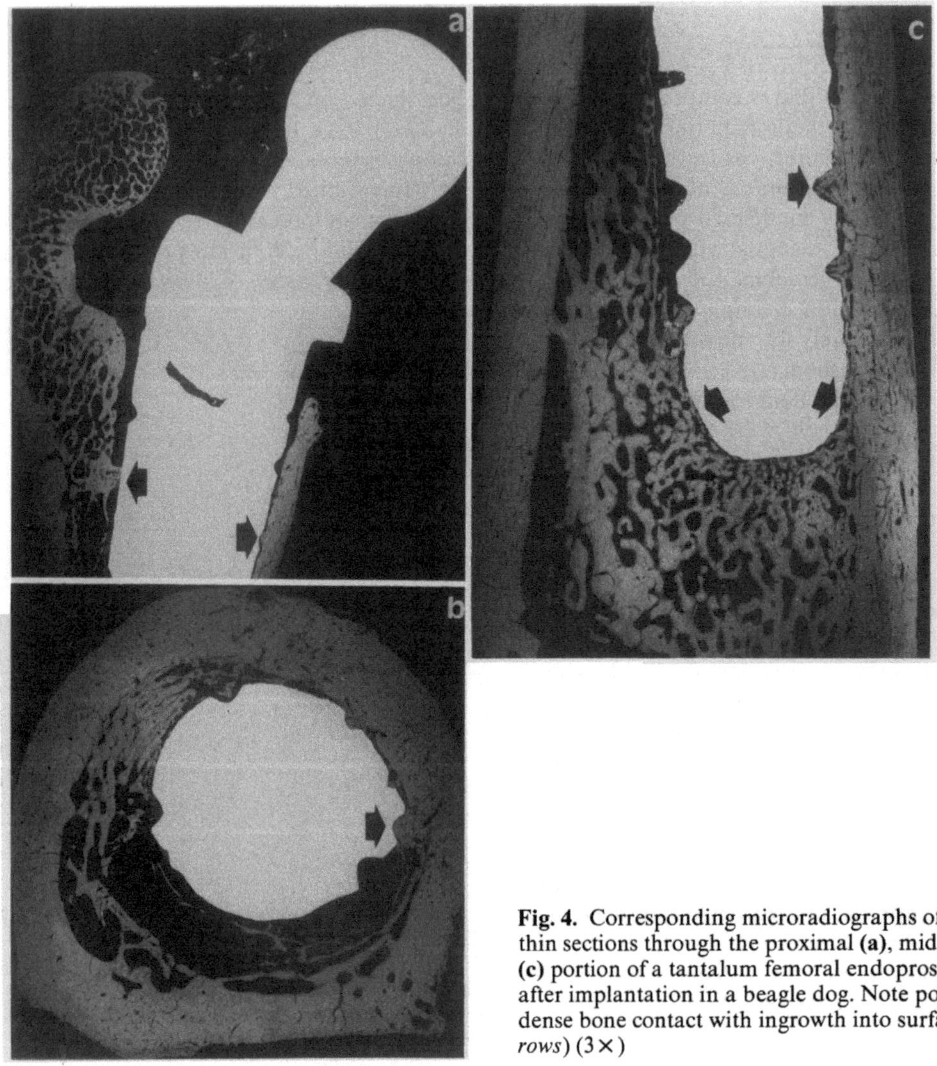

Fig. 4. Corresponding microradiographs of undecalcified thin sections through the proximal **(a)**, middle **(b)** and distal **(c)** portion of a tantalum femoral endoprosthesis 12 months after implantation in a beagle dog. Note points and areas of dense bone contact with ingrowth into surface recesses (*arrows*) (3×)

with ingrowth into the surface pits were evident in the proximal, middle and distal portions of the stem (Fig. 4a–c). In a few cases (6 out of 17), however, the proximal stem was devoid of bony contact. In all but one of these cases, loosening of the head and neck and/or the acetabular component led to unrest and an increased production of metallic wear debris. As expected, wear of the tantalum head against the polyethylene socket increased progressively with time. The wear particles were engulfed by macrophages without apparent cell damage and were deposited not only in the capsular tissue and in local and central lymph tissues, but also in the connective tissue sheath that at least partially enveloped the prosthetic stem. The presence of such macrophages interfered noticeably with the appositional growth of bone tissue, thus demonstrating the effect of wear processes on the cementless fixation of endoprostheses, even when the wear debris is inert (cf. article by Willert).

Because of these problems, we chose a more favorable combination of articulating materials for use with the niobium stems. In the 6 implants evaluated thus far, however, additional problems were encountered with the interchangeable head and neck components. The results to date are summarized in Table 1 and show 3 instances of loosening. The stable implants are anchored just as solidly as the tantalum stems. It should be noted that the dense appositional growth at the distal end of the stem, which is usually visible in x-rays and is clearly demonstrable in histologic sections, should not be interpreted as a sign of loosening if it is associated with areas of dense bony contact in the middle and proximal portions of the stem. The absence of a stable proximal anchorage despite a solid middle and distal attachment may be causally related to the elastic modulus, the E-modulus of niobium being closer to that of bone than is the E-modulus of tantalum. For the future, it remains to be determined whether the strength increase that can be produced in wires (Fig. 1) can also be achieved in larger implants such as joint endoprostheses, and whether the technique of dispersion hardening can produce tantalum and niobium materials of reproducible quality that can meet the rigorous demands of human implantation. Previous experience with animal implantations indicates that tantalum and especially the lighter-weight, cheaper niobium satisfy all major material requirements for the production of cementless prostheses.

References

Mears DC (1979) Materials and orthopaedic surgery. Williams & Wilkins, Baltimore, pp 115, 123

Pflüger G, Plenk H Jr, Böhler N, Grundschober F, Schider S (1982) Experimental studies on total knee- and hip-joint endoprostheses made of tantalum. In: Winter GD, Gibbons DF, Plank H Jr (eds) Biomaterials 1980. Advances in biomaterials, vol 3. Wiley, Chichester New York Brisbane Toronto Singapore, pp 161–167

Schider S, Bildstein H (1982) Tantalum and niobium as potential prosthetic materials. In: Winter GD, Gibbons DF, Plenk H Jr (eds) Biomaterials 1980. Advances in biomaterials, vol 3. Wiley, Chichester New York Brisbane Toronto Singapore, pp 13–20

First Experience with the PM Prosthesis

K. Walcher

The author's hospital is located in Franconia, and Franconia is the land of hip joint dysplasia. Many younger patients with severe degenerative arthritis secondary to dysplasia, in whom alternative procedures are no longer feasible, inquire almost daily about modern techniques for the surgical treatment of their disabling conditions.

Hence, we greatly welcomed the offer of Dr. Parhofer and Mönch/Memmingen and Ungethüm/Tuttlingen to join with four other hospitals (Erlangen, Freiburg, Baden-Baden and Memmingen) in the clinical testing of the new PM prosthesis. Dr. Parhofer started implantation of the PM prosthesis in July of 1980, and additional implantations were started in February, 1981, at the Center for Trauma Surgery, Reconstructive Surgery and Surgery of the Hand in Bayreuth. Thus, the present report is preliminary only and, in view of the short observation period, must be limited to questions of techniques and observations during the first 16 months.

The femoral component of the PM prosthesis consists of a stem made of the wrought implant alloy Isotan, which has a special surface relief that is receptive to bone ingrowth. Isotan is a titanium-base alloy distinguished by its excellent mechanical properties. This component was already described briefly in the report of Dr. Semlitsch.

Of all the metallic implant alloys, Isotan has an elastic modulus which most closely approximates that of natural bone.

The conical post atop the stem serves as a mount for a ceramic ball made of Biolox.

The acetabular prosthesis consists of two parts. The outer part is a conical socket constructed of titanium; the threadlike ribs on its outer surface ensure a stable anchorage in the pelvic bone. This serves as a backing for the second part, a polyethylene insert which is press-fitted into the metal socket and which receives the ceramic head (Fig. 1).

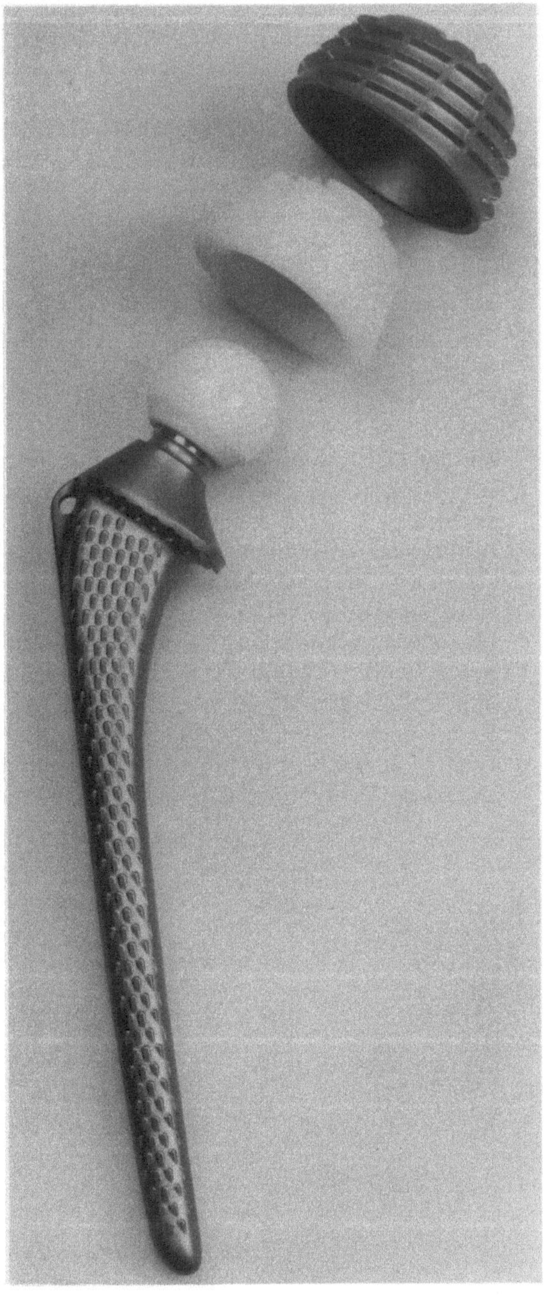

Fig. 1. The PM prosthesis

The newly designed prosthesis was tested at the biomechanical laboratory of Aesculap Instruments. Prolonged fatigue testing on a cyclic loading machine showed that the PM prosthesis is capable of withstanding millions of peak loads equal to 7 times body weight without failure.

Following some initial difficulties, a relatively simple technique of implantation has been devised:

The acetabulum is first prepared with a hammer and chisel and then widened and deepened with reamers. The smallest reamer is used first, as this will create a central guide hole for the larger reamers that follow.

Following reaming on the acetabulum, a thread is cut in the bone with a tapping instrument, and the tantalum socket is screwed in until absolutely firm. The best method is to keep rotating the socket until a slight concomitant rotation of the pelvis is elicited.

Next the polyethylene insert is press-fitted into place. In contrast to cement fixation, where care is taken to spare the subchondral layer of compact bone, we do not hestitate to allow at least one edge of the threaded socket to protrude through the dysplastic acetabulum into the lesser pelvis if this will provide sufficient bone stock for the screw thread, especially in the proximal part of the acetabulum.

With a primary perforation of this type, we have found that the acetabulum tends to become sealed off from the lesser pelvis by a new bony layer within about a year.

The radiologists at the Municipal Hospitals of Bayreuth take special lateral radiographs of the acetabulum, both postoperatively and during follow-ups, so that the bone tissue in the hollows of the screw threads can be accurately evaluated. In our view, an increase of bone density in the hollows of the threads is the best radiologic criterion for skeletal integration of the acetabular component.

Narrow seams at the base of the acetabular component should not necessarily be interpreted as resorption zones. They may result from directional adjustments made during definitive positioning of the component.

To enable good valgus positioning of the femoral stem, which is especially important in uncemented arthroplasties, a bone forceps is used to cut a groove in the trochanteric area close to the femoral neck. The appropriate rasp is then driven into the femoral canal. The rasp is withdrawn, and the stem is inserted by hand until snugly seated and then driven the rest of the way in with a hammer.

It has been our experience that with every 30th prosthesis, a crack occurs at the distal end of the stem. This appears to have no lasting consequences, and the fracture should heal completely during the 12- to 16-week period of convalescence.

The formation of a strong bony pedestal at the distal end of the stem is, we believe, a definite radiologic sign that the stem is being incorporated into the femur. This phenomenon need not be present, however, and depends largely on the amount of cancellous bone that has been introduced. Other authors interpret this pedestal as an early sign of loosening.

Pedestal formation must not be confused with a marked thickening of the lateral cortex and periosteum in response to a primary varus positioning of the stem.

Much has been written about atrophy or resorption of the calcar in connection with cemented arthroplasties. An increase in the density of the calcar apparently should be viewed as a sign of stability, implying an absence of tensile stresses at the periphery of the stump of the femoral neck. A portion of the applied load is probably transferred to the bone as a physiologic compressive stress. An enlargement of the calcar is also possible under these conditions.

If cementless implantation of the stem appears inadvisable, as in post-traumatic states with advanced osteoporosis and an unusually wide medullary cavity, the threaded socket of the PM system may be combined with the straight-stem prosthesis of Müller, using a small amount of bone cement. This is recommended only in patients over the age of 60.

It is important to realize that in severe dysplasia with deformity of the femoral head, a 2- to 3-cm lengthening of the leg may be unavoidable. If the arthroplasty is bilateral, the lengthening can easily be corrected on the second side.

Even in uncemented implantations, periarticular ossifications can occur. In one case a prior dislocation of the hip was shown to be causative.

The results of the implantations to date are as follows:

Regrettably, two infections were observed. One occurred in a 45-year-old woman with alcohol-related cirrhosis of the liver. One medial femoral neck fracture had been treated elsewhere with an Ender nail, and this had been followed by a renewed dislocation of the joint. Both prostheses had to be removed following interim suction irrigation or the implantation of gentamicin-impregnated beads. Neither failure can be ascribed to the method.

Though many criteria were used during follow-up, here we shall report on only one: bony integration of the prosthesis.

Of the 100 prostheses in the first series, 58 have been implanted for more than 6 months, and 20 for more than 1 year. Seven patients still complain of load-dependent pain in the thigh area, although definite loosening has so far been demonstrated in only one case. In 4 of these patients, difficulties were encountered during insertion of the intramedullary stem. Perhaps a stem that fits too snugly in the medullary canal is a source of eventual postoperative complaints. Other authors have speculated on this phenomenon.

Naturally, a final assessment cannot be made at this time due to the short length of follow-up.

First Experience with the PM Prosthesis

A. Reichelt and K. Bläsius

The uncemented "PM" total hip prosthesis consists of a titanium-aluminum-vanadium stem that conforms closely to the shape of the femoral shaft, a threaded acetabular cup made of the same alloy, a polyethylene insert for the acetabular cup, and a femoral ball made of aluminum oxide ceramic. Teardrop-shaped surface irregularities on the femoral stem are provided for secure attachment with the cancellous bone. The shape of the acetabular component and its external threads, which function as load-bearing elements, ensure a very stable anchorage in the pelvic bone.

Since March 30, 1981, we have used the PM system for 68 primary hip arthroplasties and 5 revision arthroplasties. The patients ranged in age from 17 to 77, with an average age of 57. The several younger patients in the series were the first in that age group in whom we had implanted hip prostheses. Nevertheless, we did not hesitate to use the system in older patients, as indicated by the relatively high average age of the population. No problems with loosening were encountered in the older age group.

Intraoperative complications consisted of 5 fissure fractures. Only the trochanteric fractures could be considered specific for the uncemented prostheses. When we first used the PM system, we occasionally had difficulty selecting the correct stem size and had to use considerable force to extract an oversized stem that had already been inserted ⅔ of the way into the shaft.

Since a template was developed to enable an accurate size estimation to be made before insertion, we have no longer had problems with fissure fractures. Shaft penetrations due to improper positioning of the leg during rasping are not specific for this prosthesis and are easily repaired within minutes. Postoperative complications (Table 1) have been limited to one dislocation. No infection or loosening has yet occurred. Trochanteric osteotomies are unnecessary as a rule. We found them necessary only in patients with exceptionally deep acetabula.

A follow-up examination was done at 3 months in 42 patients, at 6 months in 30, and at 12 months in 11.

Of the 30 patients examined at 6 months, 23 (77%) were able to walk for 60 minutes without pain. By 12 months, all patients examined had attained this walking ability. Reliance on walking aids is summarized in Table 2.

Radiographs taken some months after surgery showed no evidence of increased bone formation around the prosthesis. On comparing the postoperative radiographs with films taken later, the prosthesis, and especially the acetabular component, already appear to have their greatest investment of cancellous bone at the time of the operation. The calcar showed no evidence of osteolysis or increased porosity. On the other hand, a number of prostheses showed the periosteal thickenings and bone consolidation around the distal end of the femoral stem that have been reported by other authors.

On the whole, 32 out of 42 patients (79%) were satisfied with the surgical result when in-

Table 1. Complications with the PM Prosthesis

Intraoperative:	Shaft penetrations	1
	Fissure fractures of the greater trochanter	4
Postoperative:	Dislocations	1

Table 2. Use of Walking Aids by Patients with the PM Prosthesis

	After 6 months (n = 30) (in %)	After 12 months (n = 11) (in %)
No aids	60	73
One cane	30	27
Two canes	10	0

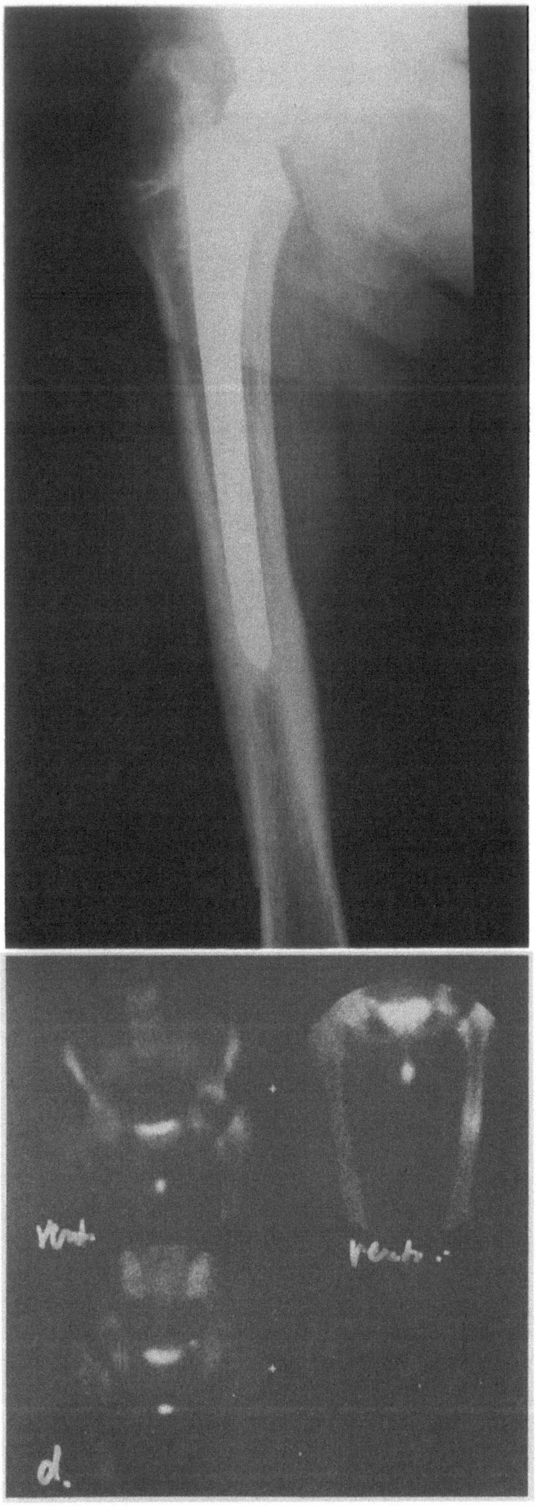

a

b

Fig. 1 a, b

Table 3. Postoperative Femoral Pain in Patients with the PM Prosthesis

After 3 months (n = 42)	31%
After 6 months (n = 30)	33%
After 12 months (n = 11)	9%

terviewed at 3 months. At 6 months this percentage was 77%, i.e., 23 out of 30. At 12 months, however, 10 out of the 11 patients questioned (91%) were satisfied with the result. This improved subjective rating is due largely to the eventual disappearance of the aching, usually in the distal femur, that was reported by many patients (Table 3).

This pain can be explained at least in part by the results of scintigraphic studies which we performed in patients who complained of persistent pain. All these patients showed, at either 6 or 12 months, an accumulation of scintigraphic indicator – a sign of increased peri- and endosteal bone formation. This bone formation could be consistently demonstrated by x-ray at 12 months and was most apt to appear when there was a varus malposition of the prosthesis causing small areas of stress concentration to develop (Fig. 1 a, b). Malpositions of this type result in micromovements that stimulate reactive bone remodeling processes, as optical stress analyses have demonstrated (Konermann).

On the other hand, if the prosthetic stem fills the medullary cavity completely and is in firm contact with the cortical bone on both sides, then no indicator buildup is apparent, and no discomfort is reported (Fig. 2 a, b).

In summarizing our results of the past 15 months, we may say that the PM total hip prosthesis is an easily-implanted system which so far has yielded some very encouraging early results.

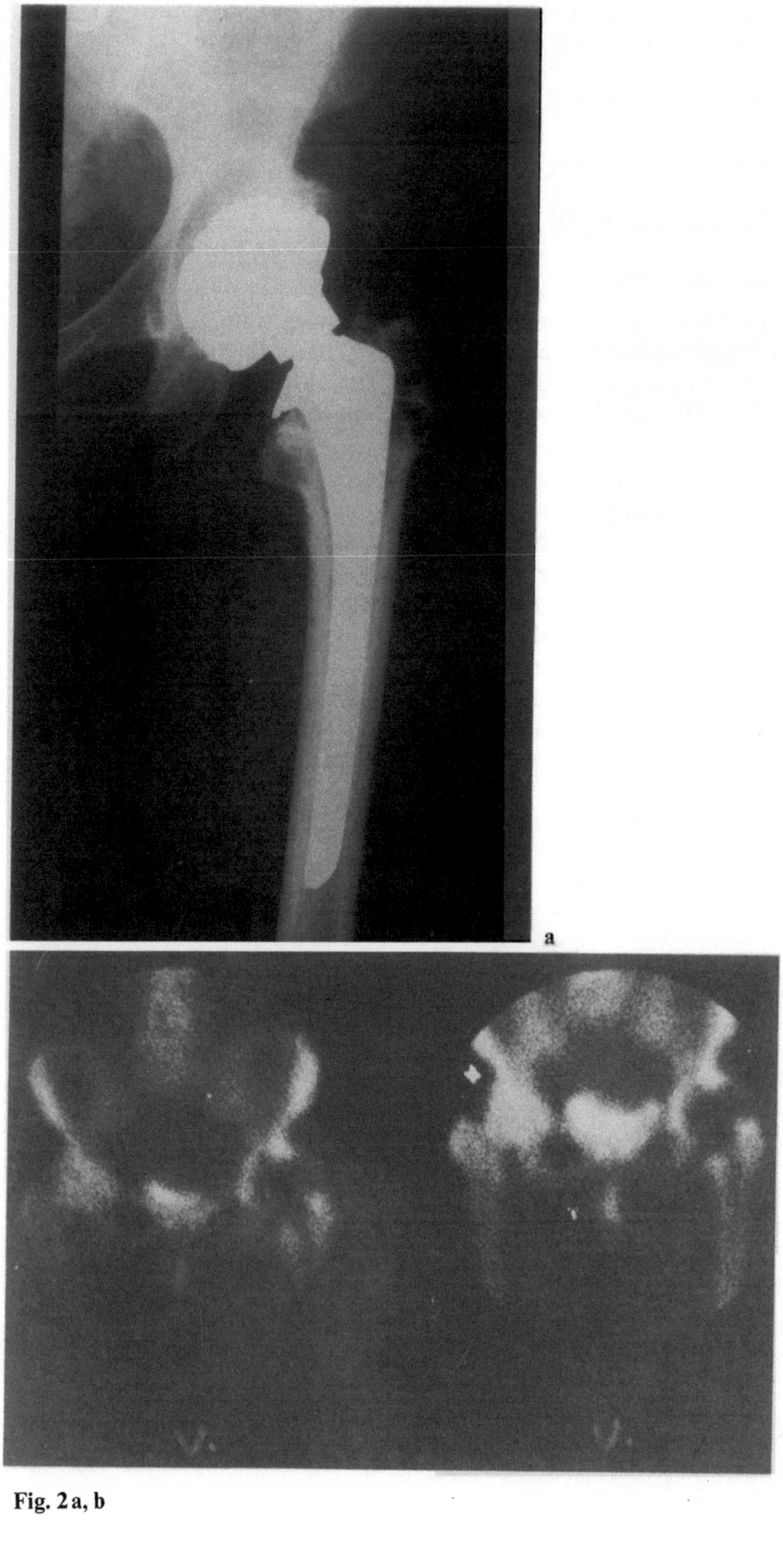

Fig. 2 a, b

Nine Years' Experience with Isoelastic Hip Endoprostheses Made of Plastic Material

E. Morscher

The concept of the isoelastic prosthesis, i.e. an implant whose elasticity and other physical properties are similar to those of the surrounding bone, is based upon the observation made during the internal fixation of fractures that rigid metal implants have a "stress-protecting" effect on the bone, causing the bone to undergo atrophy. This bony atrophy can lead secondarily to loosening of the implant.

While the "incorporation" of a hip prosthesis is comparable to the union of a fracture in many respects, an important difference must be noted: Unlike a bone compression plate, a hip endoprosthesis must transmit 100% of the forces acting upon the femur, and must do so on a permanent basis. The problem of stress protection is by no means solved in all its aspects, and changes in the blood flow through the bone are certainly responsible in part for local osteoporotic changes. It is clear, however, that the permanent incorporation of an endoprosthesis in the bone is possible only if a state of biomechanical equilibrium is established between the load and the bone structure. The implantation of a prosthesis produces significant changes in the biomechanical configuration of the hip joint, and the less the original biomechanics are altered, and the less the implant itself interferes with the

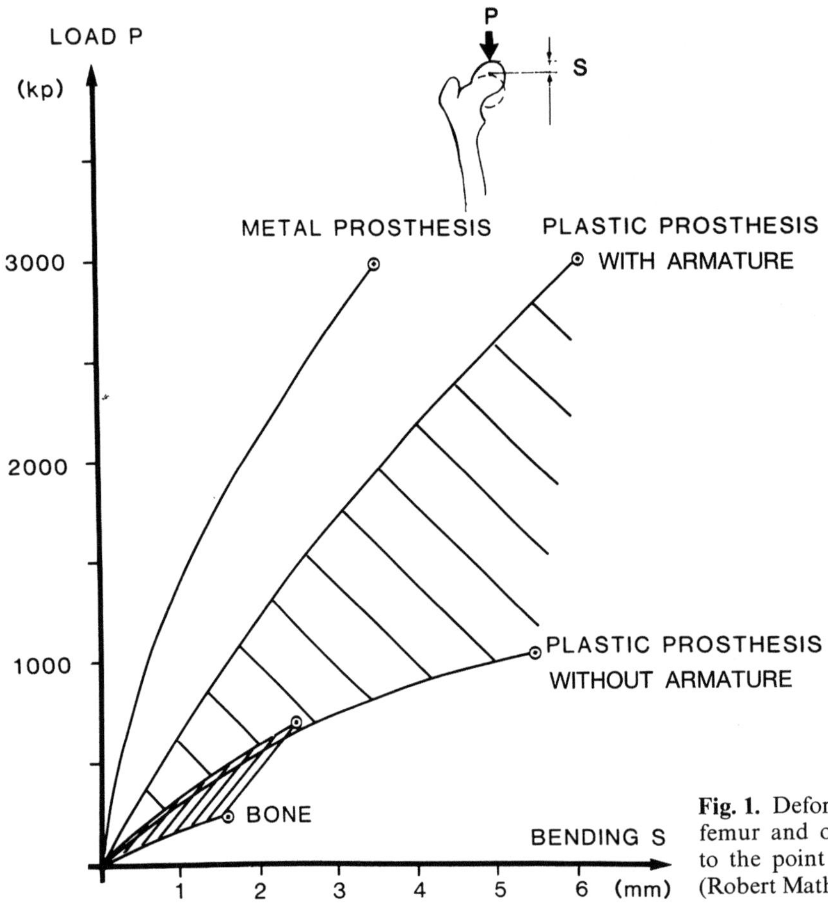

Fig. 1. Deformation of proximal end of femur and of metal and plastic prosthesis to the point of fracture.
(Robert Mathys Co., CH 2544 Bettlach)

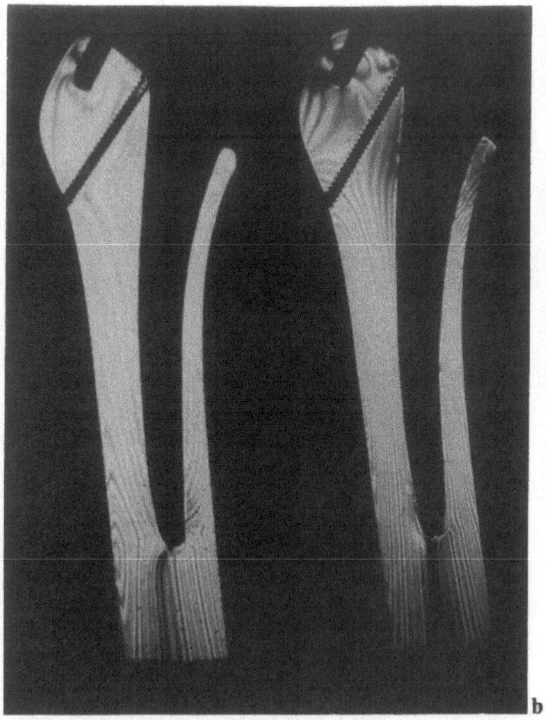

a b

Fig. 2. Optical stress analysis of the proximal femur under loading, **a** with metal prosthesis, **b** with isoelastic plastic prosthesis

Table 1. Hip arthroplasties performed from 1973 to May 1982 with the "isoelastic" hip prosthesis

THR model 1973	70
model 1975	31
Cephalic endoprosthesis	50
Cementless polyethylene cup (cemented stem)	514
Replacement of loose cups (grafting + cementless cup)	61
Replacement of loose metallic shafts	7
Double cups (cementless cup)	6
	739

pattern of force transmission and distribution across the joint, the sooner a new state of biomechanical equilibrium can be achieved.

In the early 1970s Mathys designed a hip replacement made of polyacetal resin that employed the isoelasticity principle [1].

Laboratory experiments and various tests have shown this material to be the most favorable, for in addition to other properties it has an elastic modulus that is very similar to that of natural bone. To ensure the optimum transmission of forces from the prosthesis to the bone,

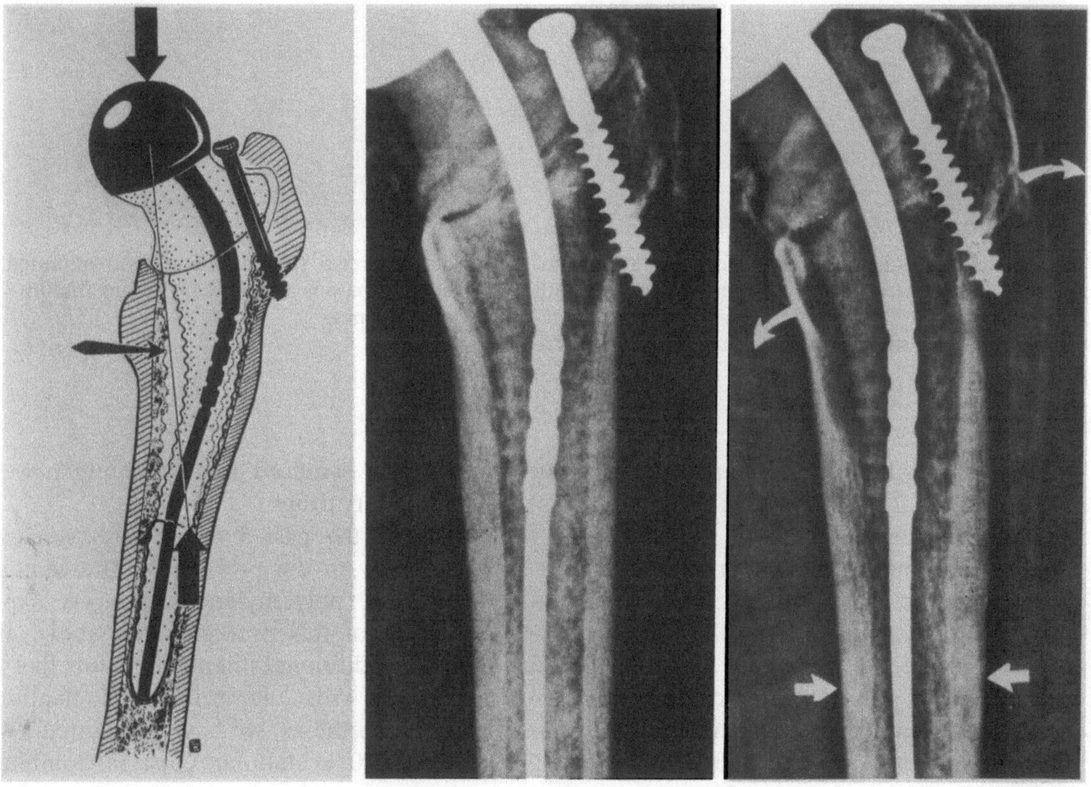

a b c

Fig. 3 a–c. Loosening of an "isoelastic" total hip replacement in the subtrochanteric area 4 years after implantation due to excessive elasticity of the neck of the prosthesis

a

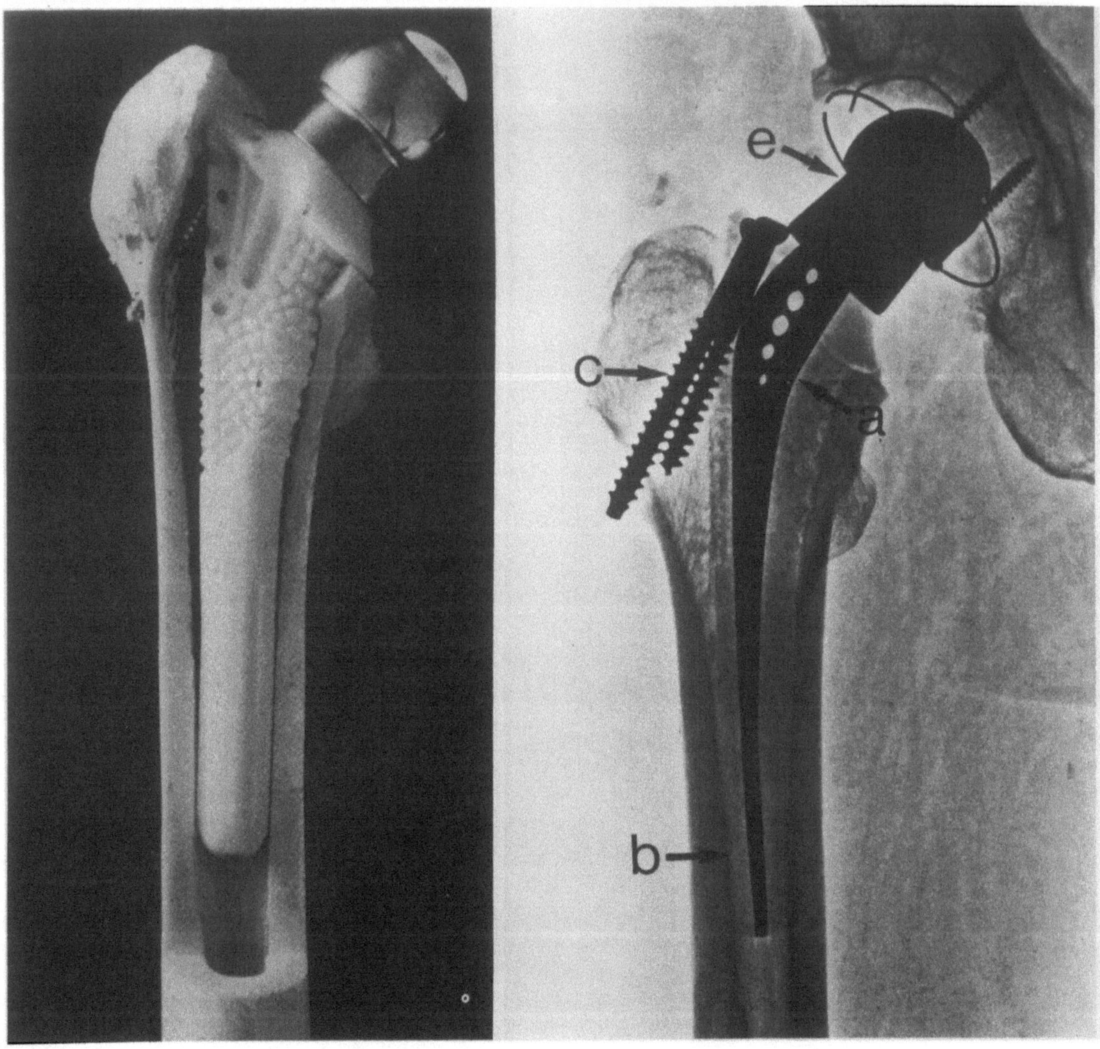

b

Fig. 4a, b. Isoelastic total hip replacement. **a** THR implanted in cadaveric femur. **b** Radiograph 2 years after implantation (1975 model). (*a*) Reinforced armature, (*b*) surface smooth in distal part of stem, (*c*) tension-band screws, (*e*) prosthetic head mounted. The polyethylene cup is attached to the acetabulum with 2 screws and 2 pegs

the prosthesis had to be implanted without cement. This also eliminated the inherent disadvantages of cement fixation.

The acetabular component of the hip replacement was also fabricated from polyacetal resin. However, this material showed an unacceptable degree of wear and has since been replaced with polyethylene. At our clinic the cementless fixation of polyethylene cups has become standard practice in recent years [8]. Polyethylene has proven so favorable, in fact, that any materials developed in the future must be measured against it, just as indomethacin serves as a standard for evaluating new anti-inflammatory drugs.

During the past 5 years we have devoted much study to the problem of the cementless fixation of polyethylene cups. To expedite resolution of this problem and, above all, to eliminate additional unknown factors like those associated with the cementless fixation of femoral prostheses, we have implanted a series of over 600 acetabular cups in combination with a conventional cemented femoral component until the end of the year 1982 (Table 1). It should be noted that throughout the develop-

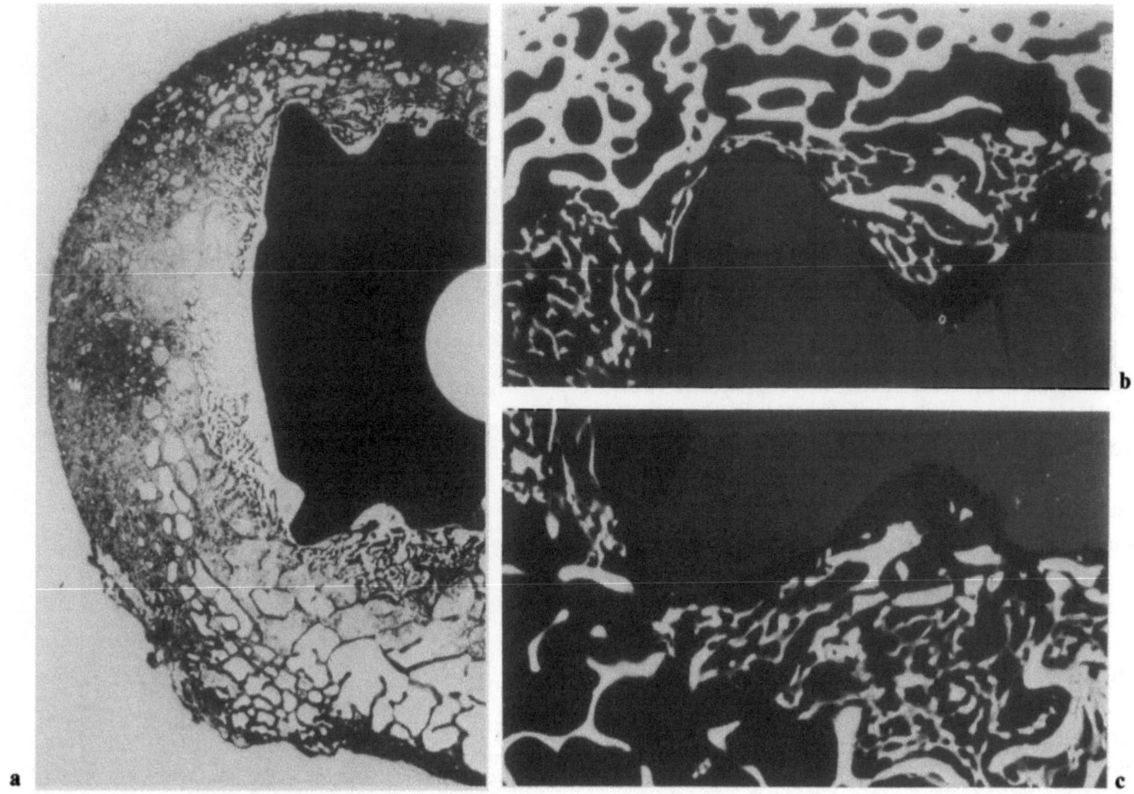

Fig. 5a–c. Histologic examination of the bed of an isoelastic femoral prosthesis 6 weeks after implantation. **a** Cross-section through trochanteric region and implant (3×). **b** Microradiograph of anterolateral edge of prosthesis with surrounding, newly-formed bony trabeculae (10×). **c** Posterolateral edge (10×) (preparation: Prof. R. Schenk, Anat. Institute, Bern)

ment of the cementless isoelastic prosthesis, we had fewer problems with the acetabular component than with the femoral component [2, 3, 4, 5, 6].

The primary goal for the femoral component was to design a stem possessing more or less the same deformation behavior as the femur itself. A femoral prosthesis consisting of a relatively thin metal armature embedded in polyacetal resin showed an elasticity very similar to that of the normal femur when subjected to stress tests (Fig. 1). Optical stress analyses of this isoelastic prosthesis also promised a significantly better stress distribution than could be obtained with metal prostheses (Fig. 2). After additional laboratory tests also showed positive results in terms of biocompatibility, surface properties, etc., we implanted the first isoelastic total hip replacement at our clinic on March 22, 1973. A total of 70 THRs of this model were implanted (Table 1). Initially, the majority of the patients had to be reoperated due to technical deficiencies, and later on due to loosening. The major cause of the failures was excessive elasticity in the proximal part of the femoral component (Fig. 3).

A prerequisite for the biomechanical incorporation of a prosthesis, and thus for its permanent fixation, is the prevention of stress concentrations and of relative movements between the implant and bone.

In contrast to the acetabular component, the femoral component must transmit forces other than pure compression: at least in its proximal portion, a bending force is also present (Fig. 3). This causes an intermittent lateral pressure to be exerted on the powerful calcar femorale. If the implant is too elastic, this intermittent pressure cannot be neutralized even by using tension-band screws and by seating the collar of the prosthesis on the calcar, as was originally hoped. Instead, the stresses lead to bone resorption and consequent loosening of the stem. The only way to eliminate such alternating loads in an intramedullary implant, and thus prevent bone resorption, is to stiffen the prosthesis in the trochanteric area. Thus, the prosthesis must be reinforced by means of a stronger metal armature in the neck-trochanteric area. A suggestion by Bombelli that the neck angle be increased from 135 to 144° has also been implemented. Additionally, "wings" have been attached to the posterior part of the prosthesis, and the component is now fixed to the bone with two cancellous bone screws instead of just one (Fig. 4a, b). The latter modifications serve mainly to enhance the stability of the prosthesis under torsional stresses.

We are currently testing a model with a beveled collar, designed to improve lateral force transmission to the femoral calcar.

As mentioned, the biomechanical integration of an implant, and thus the establishment of an intimate bond between implant and bone, is contingent upon a complete absence of relative motion at the interface. This means that a prosthesis implanted without cement must have a good primary fixation. From the very beginning, forces must be correctly transmitted from the implant to the bone, regardless of their magnitude. It has been our experience that a prosthesis may well exhibit good primary fixation as long as no weight is placed on the joint, but that the resumption of normal loading can lead to secondary bone resorption if the intermittent compressive loads are too great. Thus, it must be asked in earnest whether the permanent fixation of an implant might not benefit from a prolonged absence of weight-bearing on the operated hip. Our observations of secondary loosenings following a good primary incorporation suggest that a prolonged absence of weight-bearing can at best defer a potential loosening of the prosthesis, but cannot prevent it.

How securely can a polyacetal resin prosthesis be attached to the bone? As early as 1973, when we implanted our first model of the femoral prosthesis, we observed that in areas where conditions were ideal in terms of force transmission, primary fixation and mechanical rest (i.e., in the distal part of the stem), the prosthesis was firmly embedded in the surrounding bone, and bony ingrowth had taken place into the recesses on the prosthetic surface, creating a secure bond (Fig. 5a–c). In some cases the prosthesis was so firmly anchored that great difficulties were encountered at revision, and the prosthesis had to be chiseled out from the femoral shaft in pieces. This experience prompted us to prepare a conical-shaped cavity for the new model and omit the recesses on the distal end of the stem to simplify removal if revision should prove necessary (Fig. 4).

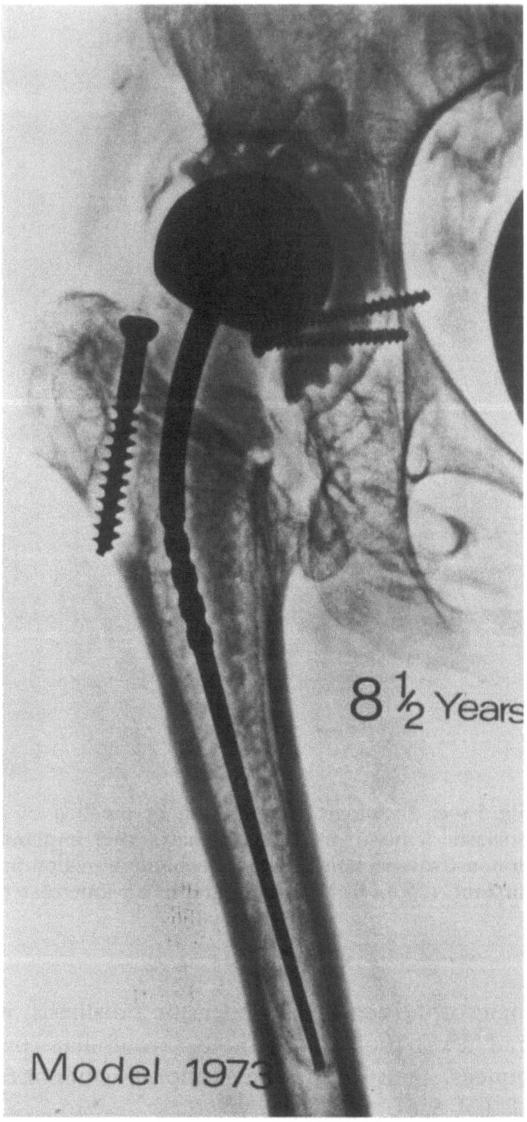

Fig. 6. Results of an "isoelastic" total hip replacement with the 1973 model 8½ years after implantation. There is heavy wear of the polyacetal resin cup. Despite the relatively high elasticity of this model, the stem of the femoral component is well incorporated. The patient is free of pain. Body weight: 45 kg. General physical activity is limited by osteoarthritis of the contralateral hip

Thus, having recognized that proximal stiffening of the implant is essential for long-term

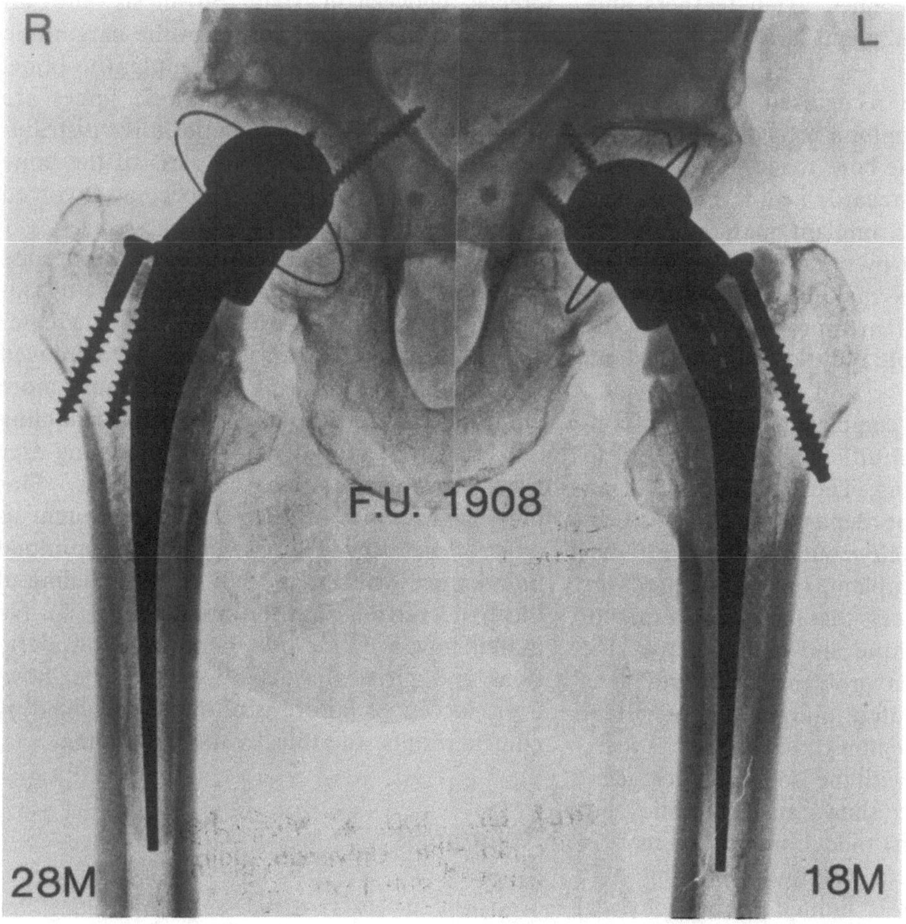

a b

Fig. 7a, b. Good result of a bilateral arthroplasty with the "isoelastic" total hip replacement, **a** 18 months and **b** 28 months after operation. There is excellent incorporation of all 4 components. The clinical result is equally good

success, what is our current concept of an isoelastic femoral prosthesis?

"Iso" means "equal," and so "isoelastic" can mean either 1) equal elasticity between a femur that is fitted with a prosthesis and one that is not, or 2) simply equal elasticity, and thus equal deformation behavior, between the bone and implant, regardless of the original deformation behavior of the bone. As mentioned, clinical results with the 1973 model clearly demonstrated that the first definition (i.e., no change in the deformation behavior of the femur) is not feasible. The second definition, however, always obtains when an implant is properly fixed to the bone and relative movements are excluded. In areas where forces are transmitted from implant to bone in the form of bending stresses, this condition of mechanical rest can be achieved only if the implant itself is not too strongly deformed under loads, i.e., is not too elastic.

But the elasticity of an implant depends as much on its overall geometry, or design, as on its elastic modulus.

Because the anchoring of a prosthetic stem in the medullary canal of the femur is somewhat like inserting a thin rod into a large-gauge tube, it is clear that the elasticity of the rod must be higher than that of the tube in areas of force application in order to obtain equal deformations under loading, and thus preclude relative movements. Galileo (1564–1642) is credited with the discovery that hollow rods offer greater resistance to fracture than solid rods of equal diameter, and that this principle explains why human and animal bones, avian feathers and the stems of certain plants are hollow rather than solid.

It also must be recognized that a plastic material exhibits a uniform mechanical behavior in all directions, while bone tissue shows marked differences in this regard, i.e., is anisotropic. The isotropy of the implant material can be corrected somewhat by modifying the shape of the prosthesis, thus making the deformation behavior of the implant approximate that of the bone. This is possible only to a limited extent, however.

An even more complex factor to be considered is individual differences with regard to elasticity and loading. The deformation of an implant or the bone depends not only on E-modulus and geometry, but also on the forces that act upon the implant. In view of the large individual differences that exist in terms of body weight, physique and activity level, the only answer to this problem is to provide a built-in upward "safety margin" of prosthetic elasticity. This is demonstrated by our 9 years' clinical experience with the isoelastic prosthesis: Fig. 6, for example, shows an "isoelastic" hip prosthesis of the first model, implanted in 1974 in a woman 154 cm tall and weighing only 45 kg. The patient is limited in her physical activity by severe osteoarthritis of the contralateral hip. After 8½ years the polyacetal resin cup shows considerable abrasive wear, but the femoral component is still firmly anchored. Thus, its elasticity was adequate for the loads imposed, taking into account the low body weight of the patient and her low activity level. The results achieved with the new model, which is reinforced in its proximal portion, give cause for optimism. Of the 40 prostheses implanted to date at our clinic, none has required revision due to loosening. It remains to be seen whether the prosthesis will stand the test of time in heavier patients.

A further limitation on the concept of isoelasticity concerns the remodeling capability of the bone. While the bone can continuously adapt to the forces acting on it, the prosthesis lacks this capability. On the other hand, there is no question that a greater elasticity than is possessed by the metal implants in wide use today is helpful in enabling the bone to undergo structural adaptation. After all, the main difference between a rigid prosthesis and an elastic prosthesis does not lie in the magnitude of the forces transmitted from implant to bone, but in the manner in which these forces are distributed to the bone. A better force distribution, in turn, will enable all parts of the bone surrounding the prosthesis to become involved in remodeling.

In summary, we are still convinced, despite the limitations attached to the concept of isoelasticity, that endoprostheses with a greater degree of elasticity than is generally employed are capable of ensuring a better and more uniform transmission of forces, thus enabling the bone to undergo natural remodeling free from abnormal stress concentrations. Our previous activities in this area have brought us much closer to realizing the goal of minimal interference with the physiologic remodeling of the bone surrounding the implant (Fig. 7). No matter how accurate our theoretical considerations and physical calculations may be, however, success or failure is ultimately decided by clinical results, and thus by the test of time.

References

1. Mathys R (1973) Stand der Verwendung von Kunststoffen für künstliche Gelenke. Aktuel Traumatol 3:253
2. Morscher E (1979) Isoelastische Prothesen. Langenbecks Arch Chir 349:321–326
3. Morscher E, Mathys R (1974) La prothèse totale isoélastique de hanche fixée sans ciment. Acta Orthop Belg 40:639–647
4. Morscher E, Mathys R (1975) Erste Erfahrungen mit einer zementlosen isoelastischen Totalprothese der Hüfte Z Orthop 113:745–749
5. Morscher E, Mathys R (1976) First experiences with a cementless isoelastic total prosthesis of the hip. In: Gschwend N, Debrunner HU (eds) Total hip prosthesis. Huber, Bern
6. Morscher E, Henche HR, Mathys R (1976) Isoelastic endoprosthesis – a new concept in artificial joint replacement. In: Schaldach M, Hohmann D (eds) Advances in artificial hip and knee joint technology. Engineering in medicine, vol 2. Springer, Berlin Heidelberg New York, p 403
7. Morscher E, Bombelli R, Schenk R, Mathys R (1981) The treatment of femoral neck fractures with an isoelastic endoprosthesis implanted without bone cement. Arch Orthop Traumat Surg 98:93–100
8. Morscher E, Dick W, Kernen V (1982) Cementless fixation of polyethylene acetabular component in total hip arthroplasty. Arch Orthop Traumat Surg 99:223–230

Experimental and Early Clinical Experience with an Uncemented UHMW Polyethylene Acetabular Prosthesis

M. Endler, Jr., F. Endler and H. Plenk, Jr.

In total hip replacement arthroplasty, the implantation of the acetabular component involves problems quite different from that of the femoral component. While the femoral endoprosthesis is inserted into a rigid, bony tube that is relatively resistant to deformation, the bony acetabulum can undergo considerable deformation on loading following the preparatory destruction of sclerotic bone that necessarily occurs during implantation of the component (Huggler et al., 1974). One means of eliminating this danger is to interpose a deformable layer at the interface between the acetabular prosthesis and the bone bed – a layer that is able to compensate for interfacial movements while serving as a medium for shock absorption. With a completely rigid implant, there is a danger that pathogenic stress concentrations will develop at the interface leading to local bone resorption and the eventual formation of a more or less thick connective-tissue membrane around the implant. Charnley (1979) always found a thick connective-tissue capsule around the acetabular prostheses in his long-term implant studies.

Based on these considerations, we may state certain basic requirements that must be satisfied by an uncemented acetabular prosthesis: Besides a stable, exercise-competent primary attachment, which is essential for successful incorporation of the implant (Griss, 1976; Swanson and Freeman, 1979), the prosthesis must be able to compensate to some extent for deformation of the bone bed without allowing significant deformation of the articulating surfaces of the prosthesis.

With regard to the implant material, it has been shown both experimentally and clinically that all bioinert materials can provide good skeletal attachment in the absence of stresses and movement, some materials becoming incorporated more rapidly than others (Galante et al., 1971; Klawitter and Hulbert, 1971; Cameron et al., 1972; Lyng et al., 1973; Spector et al., 1976, etc.). The moment a load is imposed upon the implant, its incorporation is determined by the nature of the resultant interfacial stresses and by the stability and mechanical properties of the material (Cameron et al., 1973; Biehl et al., 1975; Geduldig et al., 1975; Muhr et al., 1976; Griss, 1976; Plenk et al., 1978).

Guided by these considerations, we have developed an acetabular prosthesis made of ultrahigh-molecular-weight polyethylene which features a continuous, conical external thread (Endler and Endler, 1982). The conical thread has two functions: First, when the prosthesis is screwed into the precut thread in the acetabulum, the conical thread creates a wedge effect that sets up a good primary tension at the bone-implant interface, thus enhancing primary stability. Second, because the thread in the acetabulum can practically never be precut deep enough to receive the entire conical thread, a situation is created in which the bony acetabulum is "suspended" on the tips of the elastically-deformable polyethylene threads. This provides a shock-absorbing mechanism and also compensates for the slight deformations of the bone

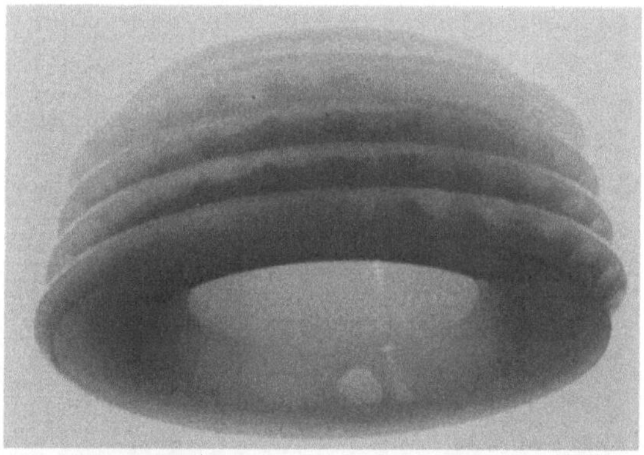

Fig. 1. Threaded polyethylene acetabular component. The drill holes that stabilize the device against rotation are clearly visible. The three holes at the socket inlet are for accommodating the seating tool

bed that are a practically inevitable consequence of surgical preparation.

To enhance the rotational stability of the prosthesis, drill holes 0.5 mm in diameter were placed in the flanks of the threads to enable bone and connective-tissue ingrowth (Fig. 1).

We felt that animal experiments were necessary to answer the following questions:

1. Does the conical thread provide the primary stability necessary for bony consolidation?
2. Does the primary interfacial tension predispose to pathogenic compressive stresses causing localized bone necrosis at the implant-bone interface?
3. In what manner does the implant-bone interface develop and what is its definitive form?
4. Does bone grow into the drill holes, or, if connective tissue ingrowth occurs, when is stability achieved by that process?

Animal experiments were conducted in 12 sheep, in which a total of 21 threaded polyethylene acetabular prostheses were implanted as part of a total hip replacement (Endler et al., 1981; Endler et al., 1982a, b). At necropsy, 2 loose acetabular components were found in 14 undislocated hips. The remaining 12 acetabular components were still clinically stable after implantation times of 1 week to 18 months and, as indicated by regular examinations with the Kistler plate, were subjected to loading during the experimental period (Endler et al., 1981).

After only a few weeks' implantation, a considerable degree of new bone formation was evident in addition to reparative processes. This bone formation was nondirectional and not only arose from bone fragments and the bone wound adjacent to the prosthesis, but was also apparent in the surrounding cancellous tissue (Fig. 2). While the new bone formation in the wound area may be interpreted largely as a biological reaction, the growth of the cancellous trabeculae in the intact acetabular bed appears to represent a functional adaptation to altered stress patterns.

This biologically-induced formation of mechanically unaligned bone tissue in the area of the bone wound is particularly evident during the first 3 months. Even large gaps between the implant and bone may become bridged during this period, assuming that the implant is stable.

Under the polarizing microscope, polychromatic optical stress phenomena can be observed in the birefractive polyethylene. Thus, up to 4 months' after implantation, isochromatic zones were frequently found at the tips of the polyethylene threads, indicating the presence of local compressive stresses. Because direct contact between the bone and implant was always found in those areas, it may be assumed that these stresses were created during the insertion of the prosthesis (Fig. 3). On the one hand, this would mean that at least a portion of the stabilizing primary tension is still present after 2 months. On the other hand, the local peak stresses do not appear to be large enough to cause bone resorption.

In the 3rd month after implantation, the definitive implant bed begins to take form. The threads of the prosthesis become invested by a

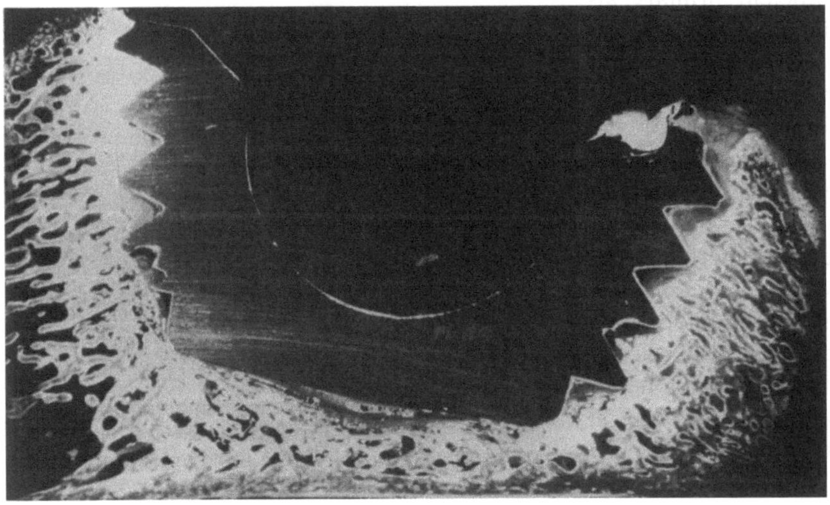

Fig. 2. Ground section of a polyethylene socket after 4 weeks' implantation. The specimen was labeled with tetracycline 2 days prior to removal. Light zones of new bone formation are present not only in the bone wound itself but also in the adjacent cancellous layer

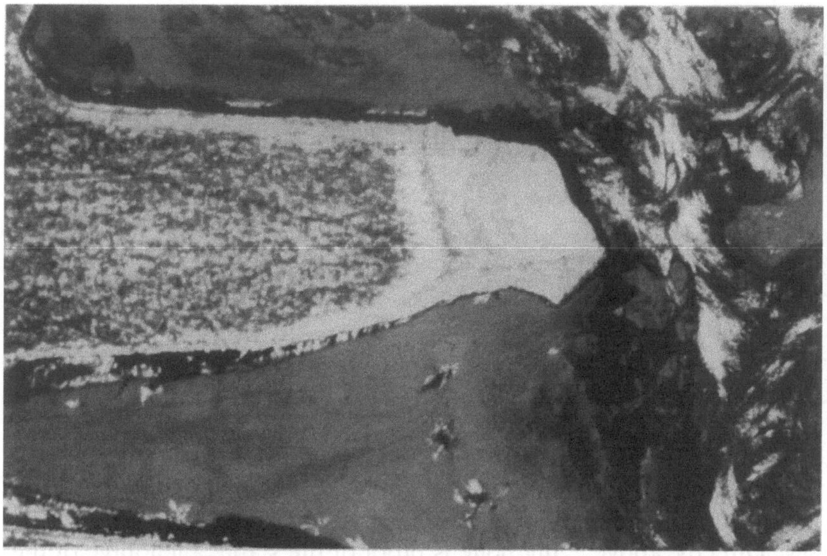

Fig. 3. Thin section through the load-bearing zone of the implant-bone interface after 4 months' implantation. In polarized light, isochromatic areas appear at sites of contact between the bone and the tip of the thread

layer of rigid collagen fibers that is markedly thinner in the load-bearing cranial region than in the unstressed caudal region. With the passage of time, there is a further ingrowth of bone into the hollows between the threads, and cartilage islands form over the tips of the threads (Fig. 4).

Almost all specimens examined showed this typical fiber-rich implant bed, with fibrocartilage pads forming over the tips of the threads and slowly spreading along the flanks. We believe that the transformation of the primary granulation tissue into differentiated supporting tissue follows the laws of causal histogenesis (Pauwels, 1960; Kummer, 1963). Between the outermost parts of the polyethylene threads and the prepared acetabulum, compressive stresses arise which create a mechanical stimulus for the formation of collagen fiber-rich tissue. As they form, the fibers become aligned in accordance

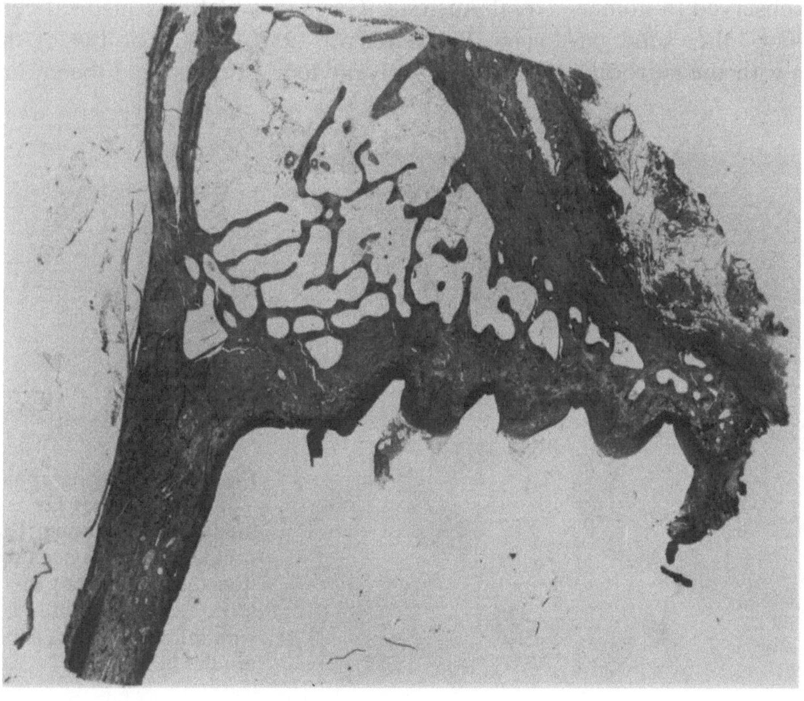

Fig. 4. Thin section in the principal load-bearing direction after 18 months' implantation (toluidine blue). A continuous bony layer has formed around the socket, and bone has invaded the hollows between the threads. Delicate cartilage pads (*dark*) are seen around the tips of the threads

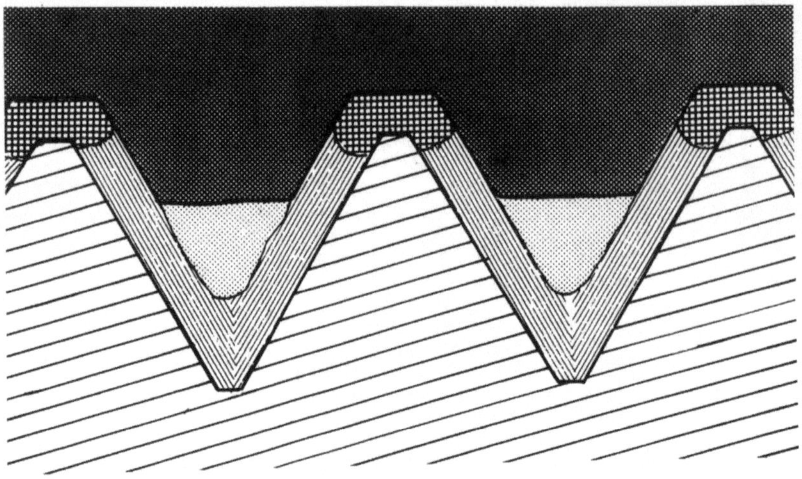

Fig. 5. Schematic representation of tissue synthesis processes around the socket (*slanting lines*). The threads of the socket are initially invested with collagen fiber-rich tissue (*parallel lines*), which is converted to fibrocartilage (*cross- hatched*) at the tips of the threads. New bone formation (*light shading*) occurs in zones of absolute rest (here: in the hollows between the threads). The new bone is in direct attachment with the preexisting bone (*dark shading*)

with prevailing tensile stresses. Directly above the tips of the threads, stabilization by the collagen fibers leads to zones of hydrostatic pressure, stimulating a differentiation into fibrocartilage, which then gradually spreads along the flanks of the threads. According to Pauwels, there is no typical mechanical stimulus which initiates formation of the bone tissue itself. It develops in zones of absolute rest on the basis of a collagen fiber-rich tissue – a situation occurring deep in the hollows of the polyethylene threads (Fig. 5).

The drill holes were found to contain granulation tissue only a few weeks after implantation. Starting in the 6th month, bone ingrowth into the drill holes could be observed in numerous specimens. In our view, the solid attachment of these ingrowths with the surrounding bone is proof of the stable anchorage of the acetabular prosthesis (Fig. 6).

Because the prostheses employed a fixation principle that already had been tested and proved effective (by Mittelmeier, in 1974, who used a ceramic socket with conical thread) and was composed of a material, polyethylene, that had been proven in conventional total hip replacements, we felt it was safe to implant the socket in selected human patients concurrently with the animal studies. After the first results of the animal experiments were made available, and a special instrumentation package had been developed, a field study was launched in which implantations of the device were started at several Austrian, German and Swiss medical centers. By March of 1982, a total of 194 of the threaded polyethylene sockets had been im-

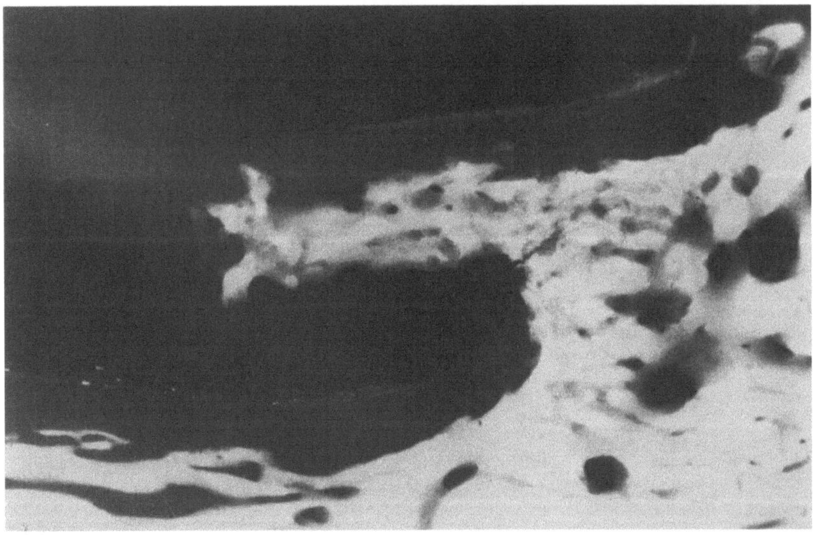

Fig. 6. Microradiograph of a thin section after 12 months' implantation. The drill hole that has been sectioned contains bony ingrowth that is continuous with the surrounding acetabular bone

planted at the Hera Sanatorium and University Orthopedic Clinic in Vienna. After some initial difficulties, no significant problems were encountered during the implantations (in 4 cases cement had to be used to attach the socket securely).

The socket is produced in 4 sizes, and so far this range has proved to be entirely adequate. On reviewing the sizes that were implanted, it is seen that the two intermediate sizes were by far the most frequently used (Table 1). From July, 1978, to March, 1981, a total of 79 threaded polyethylene sockets were implanted at the two centers indicated above. In 19 cases a Weber-Stümer stem was used for the femoral component, and in 60 cases an uncemented Zweymüller stem. Seventy-two of these patients could be followed for at least a year. The longest follow-up was 39 months, the shortest 17 months.

The arthroplasties were performed for a variety of conditions. Fifty-four patients had idiopathic osteoarthritis, 5 with associated severe polar head necrosis. Eight patients had dysplasia, 5 suffered from PCP, and 7 were treated with a prosthesis for femoral head necrosis.

Even the relatively shallow acetabula in the dysplastic hip joints provided enough stock to seat the threaded socket securely (Fig. 7). Moreover, in metabolic osteopathies secondary to treatment with cortisone, it was found that the socket was incorporated into the bony acetabulum without difficulty (Fig. 8). In the present series of 79 patients, complications relating to the joint itself arose in 5 cases (Table 2). Only 2 patients had periarticular ossifications severe enough to cause functional disability and warrant surgical removal. In one patient, a woman, the cemented Weber-Stümer stem became loose after 16 months. At revision, the acetabular component was found to be stably anchored, and the woman is now largely free of complaints. Finally, one patient in whom the socket was implanted at an excessively "open" angle complained of severe pain on weight bearing. When revision was done 8 months later (abroad), no sign of acetabular loosening was apparent. The patient was treated with a conventional cemented prosthesis and now is largely free of complaints, suggesting that the pain may have been due to a partial dislocation during weight bearing.

Table 1. Sizes of Implanted Acetabular Components

Size	Number implanted
52 mm	13
58 mm	95
64 mm	68
68 mm	18

Table 2. Complications

1 early dislocation
2 periarticular calcifications
1 loose stem
1 socket excessively open

Table 3. Evaluation of Results

Age	Hip index	
	Preoperative	Postoperative
over 90	0	29
80 – 89	0	34
66 – 71	0	6
50 – 65	16	3
under 50	63	0

The clinical results are entirely comparable to the short-term results of conventional prostheses implanted with cement. To make an overall assessment, we used the Harris index, in which pain and walking ability are the principal criteria (Table 3). A complete restoration of normal hip function could be achieved in 29 patients. The largest group, consisting of 34 patients, showed only a mild degree of disability that did not interfere with their daily activities. Three polyarthritic patients still had significant disability after the surgery, although they complained of no hip pain and had good joint motion.

The effect of the operation on pain was quite good. Again, the Harris scale was used for evaluation: 50 patients were entirely free of complaints after the surgery, 19 reported periods of weather sensitivity or mild pain after extreme exertion, and only 3 complained of severe pain after heavy exertion, though this did not limit their daily activities (Table 4).

A radiographic evaluation was somewhat difficult due to the radiotransparency of the acetabular components (only the marking wire

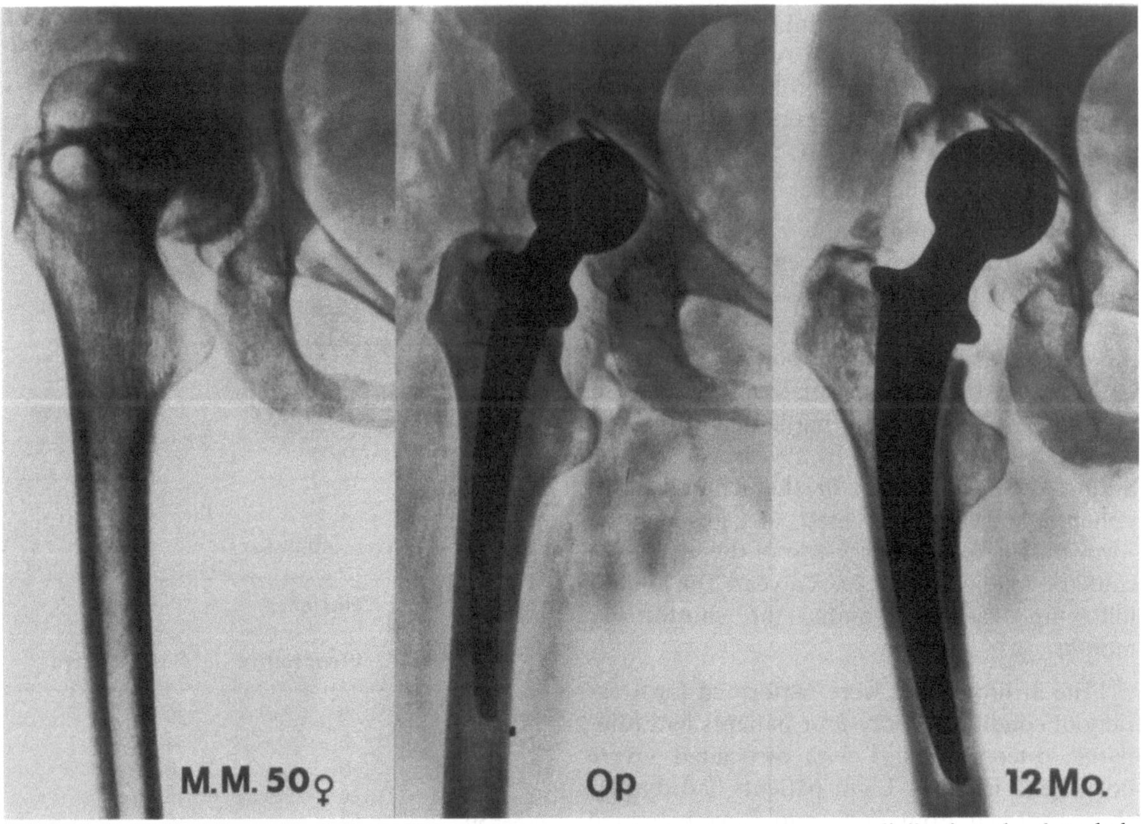

Fig. 7. Dysplasia with osteoarthritis in a 50-year-old woman. Owing to the strong medialization, the threaded acetabular component can be attached without difficulty to the thickened acetabular floor

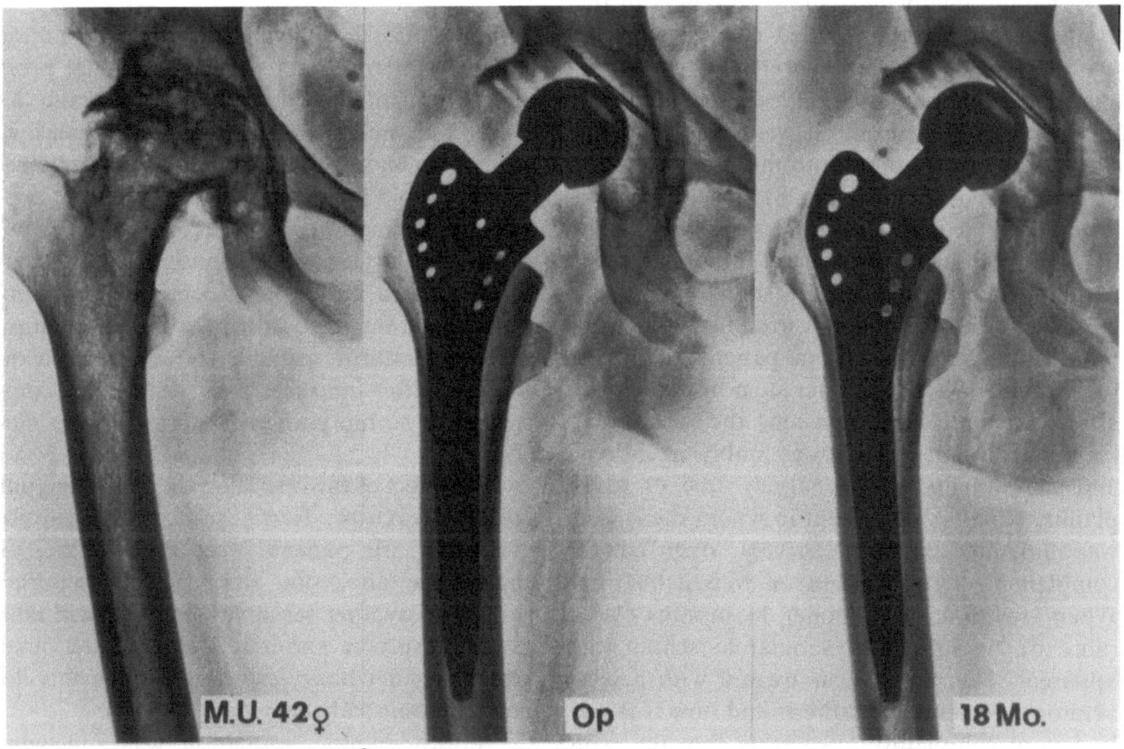

a b c

Fig. 8 a–c. Secondary, cortisone-induced femoral head necrosis in a 42-year-old woman with a kidney transplant. The disturbance of bone metabolism in no way delays the incorporation of the uncemented socket

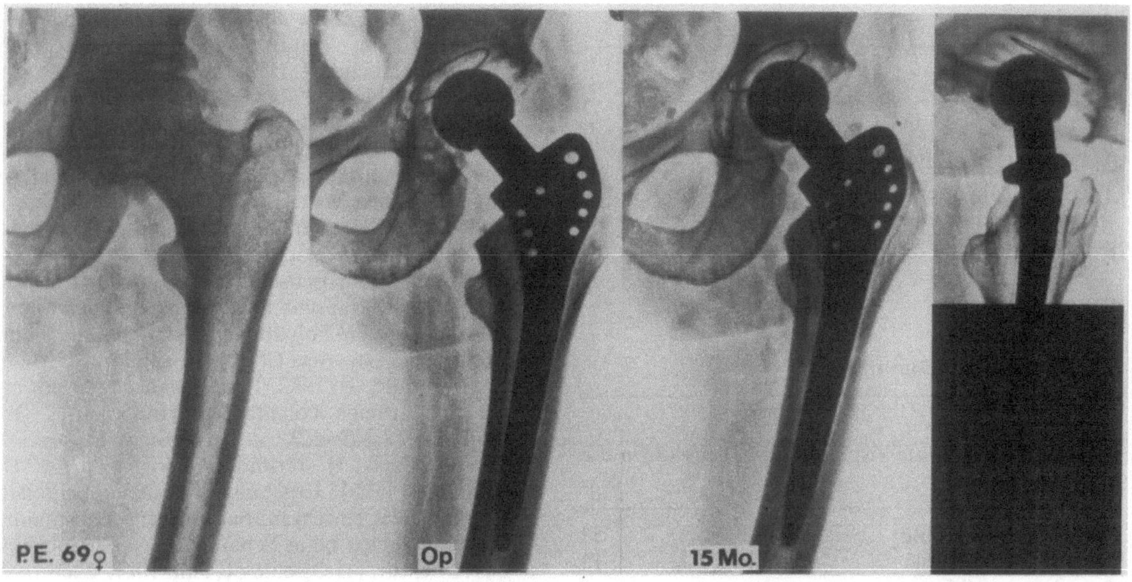

a b c d

Fig. 9 a–d. Medial osteoarthritis in a 79-year-old woman. 15 months after arthroplasty the impression of the socket threads in the bone is clearly visible, indicating good functional adaptation of the bone bed

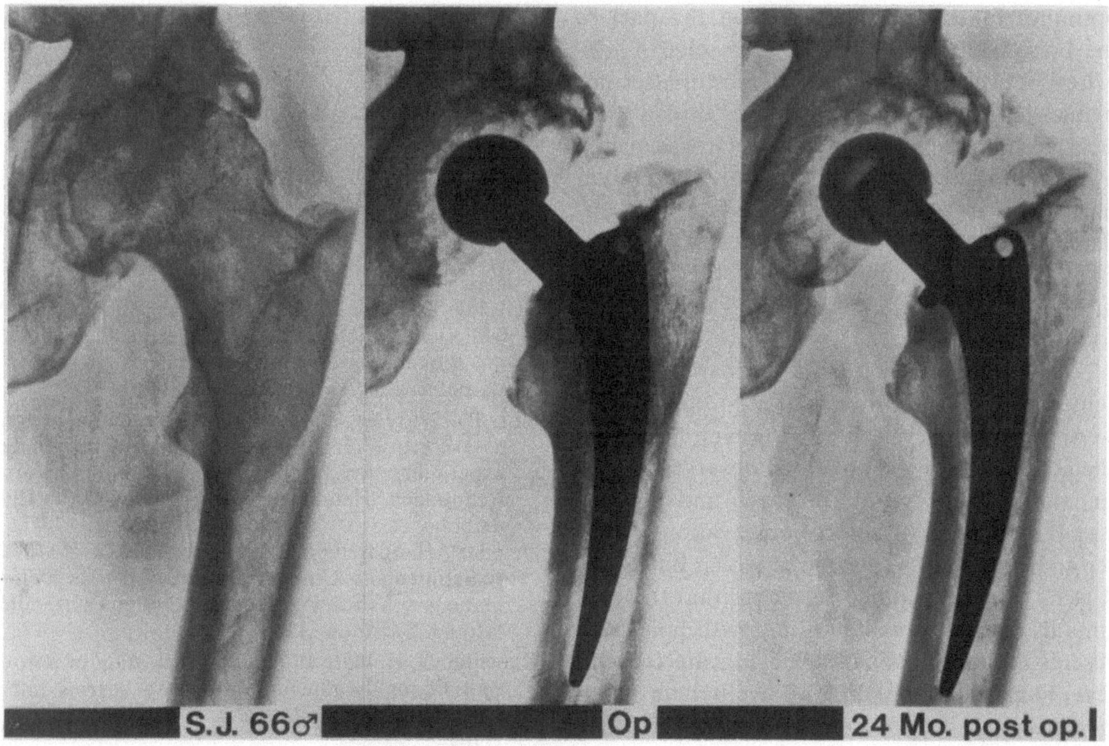

a b c

Fig. 10. a Concentric cartilage necrosis in a 66-year-old man. **b** The threads in the bony acetabulum are only faintly visible. **c** After 2 years, sclerotic bone still has not formed around the socket. However, the patient is entirely free of complaints, indicating that no loosening of the socket has occurred

Table 4. Pain

Preoperative		Postoperative
0	Free of pain	50
0	Weather sensitivity	19
2	Slight pain after prolonged exertion	3
38	Moderate pain on weight bearing	0
39	Severe pain on weight bearing	0
2	Severe, continuous pain	0

Table 5. Radiographic Visualization of Threads in the Bony Acetabulum

Threads clearly visible	53
Threads faintly visible	13
Threads not visible	6

is directly visible). In many cases a delicate zone of sclerotic bone formed around the tips of the polyethylene threads, creating an accurate "mold" of the threads that could be seen on x-rays. We believe that this process reflects an optimum functional adaptation on the part of the bone bed (Endler, 1982). This sclerosis develops between the 3rd and 9th month after implantation (Fig. 9). In 53 cases the "thread" was clearly visible on x-ray; in 13 cases it was visible over only part of the socket (mainly the cranial part), and in 6 cases no impression was apparent (Table 5, Fig. 10). Nevertheless, no socket migration was noted in any of the operated hips, nor was there any clinical evidence of socket loosening.

We realize that the short-term results presented here do not prove the long-term stability of our acetabular implant. However, based on the adaptation of the bone bed observed experimentally (Endler et al., in press) and the corresponding positive clinical observations (Endler and Endler, 1982), some of which date back 4 years, we feel justified in stating that the continuous conical thread with ingrowth holes represents a valid means of achieving the cementless fixation of UHMW polyethylene components.

References

Biehl G, Harm J, Mäusle E (1975) Tierexperimentelle und histopathologische Untersuchungen über die Anpassungsvorgänge des Knochens nach der Implantation von Tragrippenendoprothesen. Arch Orthop Unfallchir 81:105

Cameron H, McNab I, Pillar R (1972) Porous surfaced vitallium staple. S Afr J Surg 10:63

Cameron H, Pillar R, McNab I (1973) The effect of movement on the banding of porous metal to bone. J Biomed Mater Res 7:301

Charnley J (1979) Low friction arthroplasty of the hip. Springer, Berlin Heidelberg New York

Endler M (1982) Theoretisch experimentelle Grundlagen und erste klinische Erfahrungen mit einer neuen zementfreien Polyäthylenschraubpfanne beim Hüftgelenkersatz. Acta Chir Austria [Suppl] 45:1–20

Endler M, Endler F (1982) Erste Erfahrungen mit einer zementfreien Polyäthylenschraubpfanne. Orthop Prax 18:319–323

Endler M, Plenk H, Grundschober F, Girtler D, Schnabl H (1981) Ergebnisse der experimentellen Prüfung einer einschraubbaren Hüftgelenkspfanne aus Polyäthylen beim Schaf. Vortr. 6. Symposium des Arbeitskr. für Osteologie, Juni 1981, Wien

Endler M, Girtler D, Schnabl H, Plenk J, Grundschober F (1982a) Tierexperimentelle Untersuchungen mit einer zementfreien Polyäthylenpfanne. Z Orthop 120:404

Endler M, Schnabl H, Girtler D, Seebacher M (1982b) Untersuchungen mit einer Kistler-Mehrkomponentenkraftmessplatte an gesunden und hüftoperierten Schafen. Z Orthop 120:403

Endler M, Plenk H, Grundschober F, Girtler D, Schnabl H (im Druck) Ergebnisse der experimentellen Prüfung einer einschraubbaren Hüftgelenkspfanne aus Polyäthylen beim Schaf. Z Orthop

Galante JO, Rostoker W, Lueck R, Ray RD (1971) Sintered fiber metal composites as a basis for attachment of implants to bone. J Bone Joint Surg (Am) 53:101–114

Galante IO, Rostoker H (1973) Wear in total hip prosthesis. An experimental evaluation of candidate materials. Acta Orthop Scand [Suppl] 145:1–46

Geduldig D, Dörre E, Happel M, Lade R, Prüssner P, Willert HG, Zichner L (1975) Welche Aussicht hat die Biokeramik als Implantatmaterial in der Orthopädie? Med Orthop Techn 6:138

Griss P (1976) Die Aluminiumoxydkeramik – ein neuer Werkstoff für Endoprothesen. Ergebnisse der experimentellen Prüfung und erste klinische Anwendungen. Habilitationsschrift, Universität Heidelberg

Huggler AH, Schreiber A, Dietschi C, Jakob H (1974) Experimentelle Untersuchungen über das Deformationsverhalten des Hüftacetabulums unter Belastung. Z Orthop 112:44

Klawitter JJ, Hulbert SF (1971) Application of porous ceramic for the attachment of load bearing internal orthopedic applications. J Biomed Mater Res 2:161

Kummer B (1963) Grundlagen der Biomechanik des menschlichen Stütz- und Bewegungsapparates. Verh. IX. Congr. SICOT, Wien Bd 2, 60

Lyng S, Sudmann E, Hulbert SF, Suaer WB (1973) Fixation of permanent orthopedic prosthesis. Use

of ceramics in the tibial plateaus. Acta Orthop Scand 44:694
Mittelmeier H (1974) Zementlose Verankerung von Prothesen nach dem Tragrippen-Prinzip. Z Orthop 112:27
Muhr G, Stockhusen H, Müller O (1976) Die Hüftarthroplastik mit isoelastischen Totalprothesen im Tierexperiment. Arch Orthop Unfallchir 86:115
Pauwels F (1960) Eine neue Theorie über den Einfluß mechanischer Reize auf die Differenzierung der Stützgewebe. Z Anat Entw Gesch 121:478
Plenk H Jr, Locke H, Punzet G, Zweymüller K (1978) Biomechanical aspects of bone reactions on total bioceramic hipjoint endoprosthesis. Vortr. Meeting of the European Soc. of biomaterials Brüssel, 22. u. 23. Mai 1978
Spector M, Flemming WR, Kreutner A, Sauer BW (1976) Bone growth into porous high density polyethylene. J Biomed Mater Res 10/4:595
Swanson SA, Freeman MA (1979) Die wissenschaftlichen Grundlagen des Gelenkersatzes. Springer, Berlin Heidelberg New York

Cementless Fixation of a Polyethylene Acetabular Component

E. Morscher and W. Dick

As we know from the studies of Huggler et al. [5], the pelvis, and with it the acetabulum, has a relatively high elasticity and undergoes considerable deformation when subjected to loads. Moreover, because the acetabular cartilage absorbs only about 10% of the energy transmitted to it, it appears that its main function is to distribute loads [3, 6]. This function can be better maintained with an elastic acetabular component that is in close contact with the bone than with a rigid implant or a component that is coated with a layer of brittle cement.

The first acetabular cup that we implanted without cement was composed of polyacetal resin. Contrary to our expectations of this material based on the results of laboratory experiments, the implant underwent a very high degree of abrasive wear *in vivo,* forcing us to abandon the further use of polyacetal for acetabular reconstructions. In 1977 we designed an acetabular cup made of high-density polyethylene, which again was implanted without cement according to the same principles. Polyethylene is a highly favorable material for acetabular cups owing to its shock-absorbing and force-distributing properties, which derive from its high compressibility and high impact strength.

Based on the principle that the natural form and function of the hip joint should be disturbed as little as possible in order to preserve natural patterns of force transmission, we chose a hemispherical shape for the acetabular cup. The forces associated with weight-bearing are transmitted chiefly in the cortical substance of the pelvic bone and in the subchondral bone of the acetabulum. A spherical-shaped cup provides a contact surface at which the forces that develop between the pelvis and femoral head can be transmitted in a physiologic balance between compression and shear. The spherical shape also eliminates undesired stress concentrations like those that occur with cement fixation or in cups that deviate from a spherical shape (e.g., cylinders).

The fixation of an implant can be improved by enlarging its area of surface contact. In the present implant, this is accomplished with circular grooves. Because the cup is also acted upon by torsional forces caused by friction between the femoral head and acetabulum, two pegs were placed on the weight-bearing part of the outer surface of the cup to prevent rotational movements. At implantation, screws are also inserted to produce primary compression between the cup and bone and create an additional safeguard against rotation (Figs. 1 and 2).

Maximum fixation of the implant by bony ingrowth into the grooves on the outer cup

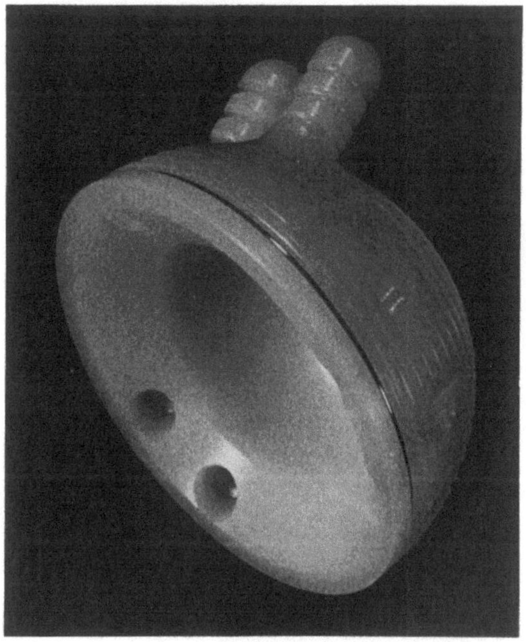

Fig. 1. Standard polyethylene acetabular cup designed for cementless fixation (manufacturer: Robert Mathys, Surgical Instruments, CH-2544 Bettlach/Switzerland)

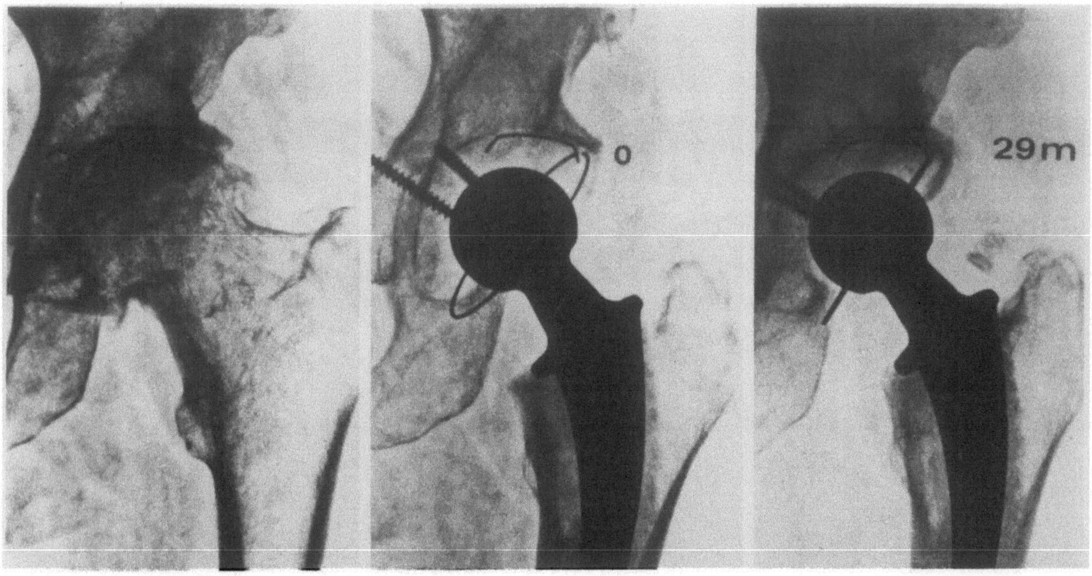

a b c

Fig. 2a–c. Cementless fixation of the polyethylene cup. **a** H.M., 68-year-old woman with primary osteoarthritis of the hip. **b** Total hip arthroplasty with uncemented polyethylene cup and cemented metal stem. **c** 29-month result. Note new subchondral bone formation in the weight-bearing area of the cup

surface takes some time to achieve. With the first cups, which had wider and deeper grooves so that bone ingrowth could be monitored radiologically, this process took approximately 6–9 months.

Movements between the implant and bone, like those that may occur with premature weight-bearing, interfere with new bone formation on the prosthetic surface [4]. Relative movements are practically eliminated, however, if the forces transmitted between implant and bone are purely compressive in nature. This is the situation at least in the cranial part of the cup. Below the equator of the cup, tensile forces occur which tend to disrupt contact between the bone and implant (Fig. 2).

Because loads from the pelvis are transmitted through the subchondral bone of the acetabulum, as mentioned above, it is important to spare as much of this bone as possible during preparation of the acetabulum. Studies by Amstutz [1] have shown, moreover, that micromovements increase when the subchondral bone is removed. In cement fixation, multiple drill holes are made in the subchondral bone to provide interdigitation between the cement and acetabulum and thus enhance the stability of the fixation. In cementless fixation, this bone stock should be preserved to the greatest extent possible. Cartilage is removed from the bone with a pneumatic drill and spherical reamer only until bleeding points appear on the subchondral bone. This will enable connective tissue from this bone to grow into the recesses on the prosthetic surface and subsequently ossify.

If the subchondral sclerotic layer has to be removed, as during the preparation of a shallow acetabulum, or if this layer is already absent, as during the conversion of an arthrodesis to an arthroplasty, it becomes necessary to anchor the cup in the cancellous bone of the pelvis. This will probably allow some degree of migration to occur until compressive forces stimulate the formation of a new subchondral bone layer.

The position of the cup in relation to the geometry of the pelvis must be such that the stresses of weight-bearing are transmitted from the pelvis to the prosthesis largely in the form of compressive forces, and the implant is in close apposition with the bone over the largest area possible.

Because the natural acetabulum is inclined 45° with respect to the horizontal plane and shows 10° of anteversion, this is the position that most orthopedic surgeons choose for the acetabular cup. However, clinical and radiologic observations as well as theoretical calcula-

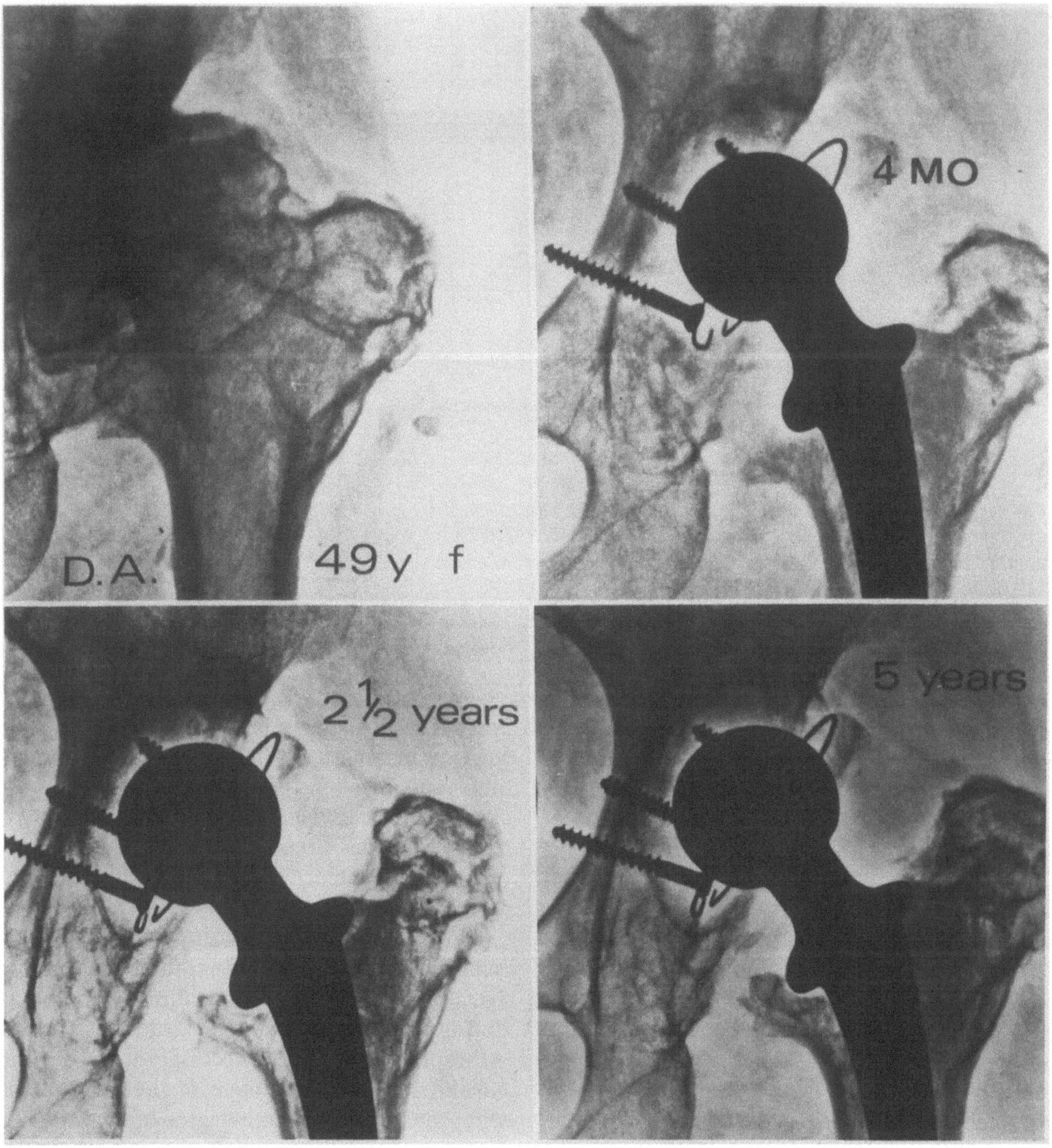

a c b d

Fig. 3a–d. 5-year result with uncemented polyethylene cup. **a** D.A., 49-year-old woman with osteoarthritis of the hip following intertrochanteric osteotomy for acetabular dysplasia. **b–d** Situation 4 months, 2½ years and 5 years after total hip arthroplasty with uncemented polyethylene cup and cemented steel stem

tions suggest that a more horizontal position would be more favorable. Thus, radiologic observations of loose cups show that, aside from cases of central migration or penetration, the cup tends to separate from the pelvis in its caudal portion and tip lateralward, the cranial part of the cup serving as a "hinge" for this displacement. One must conclude from this observation that there is a laterally-directed force acting upon the acetabular component. According to the theoretical calculations of Bombelli [2], such a force indeed exists. This force also accounts for the lateral subluxation of the femoral head in osteoarthritis of the hip. In addition, Bombelli points to the existence of a "Gothic arch" as a sign that forces are transmitted vertically to the femoral head from the body center of gravity, and not at the 16° angle calculated by Pauwels. This view is supported by our own observations with cementless polyethylene cups: cups implanted in a more horizontal position generally showed a broader zone of sclerosis formation than cups implanted at a more "open" angle.

Results

Between August 1977 and June 1982, we used our cementless acetabular cup in 534 primary total hip arthroplasties, combining it with a cemented metal femoral component. The first 250 cases, with an observation period of 6–48 months (average 19 months), were followed up in the summer of 1981. These results have been published [7]. We have not yet recognized any case of aseptic loosening of the acetabular component, either at that time or during the intervening months.

Radiographic Findings

Radiographs taken at regular intervals have demonstrated an absolutely uniform pattern with the exception of 4 cases that were complicated by infection. In many cases the subchondral bone layer is difficult to visualize in the immediate postoperative period, having been thinned during preparation of the acetabulum. However, the bone surrounding the polyethylene cup undergoes an increasing sclerosis and densification during subsequent weeks and months. This occurs almost exclusively in the cranial zone, which is the major weight-bearing area. Bone density continues to increase for about 9–12 months postoperatively. By 1 year after operation no further changes can be detected, indicating that a state of biomechanical equilibrium has been established, and thus that the biomechanical integration of the acetabular component has been achieved (Fig. 3). Below the equator of the cup, a fibrous layer generally is interposed between the polyethylene and the bone.

Postmortem Findings

To date we have conducted only two postmortem examinations of hip joints fitted with an uncemented acetabular cup. One patient was an 83-year-old woman who died of a ruptured aortic aneurysm 3 weeks after the arthroplasty was performed. The cup was in very close apposition to the bony acetabulum. Histologically, of course, there had not yet been any bone ingrowth into the recesses on the prosthetic surface. The second examination was performed in an 82-year-old man who died 3 years after operation. The cup was firmly anchored to the bone. A marked increase of bone density was evident in the weight-bearing zone, and in some places dense bone was separated only by a very thin layer of fibrous tissue from the surface of the polyethylene prosthesis (Fig. 4).

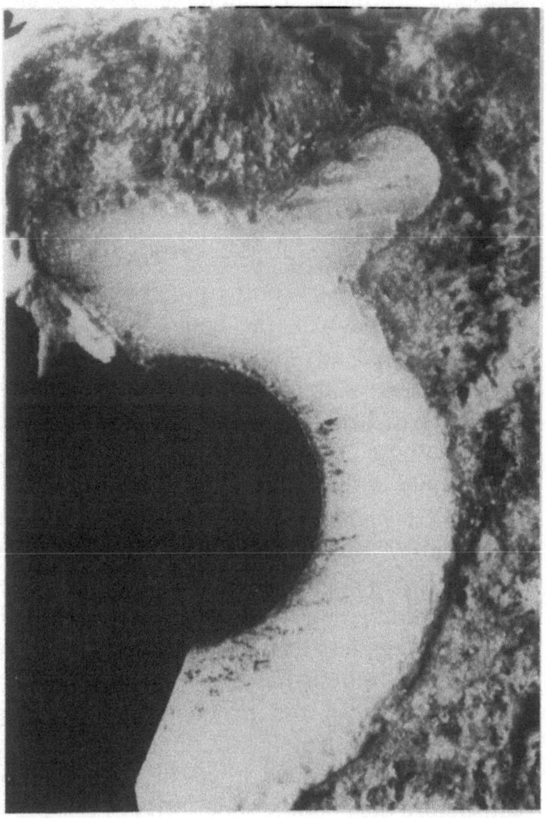

Fig. 4. Cross-section through the polyethylene cup of an 82-year-old man who died 3 years after operation

Histologic studies are also available for 4 prostheses that had to be removed and replaced on account of infection. These studies revealed a more or less pronounced osteolysis of the subchondral bony layer surrounding the acetabular cup, and a relatively thick inflammatory membrane was interposed between the bone tissue and prosthesis. In one case close contact was observed between the bone and prosthesis, but only a very mild, low-grade infection was involved. In this case depressed areas had formed on the surface of the prosthesis in its weight-bearing portion. We had observed similar depresssions and irregularities on the weight-bearing part of cemented polyethylene cups in cases where cement coverage was patchy, allowing parts of the prosthesis to come in direct contact with the bone. We have not yet encountered any problems associated with these changes in the prosthetic surface. However, the presence of polyethylene traces in the adjacent bone tissue suggests that it may be advisable in the future to coat the polyethylene with a material that would not hamper the elasticity of the cup, and that perhaps would be receptive to bony ingrowth.

In summary, we may say that experience with the cementless fixation of our polyethylene acetabular prosthesis has been entirely positive. However, because the problem of loosening does not become truly acute until 5, 8 or more years after implantation, it will be several more years before the possible superiority of this prosthetic technique over other methods can be substantiated. Nevertheless, we are already convined that for revision arthroplasties in patients with acetabular deficiencies, cementless fixation combined with bone grafting offers significant advantages over any other technique (see Dick/Jenny/Morscher: Revision Arthroplasties with the Isoelastic Total Hip Replacement).

References

1. Amstutz H (1982) Restoration of functional biomechanics in reconstructive hip surgery. NIH Consensus Development Conference, Bethesda, Maryland
2. Bombelli R (1976) Osteoarthritis of the hip. Springer, Berlin Heidelberg New York
3. Christel P, Derethe P, Sedel L (1980) Periacetabular pressure recording, using a hip simulator. Acta Orthop Belg 46:647–662
4. Ducheyne P, De Meester P, Aeroudt E, Martens M, Mulier JC (1977) Influence of functional dynamic loading on bone ingrowth into surface pores of orthopaedic implants. J Biomed Mater Res 11:811–838
5. Huggler A, Schreiber A, Dietschi C, Jacob H (1974) Experimentelle Untersuchungen über das Deformationsverhalten des Hüftazetabulum unter Belastung. Z Orthop 112:44–50
6. Meunier A, Blouet J, Christel P, Sedel L (1978) Etude expérimentale du choc avec frottement d'un contact cartilage/métal. IIe Congres de Biomécanique, Paris
7. Morscher EW, Dick W, Kernen V (1982) Cementless fixation of polyethylene acetabular component in total hip arthroplasty. Arch Orthop Trauma Surg 99:223–230

Experience with Uncemented Polyethylene Acetabular Prostheses

K. Knahr, M. Salzer and P. Frank

The introduction of bioceramics into joint replacement arthroplasty enabled the first uncemented acetabular prosthesis to be implanted in tumor patients in 1974 [4]. This prosthesis derived its main attachment from three symmetrically-arranged pegs, which enabled a mechanically stable primary anchorage to be achieved. In subsequent years uncemented acetabular prostheses of this type were implanted in 14 additional tumor patients and in 71 patients with degenerative arthritis [3].

Due to the high rate of ceramic head fractures, further use of this material was abandoned in 1978. But because the peg design had proved advantageous for the acetabular prosthesis (no revisions had been necessary due to primary loosening of the component), the attachment principle was retained, and only the ceramic material was replaced by polyethylene.

Materials

From June, 1979, to the end of May, 1982, a total of 350 pegged sockets made of polyethylene were implanted at the General Orthopedic Department of Vienna-Gersthof. The present review covers only those implants inserted between June, 1979, and September, 1980, in order that at least an 18-month follow-up could be obtained.

During that period, a total of 77 of the sockets were inserted in 76 patients. These consisted of 24 men and 52 women ranging in age from 34 to 79. The average age at the time of the operation was 60. The only exception was an 8-year-old boy who sustained a pathologic fracture of the proximal femur secondary to radiation therapy for an Ewing sarcoma. In this case the affected part of the femur was resected and replaced with a total endoprosthesis. Until his death from generalized metastasis 18 months postoperatively, the patient had full motion and weight-bearing ability in the operated limb.

Table 1. Cement-Free Implantations of Pegged Polyethylene Acetabular Prostheses from June, 1979, to September, 1980 (n = 77)

Diagnosis	
Idiopathic osteoarthritis	49
Osteoarthritis sec. to dysplasia	8
Malignant bone tumor	12
Radiation necrosis	3
Revision THR	3
Chronic polyarthritis	1
Bekhterev's disease	1
Sex distribution	
24 men : 52 women	
Age distribution	
(8) 34 – 79 years (average = 60.0)	

Forty-nine patients were diagnosed as having idiopathic osteoarthritis of the hip. Eight patients had osteoarthritis secondary to dysplasia, 12 had a malignant bone tumor, and 3 had severe femoral head damage secondary to radiotherapy for a gynecologic malignancy. Additional indications were 3 revisions of primary total hip replacements, 1 chronic polyarthritis, and 1 degenerative arthritis associated with Bekhterev's disease.

Surgical Technique

The implantation of a pegged socket is somewhat involved from a technical standpoint and requires careful preparation of the acetabulum. First the acetabular inlet should be freed of troublesome capsule remnants about its entire circumference. After the acetabulum has been reamed down to the inner cortex, the peg template is applied. This should have a stable primary seating within the acetabulum. The template is additionally secured with a Kirschner

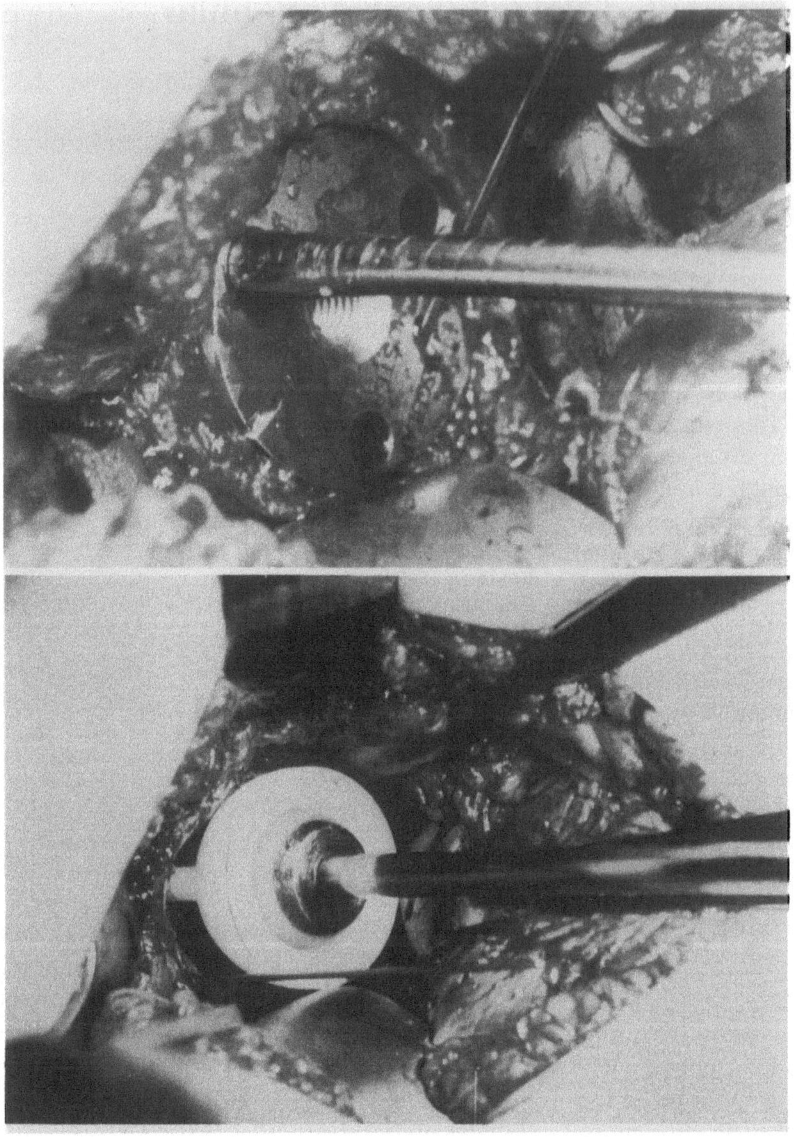

a

b

Fig. 1 a, b. Implantation technique for uncemented, pegged acetabular prosthesis. **a** The template is inserted, and the anchoring holes are cut with a flexible drill. **b** Marking the rotational alignment makes it easier to fit the pegs accurately into the anchoring holes

wire, and then the anchoring holes are cut using a drill with a flexible shaft (Fig. 1a). It is usual for the inner cortex of the pelvis to be perforated at this time. After the rotational position of the template has been marked with a Kirschner wire (the marking on the template corresponds to that on the prosthesis), the template is removed, and the polyethylene cup is inserted using the marking as a guide (Fig. 1b). The cup is driven in firmly with the aid of an impactor to achieve a mechanically stable primary seating.

Results

Of the 76 patients with 77 implanted acetabular prostheses, 8 died before the minimum follow-up period of 18 months had elapsed. The remaining 69 hips were examined clinically and radiologically after a period of 18–33 months (average 24.2 months).

The clinical results were evaluated according to the Harris scale [1]. It is important to note that the present study represents an overall assessment of the hip prosthesis and does not permit specific inferences to be drawn with regard to the acetabular component. Of the 69 hip joints that were reviewed, 43 showed an excellent or good result (more than 80 points). The result was rated as fair (70–79 points) in 16 cases, and as poor (less than 70 points) in 10 cases. Most poor results were due to problems of functional rehabilitation (poor walking ability, reliance on walking aids, restricted motion). Only one patient required revisional surgery due to a severe protrusio acetabuli (see below).

The radiologic follow-ups showed that adequate positioning was achieved in 65 of the sockets (40–50° varus). The socket had been implanted at an excessively "open" angle in only 4 patients. A total of 2 dislocations were recorded, both in the same patient. On one side the socket had been positioned normally, while on the other it was in a marked valgus position. Both operations were performed within a one-month period during a single hospitalization. After the 2nd operation the patient had to be moved to a special unit because of acute cardiac decompensation. When the patient was returned to the orthopedic unit, both hip joints were found to be dislocated. A permanent, stable reduction was achieved by reducing the hips under general anesthesia and then immobilizing them for 6 weeks.

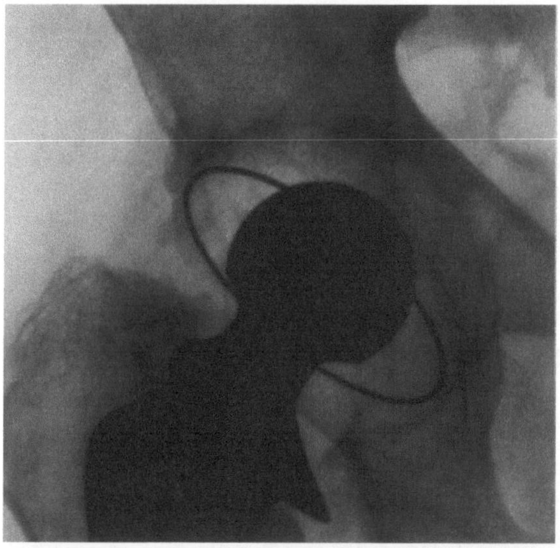

Fig. 2. 67-year-old woman (Z.A.) 31 months postoperatively. The implant is stably anchored, and a fine seam of sclerotic bone is visible around the pegs

After the minimum follow-up of 18 months, a sclerotic zone was clearly evident in the weight-bearing portions of the acetabular floor and around the anchoring pegs in all but 2 of the 69 acetabula (Fig. 2). A "seam" of the type that generally develops around bone cement or ceramic was not observed in any case. The more favorable elastic behavior of the polyethylene presumably accounts for this. Similar results were seen with the socket described by Morscher, in which pegs were supplemented by fixation screws [2].

Special Indications

With a *dysplastic acetabular roof,* it usually is not possible to obtain sufficient bony coverage in that area, even when the socket is deeply im-

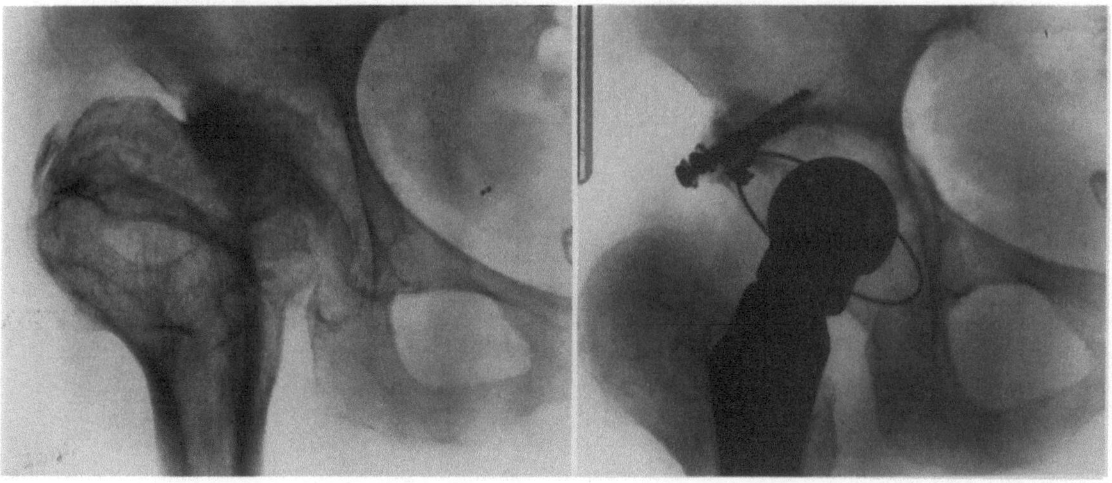

a b

Fig. 3 a, b. 54-year-old woman (S.E.) **a** with osteoarthritis of the right hip secondary to dysplasia. **b** The pegged socket is stably implanted following augmentation of the acetabular roof with corticocancellous bone from the resected femoral neck planted in a normal position. However, it is always possible to anchor at least 2 pegs securely in the pelvis despite the dysplasia. The roof can be augmented by applying a corticocancellous bone graft from the resected femoral neck and transfixing the graft with screws (Fig. 3). Even a steep acetabular roof can be augmented in this manner. This method proved very useful in all 8 dysplastic hips [3].

Even after *local radiation therapy* in the pelvic region, it should be possible to perform an uncemented implantation despite preexisting damage to the acetabular stock (Fig. 4a, b). In addition, we were able to anchor a pegged socket stably in patients with acutely painful femoral head necrosis associated with a *primary chronic polyarthritis,* even though the acetabular roof was badly deficient as a result of cystic degeneration. The socket can also be securely implanted without cement during the *revision* of loose cemented sockets.

The only failure to data occurred in a woman with psoriatic arthritis. The patient had also undergone a hysterectomy with local radiation therapy six years previously (Fig. 5a, b). Several months after the arthroplasty, a markedly progressive protrusio acetabuli became apparent, and increasing pain made it necessary to remove the prosthesis at 15 months postoperatively (Fig. 5c, d). Apparently the combination of both factors – acute psoriatic arthritis and the sequelae of local irradiation – caused such severe damage to the bony acetabular roof that a prosthesis could no longer be stably supported.

Discussion

Experience shows that peg attachment is a useful principle for the cementless fixation of acetabular prostheses. Given suitable exposure of the acetabular inlet, the implantation of the

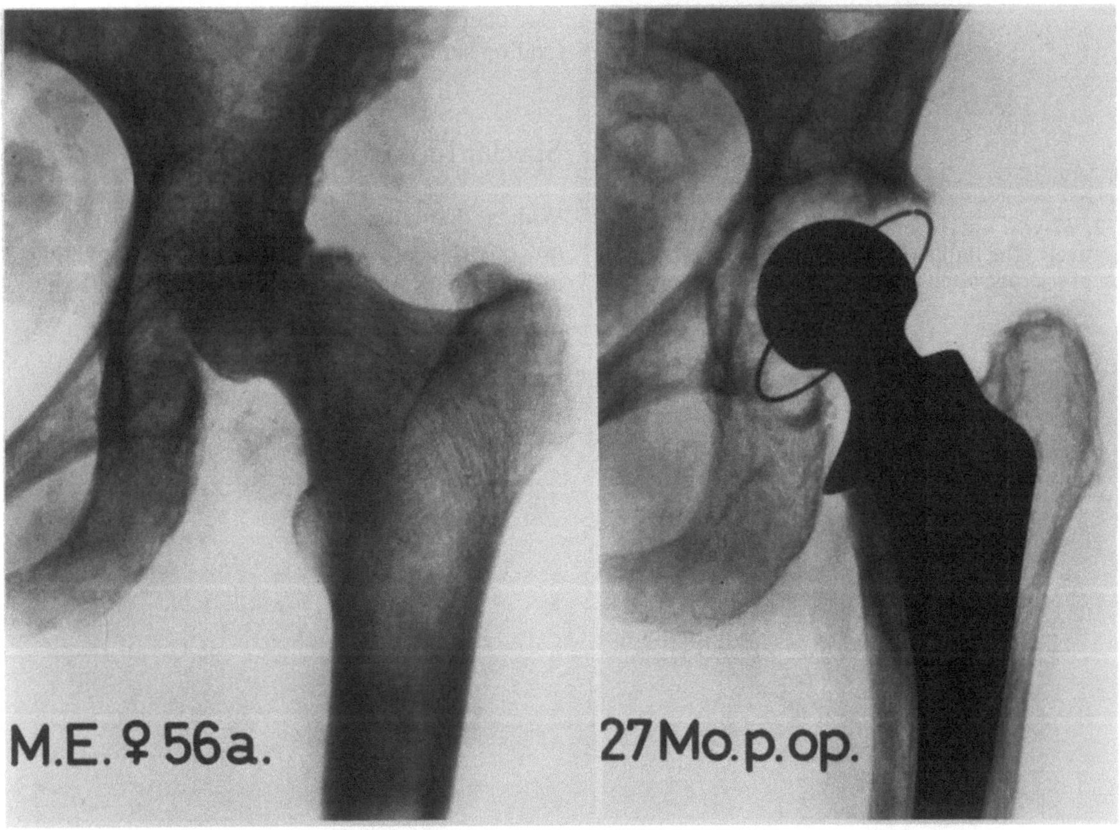

a b

Fig. 4a, b. 56-year-old woman (M.E.) **a** with radiation necrosis of the left hip following radiotherapy for a uterine carcinoma. **b** 27 months postoperatively the polyethylene socket is stable; the patient is entirely free of complaints and is able to walk without aids

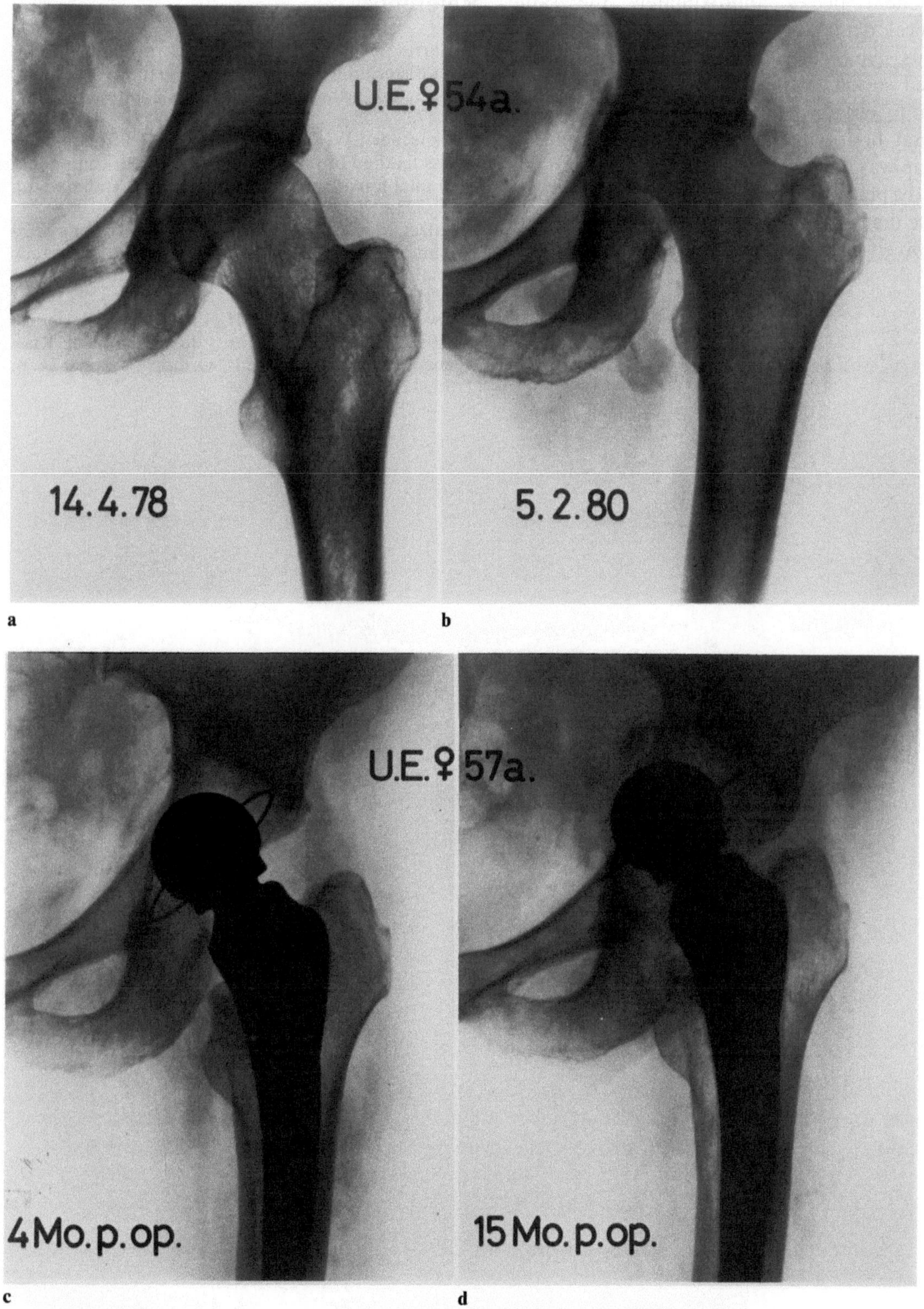

Fig. 5a–d. 54-year-old woman (U.E.) with radiation necrosis of the left hip and concomitant psoriatic arthritis. **a, b** Rapidly progressive destruction of the hip joint. **c, d** Increasing protrusio with severe pain and restricted motion

component places approximately the same technical demands on the operator as do the various types of screw-in socket. With the pegged socket, in fact, it should be somewhat easier to obtain a deep seating with good peripheral bone coverage. Valgus positioning of the cup was done only in exceptional cases. Even with dysplasia of the acetabular roof, the pegs enable the cup to be attached without cement in a relatively straightforward manner.

References

1. Harris WH (1969) Traumatic arthritis of the hip after dislocation and acetabular fractures: Treatment by mold arthroplasty. J Bone Joint Surg [Am] 51:737–755
2. Morscher EW, Dick W, Kernen V (1982) Cementless fixation of polyethylene acetabular component in total hip arthroplasty. Arch Orthop Trauma Surg 99:223–230
3. Salzer M, Knahr K, Plenk H Jr (1981) Long-term clinical and histological evaluation of bioceramic total hip endoprostheses. Orthop Clin North Am 4/11:1231–1240
4. Zweymüller K, Locke H, Plenk H Jr, Salzer M (1976) Endoprothesen aus Biokeramik bei Knochengeschwülsten. Med Orthop Techn 96/6: 169–171

Cementless, Isoelastic Total Hip Prosthesis: Preliminary Report on the First 215 Consecutive Cases

R. Bombelli and R. F. Santore

Abstract

Two hundred of the first 215 (93%) consecutive cementless, "isoelastic" total hip replacements performed personally by the senior author have been reviewed.

Average length of follow-up was 17 months and minimum length was 6 months. Maximum follow-up was 25 months.

No cases of femoral or acetabular component loosening or component breakage have been observed.

Introduction

The "isoelastic" prosthetic system (R. Mathys) has been designed to approximate closely the physiologic transmission of forces to the bone. This has been achieved 1) by eliminating the acrylic cement interface between the prosthetic components and bone, 2) by using biomaterials which approximate the elastic modulus of bone, and 3) by employing design features which enhance early stability and facilitate eventual stable incorporation into the host bone.

Experience with the femoral stem was acquired by the cautious use of the component for endoprosthetic femoral head replacements in elderly patients with femoral neck fractures. The first case was performed in 1974. To date, 84 such cases have been performed. An example of a case done in 1978 with a three-year X-ray follow-up is shown in Fig. 1. In the 77-year-old patient a 12-mm shaft hip endoprosthesis was used. Clinical results were uniformly satisfactory.

The use of an uncemented stem with a 32-mm diameter head and corresponding uncemented acetabular component as a complete total hip replacement system commenced at this institution in 1979.

Components

The femoral component combines a flexible stainless steel core with a circumferential polyacetate shell. The original femoral component had a very thin stainless steel core which was subsequently modified to larger dimensions because of excessive flexibility of the first-generation design. No patient in this follow-up group had the first-generation unit. Initially, the maximum available total stem width was 14 mm. In late 1980, widths of 16 and 18 mm were introduced.

A modularly designed head-neck unit attaches to the neck of the femoral stem via a snap fit. The same femoral stem can thus be used both for total hip replacement and endoprosthetic replacement. The hemispherical acetabular component, made of ultrahigh-molecular-weight polyethylene, has a 32-mm inside diameter and outside diameters which range from 46 to 64 mm in 2-mm increments. Two pegs are located on the superolateral surface to enhance the stability of the press fit, as well as provide an anti-rotational effect.

Three supplemental screws are then used along the lateral and posterior aspects of the rim to provide a stable, five-point fixation. There have been no design modifications of this component.

Clinical Material

Between April, 1979, and May, 1981, 215 consecutive, cementless, "isoelastic" total hip replacements were performed by the senior author. Ninety-three percent of cases have been seen in follow-up, a minimum of 6 months and a maximum of 25 months having elapsed from the time of surgery.

Of the 15 patients not available for follow-up, 3 were perioperative fatalities (1 pulmonary embolism, 1 cerebrovascular accident and 1 cardiac failure), 5 died between 6 and 10 months after surgery (3 malignant tumors, 1 myocardial infarction and 1 cerebrovascular accident), and 7 were lost to follow-up.

This paper is submitted as a preliminary report only, since insufficient time has transpired for definitive evaluation of a novel prosthetic technology.

The average age of all patients was 66 years. Diagnoses included osteoarthritis in 72 percent (155 cases), femoral neck fracture in 14 percent (30 cases), osteonecrosis in 8 percent (17 cases) and rheumatoid arthritis in 3 percent (7 cases). There were five cases of pseudoarthrosis and one case of conversion of a loose, cemented total hip replacement to an "isoelastic," cementless THR. Of the 155 cases of osteoarthritis, 7 represented cases of recurrent arthritis after a prior osteotomy.

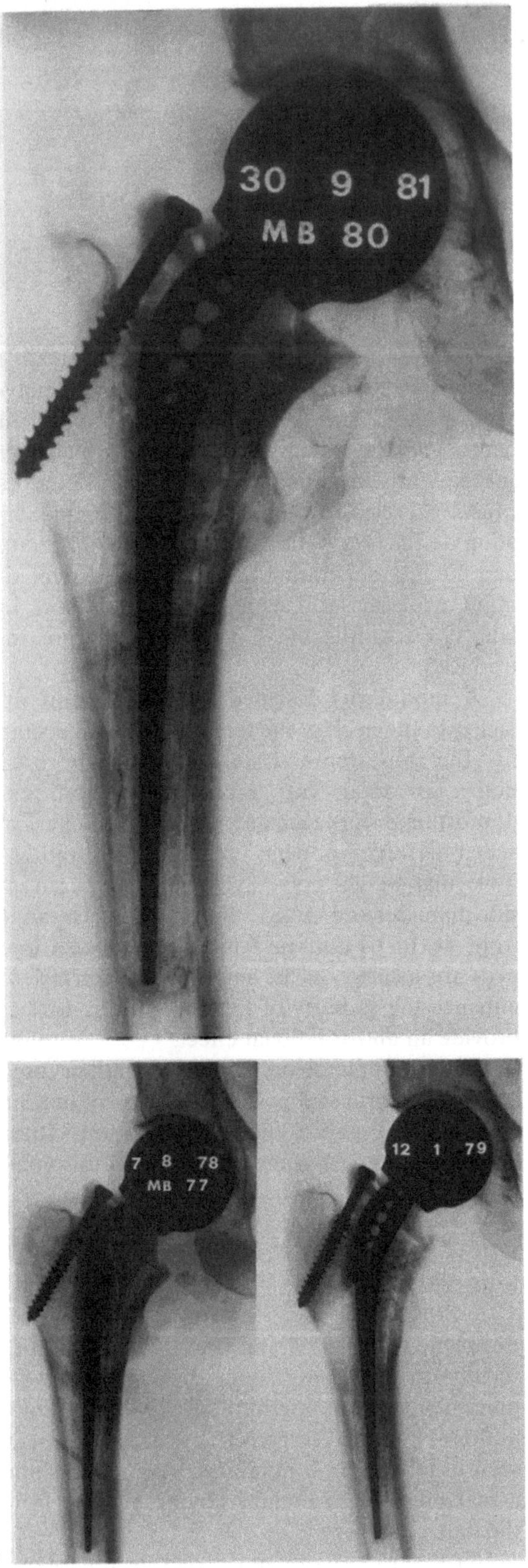

a

b

Fig. 1 a, b. (see text)

Surgical Technique

The initial 26 cases were performed from a posterolateral approach. Later the routine use of the Müller modification of the Watson-Jones incision was adopted, for two reasons. One was the occurrence of several troublesome dislocations after the posterolateral approach, and the other was the conviction that the lateral approach affords a more complete view of the acetabulum that is of particular value in cases of dysplasia.

Relaxing incisions are made both in the tendon of the gluteus minimus and the anterior muscle fibers of the gluteus medius just proximal to their insertions. A total capsulectomy is performed. The acetabular component is inserted in 25–30° of abduction and 10–15° of flexion. Two fixation screws are placed inferioposteriorally and one laterally. The screws are deliberately not placed diametrically opposite one another, as in true anterior and true posterior positions, for example, in order not to block slight deflection of the HDP component in gait. The need for secure anchorage is thus balanced with the objective of force transmission to the acetabular bone. This technical compromise theoretically permits micro-movement of the HDP component which mimics the function of the facies semilunaris-transacetabu-

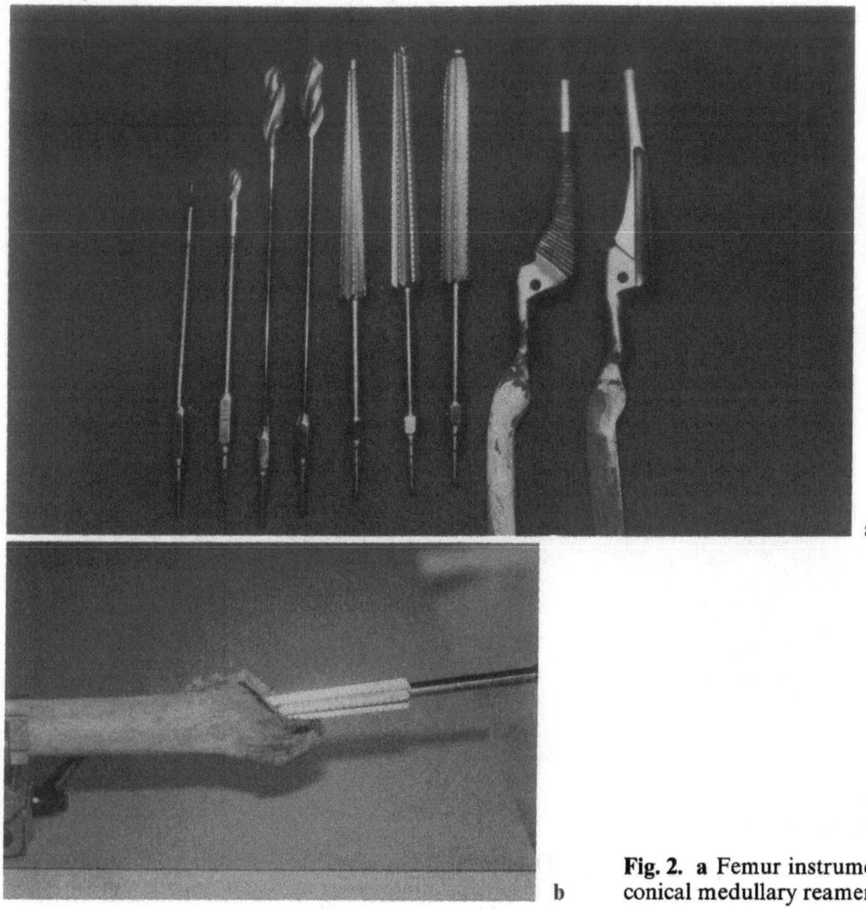

a

b

Fig. 2. a Femur instrumentarium, b side view of conical medullary reamer

lar ligament complex in the dispersion of forces in the normal adult acetabulum.

Extensive femoral reaming with standard and conical reamers and rasps, as shown in Figs. 2 a and 2 b, is performed to permit insertion of a component of maximum possible width. Cancellous bone fragments removed from the metaphysis and bone debris recovered during power reaming are reintroduced at the time of femoral component insertion and serve as a form of bone paste.

Two 6.5-mm cancellous screws anchor the proximal lateral portion of the component to the greater trochanter. These serve two purposes. One is to resist rotation and the other is to buttress the lateral portion of the prosthesis from excessive tension in a fashion analogous to that of a tension band.

A head-neck unit of appropriate size is used. The modular design with lengths of 28 – 34 – 40 – 44 mm both simplifies soft tissue length-tension adjustments and reduces the necessary component inventory.

The anterior abductor tenotomies are repaired with dexon sutures, and multiple suction drains are placed.

In late 1981 (not available for use in the first 215 cases) femoral components of longer lengths were introduced (180 mm versus 140 mm). These are now used as components of choice because of further enhancement of early stability and protection against varus malposition.

Postoperative Management

In the recovery room the ipsilateral leg is placed in a foam pillow splint in abduction and slight flexion. Patients rest in standard hospital beds without traction. Active exercises in bed commence on the first postoperative day. Passive physiotherapy is not permitted. On the fourth or

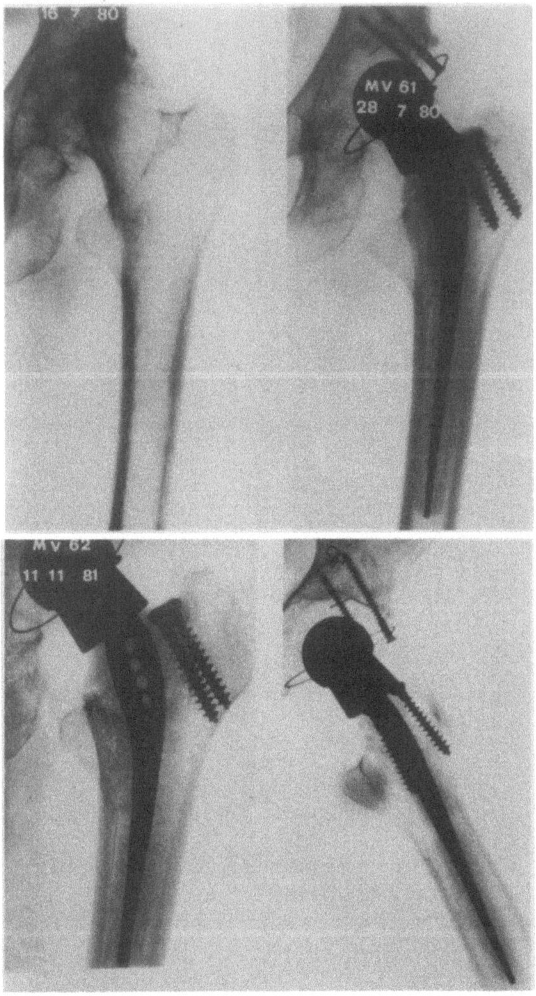

a

b

Fig. 3 a, b. 61-year-old patient with a cementless iso-elastic hip endoprosthesis

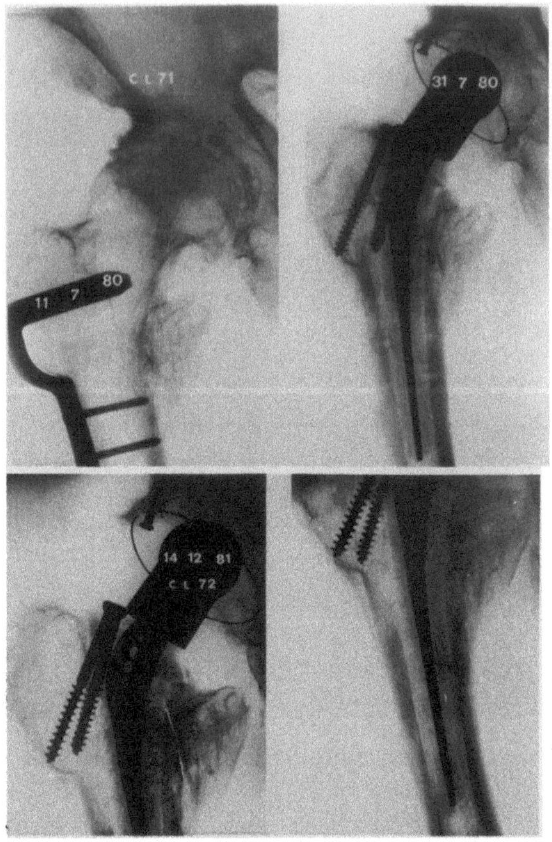

a

b

Fig. 4 a, b. X-ray control 17 months after total hip arthroplasty, in a patient who had undergone an osteotomy 11 years previously

fifth day after surgery ambulation in an axillary support walker is begun. Patients normally are discharged with two Canadian crutches in two weeks' time.

Patients are advised to use two crutches for six months and one for three months. The actual average time of crutch support as reported by patients on follow-up exam was 4.5 months for two crutches and 2.5 for one.

Patients generally abandon crutches when discomfort associated with ambulation ceases, regardless of recommendations to the contrary. In the follow-up of the early cases, an aching discomfort along the anterolateral thigh lasting many months was reported by most patients in whom small femoral components (12 and 14 mm) had been inserted in relatively large femora. The eventual cessation of discomfort has been used as a rough clinical gauge of the stabilization of the prosthesis in bone.

The current use of wide and long femoral components has produced a dramatic reduction in the duration of such symptoms.

Complications

Complications in the first 215 cases included three perioperative mortalities (1.4%), three deep infections (1.4%), four dislocations (1.9%), nine cases of heterotopic bone formation (4.1%) and one case of transient femoral nerve paresis.

Intraoperative fractures included 45 (21%) longitudinal or segmental violations of the femoral neck, 2 femoral shaft fractures (0.9%) and 9 (4.2%) fractures of the greater trochanter.

Seven broken screws on the acetabular side and one on the femoral side have been seen on review of the X-rays. None of these has migrated intraarticularly.

Management of Complications

Dislocations are managed by closed reduction under i.v. medication (three cases) and application of a 1/2 spica walking cast. If necessary, as in one of these cases, open reduction is performed.

Infection is managed aggressively by reoperation, resection of necrotic tissue and copious irrigation with betadyne solution. If early, the components are retained and the wound closed primarily. If late, and evidence of osteomyelitis exists, the components are removed and the wound closed primarily. Systemic antibiotics are administered.

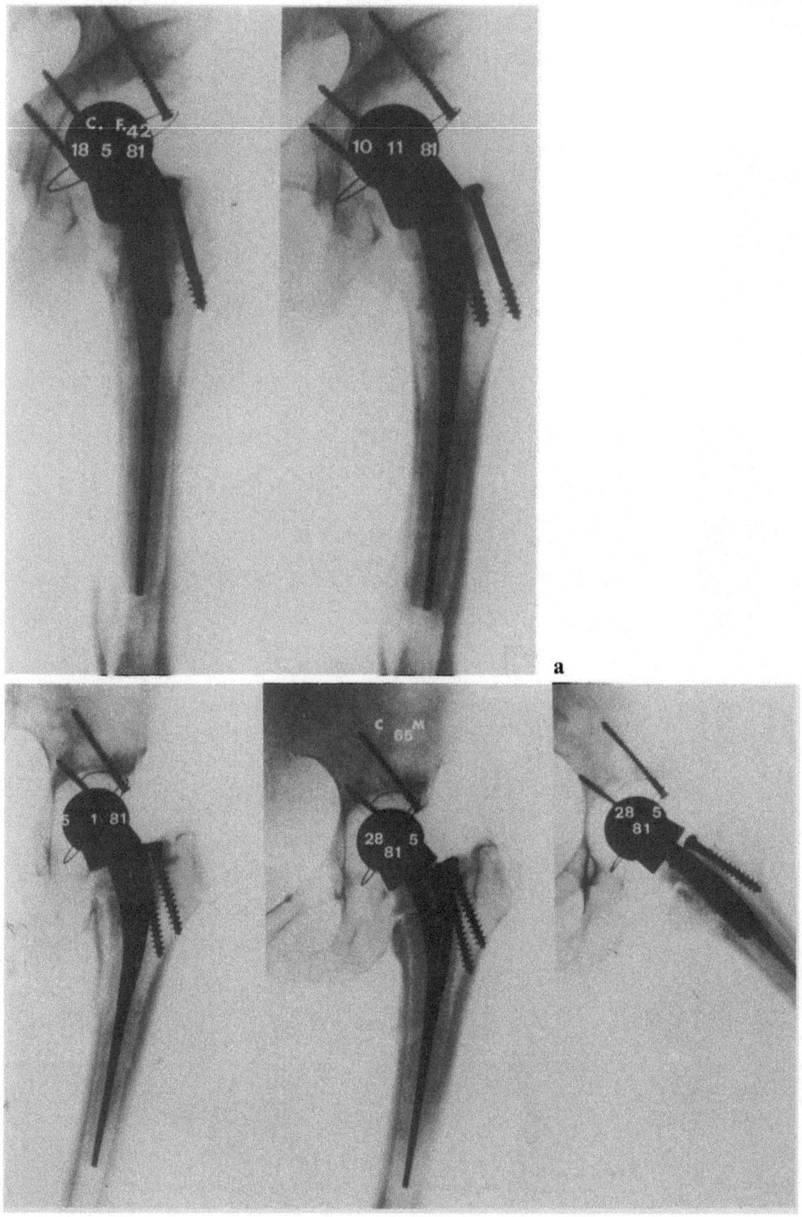

Fig. 5a, b. (see text, p. 217)

So far, no instance of heterotopic ossification has resulted in severe restriction of motion or required further therapy.

Shaft fractures are managed by cerclage wiring, trochanteric fractures by figure-of-eight wire reattachment, and neck fractures by grafting cancellous bone into the defects.

Radiologic Assessment

Radiologic evaluation of the 200 cases in the study has revealed no evidence of gross or radiologic loosening of acetabular or femoral components. In Fig. 3a representative case with follow-up of 16 months after surgery is shown to demonstrate the characteristic appearance of the component-bone interface and component positioning.

Additionally, no radiologically discernable bone resorption has been seen in either the calcar region, the anterior, posterior, medial and lateral aspects of the shaft, or the greater trochanteric region.

On the contrary, where an egg-shell thin cortex was present before operation, a thickening of the bone has been seen on postoperative X-rays. Where holes in both the medial and lateral cortices were present at sites of previously indwelling screws, as in the case of the seven failed osteotomies that were converted to THRs, these holes filled in uniformly with bone. In Fig. 4

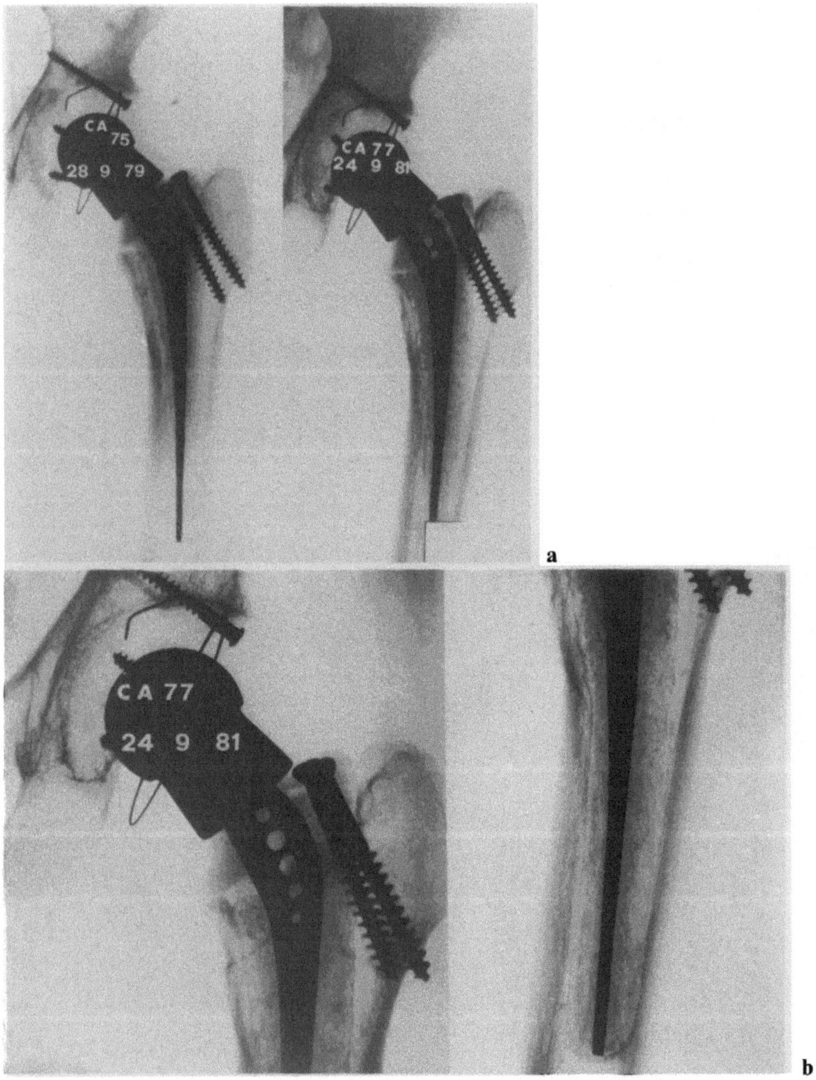

Fig. 6a, b. Varus position of prosthesis, 2 years after total hip arthroplasty

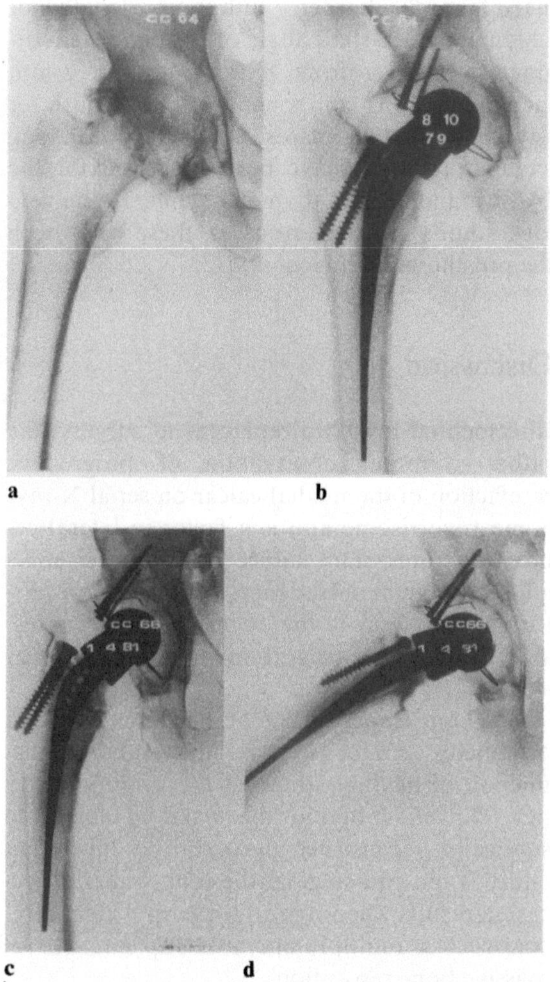

Fig. 7a–d. Condition of acetabulum **a, b** before and immediately after surgery, **c, d** 18 months later

note the thinned cortex where the plate was previously located and the visible screw holes on the early postoperative film. Seventeen months later the cortex has remodeled and the screw holes have filled with bone.

Where fractures have been sustained intraoperatively, regardless of location, rapid healing has ensued. There has not been one instance in the reviewed cases of delayed healing or nonunion of fractures or greater trochanteric osteotomies. In Fig. 5a, a case of a burst-type diaphyseal fracture adjacent to the tip of the prosthesis is shown. This fracture was first noted one week after surgery on routine X-ray. Ambulation with two crutches was permitted. Full healing is seen six months later. Fig. 5b demonstrates a fracture of the medial femoral

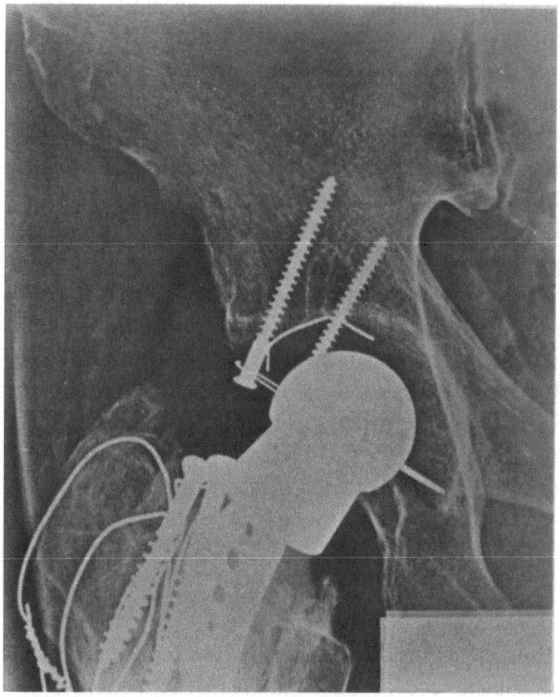

Fig. 8. Photographic negative showing sclerotic halo

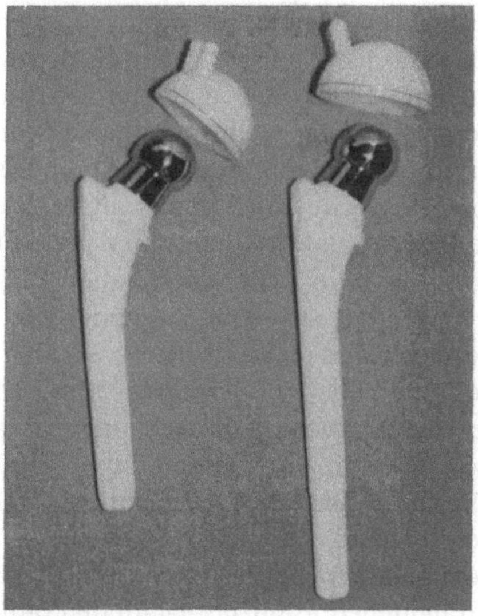

Fig. 9. New form, used since 1982 (*right*)

cortex with full healing four months later, again after routine postoperative ambulation.

Where inexact fitting of the collar of the prosthesis to the bony calcar has been witnessed intraoperatively and visualized on the immediate postoperative X-ray, obliteration of the gap by bone formation has been observed.

In addition to an ache in the thigh in the early patients in whom proportionately small femoral components were inserted, varus malposition was consistently observed (Fig. 6a and b). This was associated with a void at the proximolateral aspect of the femur adjacent to the component, and a distal "windshield-wiper" effect at the tip of the component. In follow-up films dense trabecular bone reinforcement at the tip and gradual filling of the proximolateral gap were observed.

On the acetabular side (Figs. 7, 8), a thin sclerotic "halo" is seen to form immediately adjacent to the perimeter of the component. No lucent lines have been observed nor has there been any instance of component migration. Bone is seen to form regularly over any uncovered portion of the far lateral rim.

Component Design

Current component design and surgical technique have evolved both from theoretical considerations and from experience in the early cases.

It is felt that components of maximum length and thickness should be employed, even though this requires extensive reaming of the proximal femur. Since the diameter of the proximal femur is larger in the AP than in the mediolateral direction, considerable reaming is required to achieve circumferential contact (see Fig. 4, page 186). A solid circumferential press fit enhances early stability. The combination of a wide and long stem size and circumferential press fit prevents varus malposition.

Most of the femoral fractures reported among the complications were sustained as a consequence of efforts to implant large components. The clinical status of these patients was not adversely affected.

The proximolateral border of the prosthesis has been straightened to further facilitate eradication of any bony void.

An increase in the valgus of the neck-shaft angle has been adopted, from 135° to 144° (Fig. 9), in order to enhance the vertical component of abductor tension and thereby increase the likelihood of a secure press-fit. As a direct consequence, the acetabular component is now placed in less abduction to increase contact surface area between the components.

The current femoral component has a thick yet compliant stainless steel core, straight proximal femoral border, minimum length of 140 mm, a neck-shaft angle of 144° and stem diameters ranging from 8 to 18 mm in 2-mm increments. This component was not in use for any of the first 215 cases. Since late 1981, long lengths (180 mm) have been produced for the 14-, 16- and 18-mm diameter stems. In the senior author's most recent cases, these have been the prostheses of choice.

Discussion

In cemented total hip replacement surgery, the rather common observation of progressive rarefaction of the medial calcar on serial X-rays is most worrisome and is a factor in lateral cement fractures, stem failure via cantilever effect and component subsidence. An even more disturbing situation is the occurrence of progressive lucency and migration on the acetabular side.

William Harris of Boston has remarked that orthopedic surgeons have the dubious distinction of having witnessed the evolution of a new clinical entity in the wake of efforts to surgically reconstruct the arthritic hip. That entity is the end-stage girdlestone which on occasion results when it is no longer possible to reconstruct a multiply-operated hip because of massive bone resorption.

The issue of whether to eliminate the use of bone cement or to perfect its use has emerged as one of the great debates in the orthopedic world. This debate has been fueled by the problem of loosening of conventionally cemented prostheses, particularly when these operations have been performed in young patients.

No single variable, whether it be pressurization of cement, metal backing of HDP, sintering of stems or the use of carbon or ceramic materials is likely, in itself, to provide a comprehensive solution to the problem of loosening.

Any one particular technical modification must be viewed in the context of the biocompatibility of the entire system in use, i.e. biomaterials, component design and fixation method. We prefer the deliberately vague term "biocompatibility" because it is not yet clear whether rigid fixation, with or without cement, should be the objective of implant surgery. Rigid fixation, however achieved, may lead to bone resorption regardless of design features or biomaterial properties of the components. Our overall goal must be long-term tolerance by bone of the prosthesis, consistent with enduring good clinical function and a minimum of adverse sequelae of the technology.

Revision Surgery

In 1981 the first attempt was made in this institution to apply the cementless isoelastic theory and technology to the difficult problem of the loose cemented THR. The inherent capacity of bone to reconstitute and remodel provided the inspiration for this attempt to reverse the vicious cycle of progressive bone resorption and destruction witnessed in cases of loosening.

Use of large components, particularly on the acetabular side, and extensive simultaneous iliac crest autogenous bone grafting are required in difficult cases.

Eleven revisions have now been performed, with encouraging early results. Follow-up is too short, however, for even preliminary conclusions to be drawn.

Summary

The principal goal of the cementless, "isoelastic" concept is the achievement of a stable incorporation into bone of durable, mildly flexible components which transmit stresses to bone in a more or less physiologic range. As of this date, the extensive remodeling of bone which has been observed on follow-up of the cases, together with the absence of any evidence of radiologic or gross loosening, provide early substantiation of the validity of the concepts.

Critical long-term follow-up will be needed before definitive conclusions can be drawn.

Four- to Eight-Year Postoperative Results of the Partially Uncemented Lindenhof-Type Ceramic Hip Endoprosthesis

P. Griss

During the period from September, 1974, to October, 1978, 95 hip endoprostheses of the Lindenhof type were implanted at the Lindenhof Orthopedic Hospital. To date this has permitted a follow-up of 4–8 years (average about 5 years). For a general statistical review of this series, the reader is referred to an earlier paper (Griss and Heimke, 1981). Here I shall note only that the majority of patients were in the 40–60 age group, and that the arthroplasties were most often performed for early osteoarthritis of the hip, femoral head necrosis and PCP.

In each case the acetabular component consisted of a cylindrical, screw-type socket with a wide rim. This socket is available in 3 sizes and, with the aid of precision reaming and cutting instruments, can be accurately implanted without cement by a press-fit technique (details in Griss et al., 1975). The socket and head are constructed of dense Al_2O_3 ceramic. The cemented stem was initially made of stainless steel (Charnley type) or chromium-cobalt cast alloy (Weber type), but Endocast alloy has been used since 1976 (see Griss et al., 1978, for description). The head and metal stem are interconnected by means of a self-locking cone.

During the last systematic follow-up examinations of all operated patients in 1980, 84.2% of the patients were satisfied with the result. 15.8% had residual complaints or new complaints of varying degree that impaired the function and weight-bearing ability of the artificial joint. Since then 2 more years have passed, and a number of patients, though not all, have again presented for routine follow-up, providing statistics that enable the following picture, as yet incomplete, to be drawn.

The most favorable situation is one in which primary contact between the acetabular bone and ceramic socket is established during implantation. If the socket can be screwed securely into an accurately prepared bed, generally this intimate bony contact will be maintained for years afterward, as the component becomes invested by a sharply-defined layer of sclerotic bone (Fig. 1a, b).

In most cases it will not be possible to prepare a perfectly congruent bed to receive the prosthesis, and a soft, unsharp interfacial zone will be visible on the early postoperative radiographs. Subsequent weight bearing, however, will lead relatively quickly to a biomechanical adaptation of the pelvic bone; the unsharp, poorly-mineralized interfacial zone will become more dense, and the implant will become permanently integrated.

Large gaps around the implant resulting from improper reaming or imperfections of prosthetic shape should be sealed with autologous bone grafts at the time of the operation. These grafts generally will become well incorporated within a year, frequently accompanied by a noticeable settling of the prosthesis. This settling process should not be confused with loosening, however, for it is not associated with clinical symptoms and continues for no more than 1–2 years after implantation (Fig. 2a, b).

Based on our own experience, it appears that these adaptation processes contribute positively to the long-term success of most implants. In the last 4 years, however, we have also ob-

Table 1. Serious Complications Associated with the Ceramic Screw-In Acetabular Prosthesis System (Lindenhof Type, n = 95)

Complications	Prevalence
1) Ceramic head fractures	6 = 6.3%
2) Acetabular loosening	8 = 8.4%
3) Stem loosening	4 = 4.2%
4) Stem fracture (Charnley)	2 = 2.1%
5) Periarticular calcifications (2nd-degree)	2 = 2.1%
6) Acetabular settling (pain) (loosening?)	2 = 2.1%

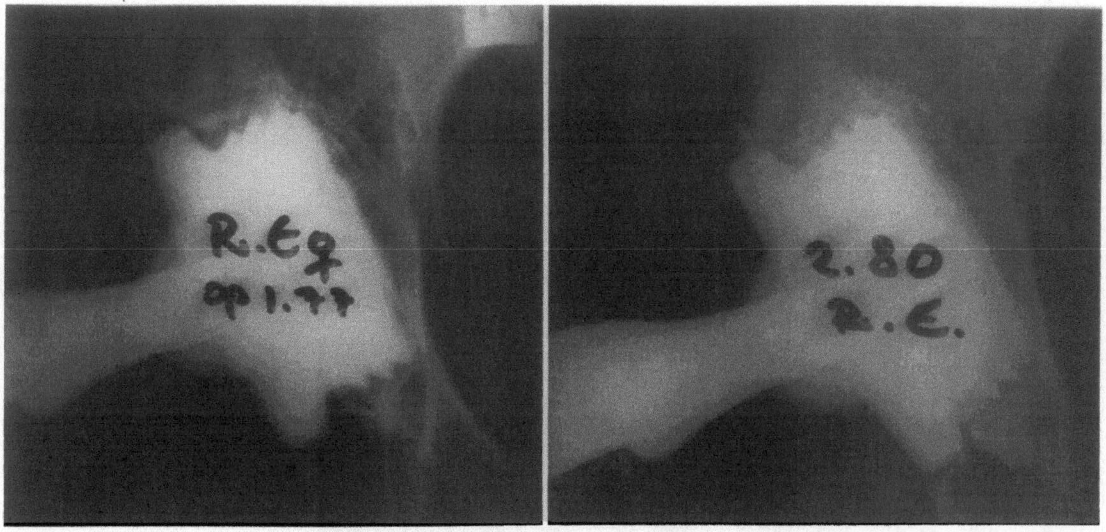

a b

Fig. 1 a, b. Radiographs of the right hip in a 56-year-old woman. D'Aubigne hip score = 18. Good result of an uncemented acetabular prosthesis. **a** 1 month after implantation; **b** 3 years after implantation

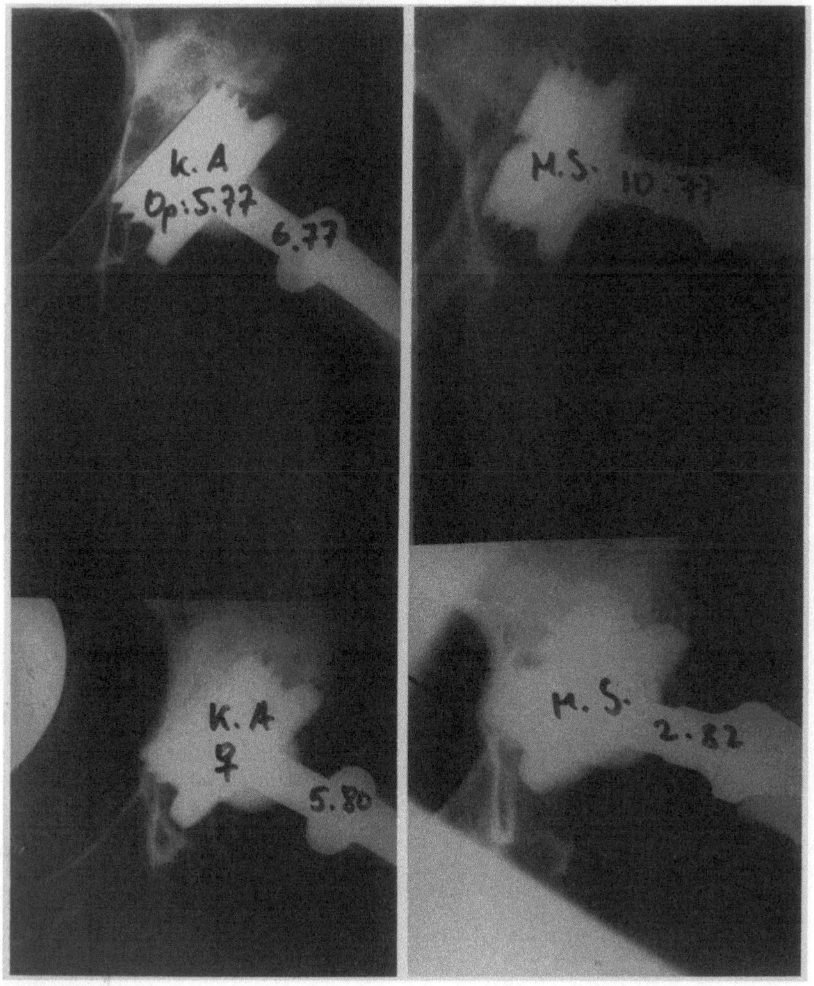

a b

Fig. 2 a, b. Comparative radiographs of two acetabular migrations: **a** 57-year-old woman with increasing load-dependent pain; **b** 56-year-old woman with load-dependent pain that is presently in remission. (**a** = Example of protracted acetabular loosening. **b** = Example of acetabular settling, so far with good result. Neither case has yet been revised)

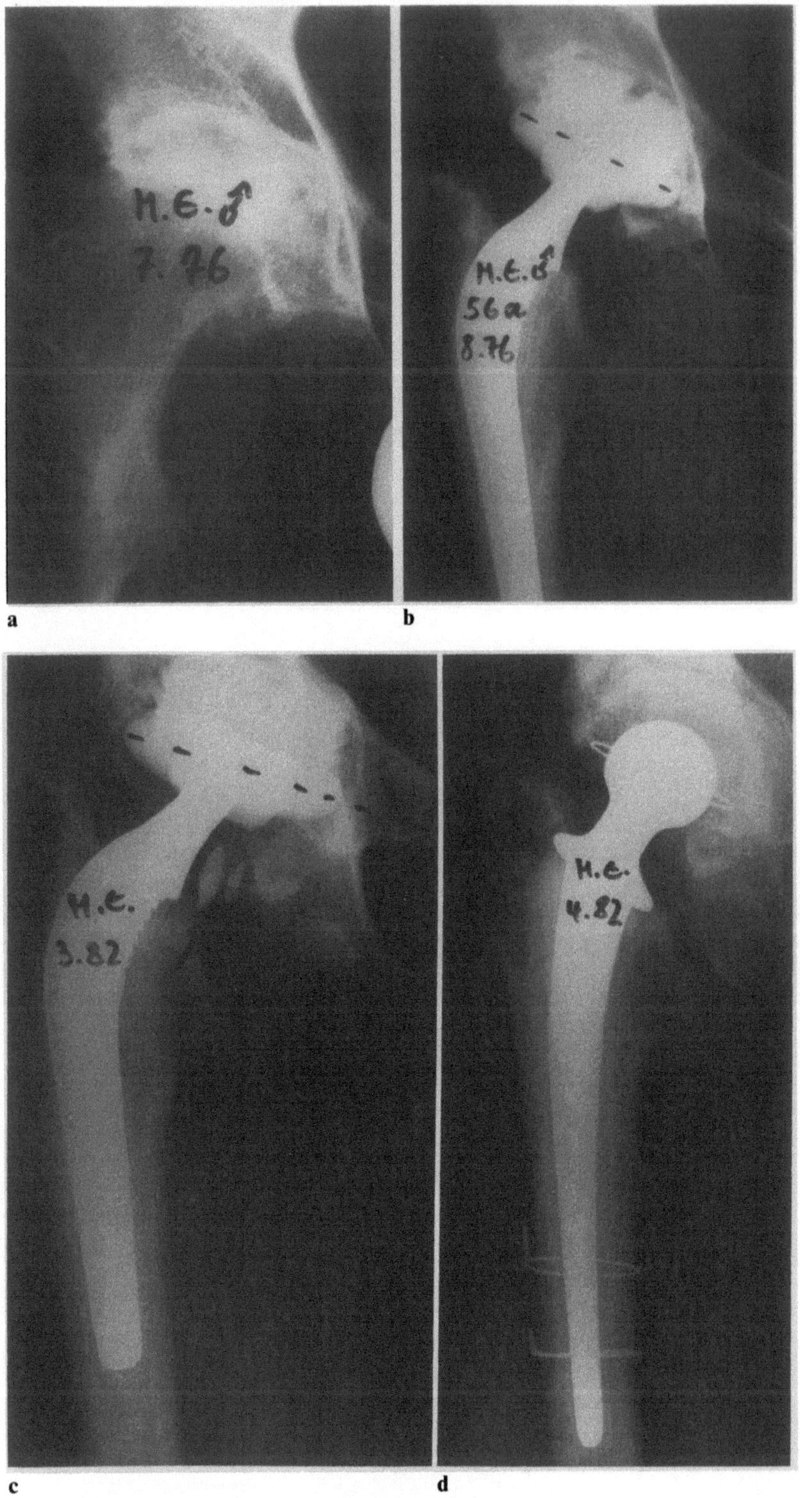

a b c d

Fig. 3a–d. Series of radiographs documenting acetabular loosening with a cracked ceramic head in a 56-year-old man. **a** Preoperative film. **b** Immediate postoperative film. **c** 5 years 7 months later: acetabular migration and tilting, 2 head fragments in joint space (*arrow*). **d** Revisionary prosthesis

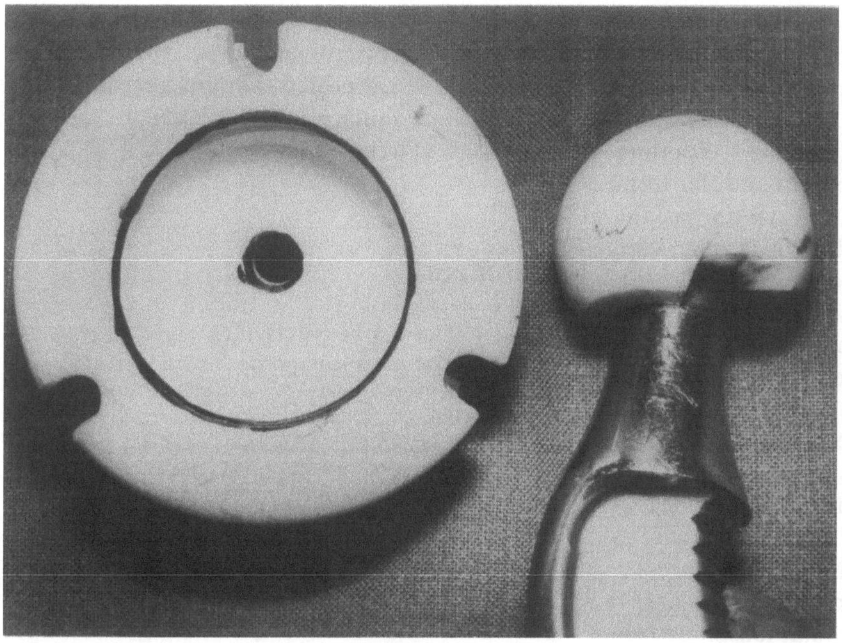

Fig. 4. Photo of the components removed from the patient in Fig. 3. There is gross wear of the acetabular component, despite correct implantation of the endoprosthesis (cf. Fig. 3). Small fragments are broken from the ceramic head. The dark scratches occurred at operation (rim of socket has been marked with black ink for better contrast)

served a number of radiographic complications and changes that demand closer attention.

The overall statistics relating to complications are as follows: We observed serious complications in 25.3% of the patients. In 14.6% they were severe enough to warrant revision, which usually consisted of replacing the prosthesis. These complications are listed in Table 1. In 6 cases a ceramic head fracture occurred from 2 weeks to 5 years postoperatively. Generally these fractures were not associated with additional trauma. A damage analysis of removed components pointed to inhomogenous grain size in the ceramic and a suboptimum cone geometry as the probable causes of these failures. These flaws were corrected in subsequent implants.

We witnessed 8 cases of acetabular loosening and 4 cases of stem loosening. Thus, loosening of the uncemented socket was twice as prevalent in our series as loosening of the cemented stem. What is more, the loosening of uncemented sockets is a phenomenon which we have observed only in the last two years. In some patients both components were loose (Fig. 3a–d).

In cases of acetabular loosening, varying degrees of wear of the ceramic head and socket were frequently seen at revision. In the simplest case, shallow wear grooves were visible about the circumference of the ceramic head in the area where the head was subject to large, sustained loads. Heavier degrees of wear involving losses of up to 2 mm from the head and socket were also found (Fig. 4). None of the worn components showed any abnormality of position that might have pointed to a subluxation or marginal loading of the head and socket as the cause of the excessive wear. Our series, in fact, included 3 cases in which the socket had been implanted in considerably more than 50° of abduction. These components became incorporated into the bone without a seam and have been functioning for up to 7 years without difficulty. We also have the components from a patient who had undergone a bilateral THR and in whom both intramedullary stems (Charnley type), made of stainless steel, fractured consecutively at 8-month intervals 5 years after the operation. The patient was a manual worker by trade and is known to have played tennis for up to 4 hours a day. The left side showed a concentric wear of several hundred micrometers, while the wear on the right side was smaller but still visible. These contradictory phenomena cannot be explained simply by variations in the quality of the ceramic. We believe, rather, that the tolerance limits of ceramic-on-ceramic combinations for daily use are actually much closer than we are accustomed to from the traditional polymer-on-metal combinations used in cemented systems. Apparently, unexpected wear situations can arise in which the ceramic wear debris is not adequately removed from the articulating surfaces of the components, creating a danger that individual grains will become wedged between surfaces of equal hardness (Plitz and Griss, 1981). This sets up a grinding action which causes abrasive wear and, far from abating, actually tends to increase with passage of time. As the components lose their sphericity, this mechanism becomes increasingly more active, ultimately leading to a catastrophic wear situation. Histologic examination in such cases reveals ceramic wear particles up to 40 μm in diameter, some of which are embedded in giant cells, but most of which are stored in the cytoplasm of mononuclear macrophages and are transported away from the area by local mechanisms. The tissue burden of wear debris can become so large that the histologic picture resembles that characteristic of polyester wear. It is conceivable that the acetabular loosenings observed by us in the last two years may be related, at least in part, to abnormal ceramic wear situations of this type. If so, this would represent a significant late complication requiring further intensive observation and study.

Progress, especially in the ceramic sector, has led to the development of a new aluminium oxide ceramic, in clinical use for 2 years, which has a smaller and far more uniform grain size than the material previously used (Heimke and Griss, 1981). It is expected that this new ceramic will contribute much toward solving the problems described here.

References

1. Griss P, Heimke G (1981) Five years experience with ceramic-metal-composite hip endoprostheses. I. Clinical evaluation. Arch Orthop Trauma Surg 99:157–164
2. Griss P, Heimke G, v. Andrian-Werburg H (1975) Die Aluminiumoxidkeramik-Metall-Verbundprothese. Eine neue Hüftgelenktotalendoprothese zur teilweise zementfreien Implantation. Arch Orthop Unfallchir 81:259–266
3. Griss P, Jentschura G, Heimke G (1978) Zur Technik der Pfannenimplantation bei dysplastischem Acetabulum. Arch Orthop Trauma Surg 93:57–63
4. Heimke G, Griss P (1981) Five years experience with ceramic-metal-composite hip endoprostheses. II. Mechanical evaluations and improvements. Arch Orthop Trauma Surg 98:165–171
5. Plitz W, Griss P (1981) Clinical, histo-morphological and material-related observations on removed alumina-ceramic hip joint components. Conf. Proc.: Implant retrieval: Material and biological aspects. Gaithersburg, MD 1980, U.S. Dept. of Commerce, pp 131–147

Total Hip Replacement with the Autophor Cement-Free Ceramic Prosthesis

H. Mittelmeier

Our total hip system is based not only upon the use of aluminium oxide ceramic, but also upon a return to the principle of cementless fixation. The importance of this principle was demonstrated by our histopathologic studies of the first Judet prosthesis made of polymethylmethacrylate (PMMA) (Mittelmeier and Singer, 1956). We discovered the importance of fatigue fractures and surface wear of this prosthesis, resulting in marked foreign-body reactions to the wear debris, as well as the significance of biomechanical effects, which not only stimulate the formation of a new load-bearing bone layer, but also create excessive stresses on the new bone with consequent loosening as a result of resorption. Thus, some 25 years ago we suggested increasing the surface area of the implant as a means of solving the problem of endoprosthetic fixation, reasoning that this would promote adaptation of the bone, improve the distribution of stresses, and reduce compressive forces below the critical resorption threshold, thereby effecting a balance between load and structure and preventing prosthetic loosening. We proposed to accomplish this by incorporating projections and recesses into the prosthetic surface, and by replacing PMMA with a fracture- and wear-resistant biomaterial.

These proposals were largely neglected due to the development of Charnley's total hip replacement in 1960, which employed a metal-on-polyethylene combination to reduce friction and self-curing bone cement to provide good primary fixation and an enlarged area of bone contact. Owing to its initial success, this prosthesis achieved a worldwide popularity both in its original form and in numerous modifications. But the Charnley system and its modifications had some serious disadvantages. One was an unacceptable rate of wear (about 200 m/year on the average) caused by projecting carbide spicules on the surface of the metal head and resulting in an increasingly severe foreign-body reaction in the prosthetic bed. The main problems, however, related to the bone cement, which not only exerted a toxic effect on the implant bed, but also was prone to fatigue fracture, possibly leading to stem breakage and to a high rate of aseptic loosening requiring revision. Thus, the relatively poor longevity of these prostheses prompted Charnley himself (1979) to recommended that they be used only in older patients with a limited life expectancy. They could not solve the problem of the severely damaged hip in younger patients, for which a functionally-unsatisfactory salvage operation (arthrodesis, Girdlestone) remained the only recourse.

The somewhat controversial problem of "cement aging" due to fatigue has been demonstrated beyond question in alternating bending tests at our biochemical laboratory. The Woehler curves from these tests indicate a steady decline up to about 15 million load cycles (1 million cycles = about 1 year of use), which accounts for the frequent failure of cemented prostheses after several years of service.

Perhaps these problems can be solved one day by the use of improved cements. We personally have suggested carbon fiber reinforcement and bioactivation with apatite for this purpose (Mittelmeier et al., 1980), but more work needs to be done before improved cements become a reality.

The problems with the Charnley prosthesis and its modifications prompted us in 1969 (H. Mittelmeier in collaboration with Osteo AG of Switzerland) to begin development on a new cement-free total hip prosthesis based upon the surface-enlargement principle. The distinguishing feature of this prosthesis, which we call the Autophor system, is its distinctive "bearing ribs," a series of cross-ridges which are machined into the surface of the high-strength material, and which significantly augment the surface area of the implant. The components are tapered or given conical shapes so that a pri-

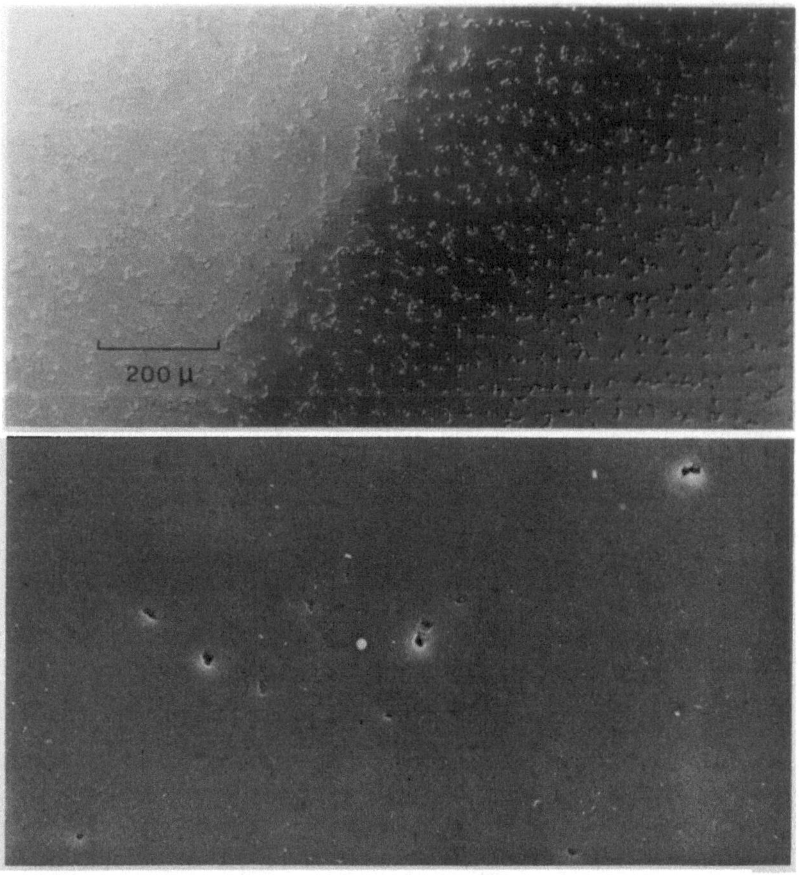

a

b

Fig. 1. Scanning electron micrographs of **a** a highly polished CoCrMo femoral prosthetic head with projecting carbide spicules and **b** a polished aluminum oxide ceramic head (same magnification)

mary tension is created during press-fitting of the implants, and a good primary fixation is obtained. Our original intention was to use metal-on-polyethylene, and this combination was first used clinically in 1973. However, studies since then have compelled us to abandon this combination in favor of aluminium oxide ceramic.

The use of aluminum oxide ceramic for joint prostheses was first proposed by the German inventor Rock in 1934. Eyring of the U.S. made first practical use of this material for an elbow prosthesis in 1968, and Boutin (1972) of France used it for a total hip replacement in 1970. Initially Boutin cemented the femoral and acetabular components in a conventional manner, but later he used a self-retaining design.

In the early 1970s, various groups of manufacturers and orthopedic surgeons in Germany began intensive research on the use of aluminum oxide ceramic as a prosthetic material (Griss et al., 1973; Dorre et al., 1975; Mittelmeier et al., 1980, 1981; Salzer et al., 1975). Our own research has centered on the "Biolox" ceramic (Feldmühle AG).

Biolox is an aluminum oxide ceramic with an Al_2O_3 content of 99.7% and a maximum grain size of 4 µm. The principal advantages of the material relate to its purity, density, and small grain size (Dorre et al., 1975). The prosthetic components are produced from polycrystalline powder by sintering.

Of particular importance are the excellent tribologic properties of the ceramic, for, in contrast to metallic surfaces, the ceramic surface can be polished to a perfect smoothness.

In simulator tests (Dorre et al., 1975), the Biolox ceramic showed an initial friction coefficient comparable to the "low-friction" metal-on-polyethylene combination of Charnley; this coefficient even surpassed that of Charnley's prosthesis as wearing time increased. But the most important property of the ceramic is its extremely low wear, which is only about $1/10$ to $1/20$ that of the metal-PE combination (assuming a perfect surface roundness and polish). The simulator tests indicate that the ceramic should retain its excellent wear resistance for several decades and perhaps for a lifetime.

A ceramic-polyethylene combination also shows low friction and significantly less wear than the metal-PE combination, although the ceramic-ceramic design shows the lowest degree of wear (Semlitsch).

The reason for the excellent wear properties of the ceramic lies in the attraction of hydrogen atoms in the dipole water molecules to the oxygen atoms in the aluminum oxide. As a result of this reaction, a lubricating film is formed. The superiority of the aluminum oxide ceramic to other biomaterials in this regard (stainless steel, cobalt-chronium alloys, polyethylene) is most clearly demonstrated in the "drop test," in which the ceramic shows the flattest tangent angle (Semlitsch).

A further advantage is the high corrosion stability of the ceramic and of its wear particles, for the aluminum oxide molecules are highly stable and release practically no chemically active metal ions. This is the basis for the excellent biocompatibility of the material.

Another clinical advantage of aluminum oxide ceramic is its good radiocontrast with respect to bone, polyethylene, bone cement and metal. Moreover, unlike polyethylene, it can be autoclaved repeatedly (at 138 °C) without damage.

Numerous biocompatibility experiments of the ceramic involving cell cultures and test implantations in rats and rabbits (including powdered specimens) have demonstrated the excellent tissue compatibility of the material (Griss et al., 1973; Willert et al., 1974; Harms et al., 1980). Unfortunately, the ceramic has an intrinsically low bending strength, and so this material is not ideal for the production of intramedullary stems. This has prompted the development (by Krupp AG) of the high-strength cobalt-chronium cast alloy known as "Endocast," which has twice the fatigue strength of traditional Co-Cr alloys and in electrocorrison tests displays a corrosion resistance superior to that of stainless steel, conventional Co-Cr alloys, and even the much-publicized titanium alloys (Müller). These properties are achieved through a special heat treatment and

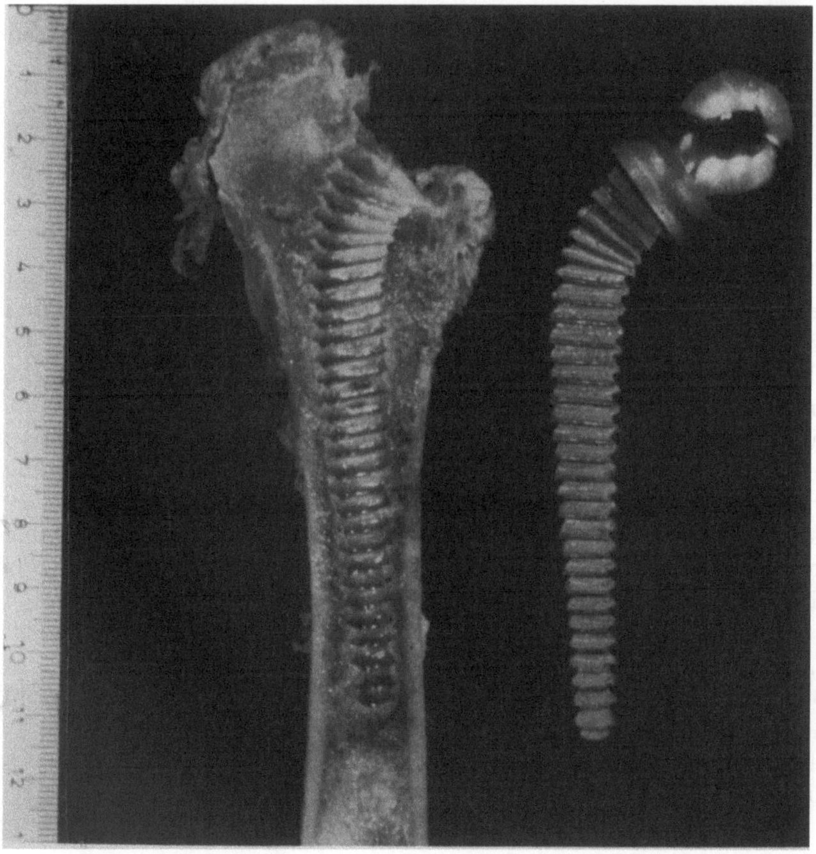

Fig. 2. Preparation of a dog femur showing pronounced "molding" of the bone to the stem of a bearing-rib prosthesis

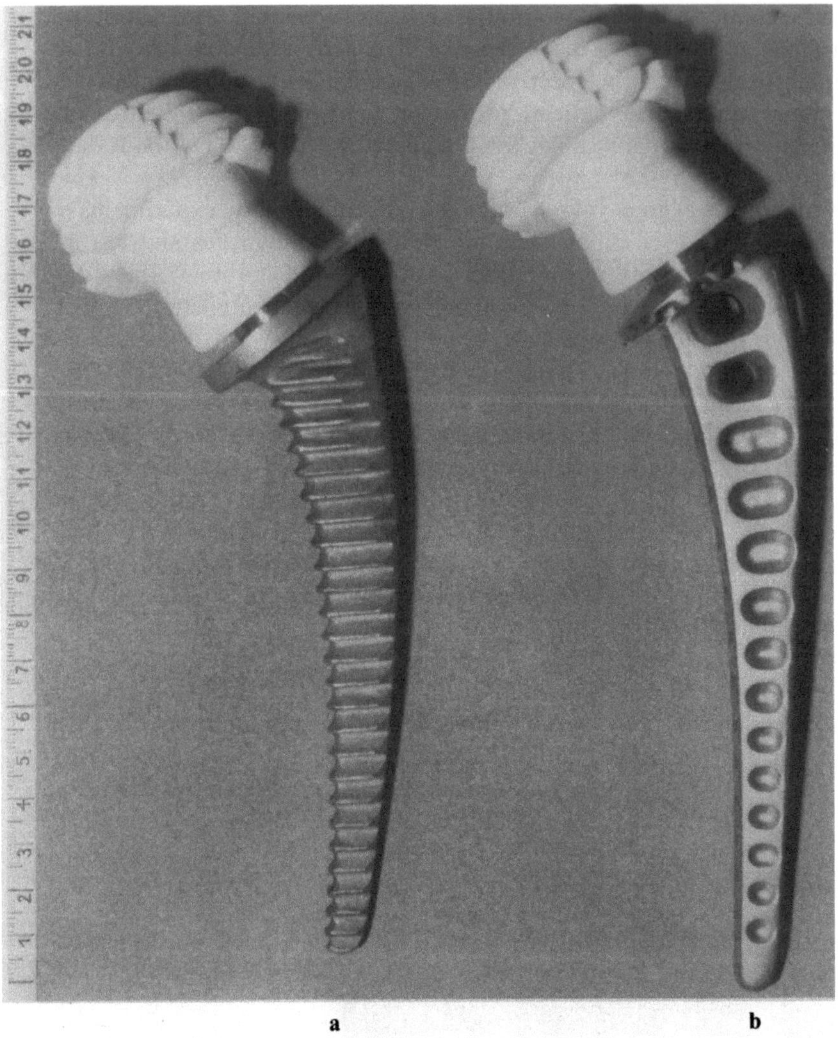

Fig. 3. "Autophor" ceramic hip prostheses with conical screw-in acetabular component and ceramic head that is press-fitted onto the conical post atop the metal stem. **a** Type-I stem with transverse bearing ribs constructed of conventional CoCr cast alloy; **b** type-II stem constructed of new Endocast alloy

by binding nitrogen into the alloy. Biocompatibility experiments conducted at our clinic also have demonstrated an outstanding tissue compatibility (Harms and Mäusle, 1980).

Owing to the excellent mechanical and biological properties of the aluminum oxide ceramic and of Endocast, we have used both of these biomaterials since 1974 for the construction of bearing-rib prostheses.

Miniature bearing-rib prostheses implanted experimentally in dogs showed an excellent "molding" of the bone to the ridged implant surface through ingrowth, producing a permanent, stable retention (Biehl et al., 1975). On the basis of these results and others, we felt that all essential prerequisites had been met for a successful clinical application of the total hip system.

Initially, the stem of the Autophor femoral component featured simple circumferential bearing ribs (type I stem), but this model did not show optimum rotational stability during clinical testing and so was abandoned in late 1976 after 2 years' use. It was replaced with an improved stem (type II) with extra longitudinal ridges along its edges, resulting in a honeycomb-like surface profile with an offset double-Y cross-section. Also, an extra stabilizing wing was placed on the craniolateral part of the component, and ridging was placed on the undersurface of the collar.

The femoral heads are available in diameters of 32 and 38 mm, each with 3 different neck lengths (length difference 8 mm). The head is press-fitted onto a conical post atop the metal stem. This "self-locking cone" creates a wedging effect that holds the head securely in place, yet enables the head to be replaced without difficulty should the need arise.

The acetabular component of the Autophor system was fashioned in the shape of a truncated cone to prevent tilting (analogous to the famous "egg of Columbus") and was threaded externally so that is could be screwed into the acetabulum.

Like the other components, a range of sizes is also offered for the acetabular sockets and intramedullary stems.

The external thread on the acetabular component increases its surface area by an average of about 50 cm^2. The bearing ribs on the femoral component increase the surface area by an average of about 20 cm^2.

The truncated conical shape of the socket and the tapered shape of the stem create a good primary tension at implantation and provide for a solid primary anchoring of the components.

With regard to the surgical technique of implanting the Autophor system, several points should be noted: The bony acetabulum is shaped to receive the truncated conical socket, and threads are precut in the bone with a special tap (the screw-in socket also has a self-tapping action when inserted). In the femur, the ribbed stem is implanted together with small pieces of autologous bone, which are pressed into the hollows on the stem and into the wall of the femoral canal as an aid to fixation. They serve as an "autologous bone cement," but one which cannot cause foreign-body reactions and which will promote and hasten the bony attachment of the prosthetic stem.

It should be mentioned that besides the uncemented Autophor prosthesis, we have also developed (again in collaboration with Osteo AG) a cementable ceramic implant system of conventional design ("Xenophor") that is compatible with the same heads used in the Autophor system, but which can use either ceramic or polyethylene acetabular components. The compatibility of the head components makes it possible to combine a cemented socket with a

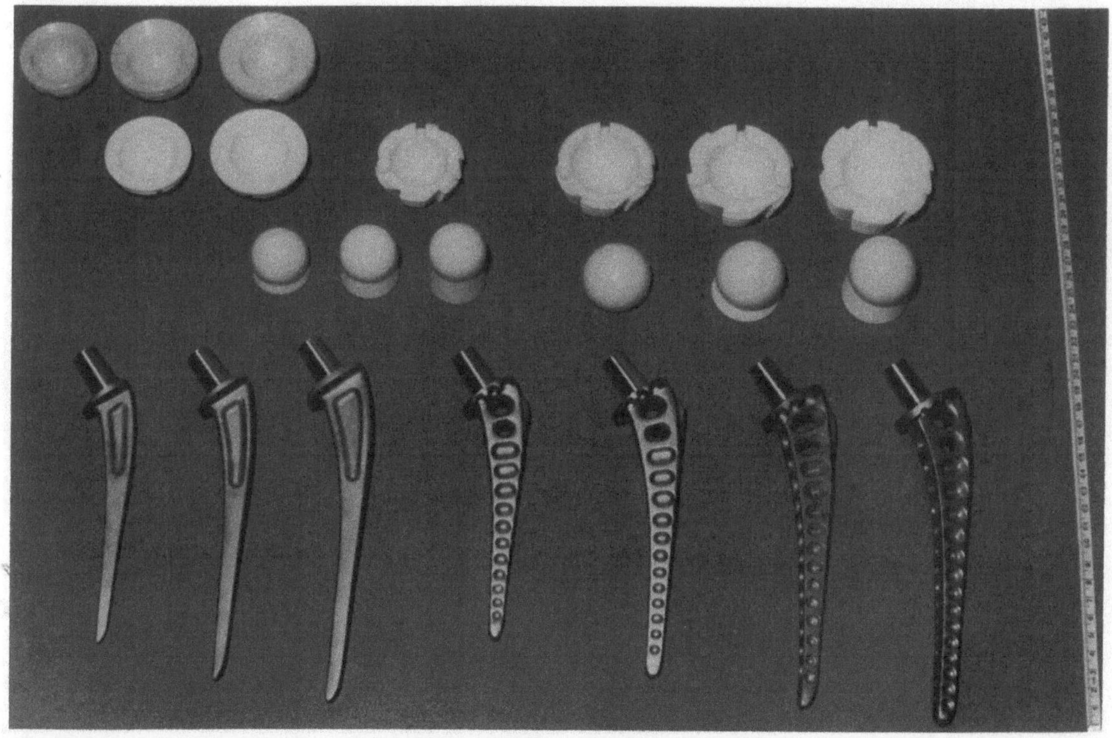

Fig. 4. Full set of ceramic hip prostheses showing range of available sizes. On the left is the cementable Xenophor type with smooth stems and hemispheric acetabular components (available in ceramic or polyethylene). On the right is the "Autophor" system with the improved type-II bearing-rib stems and ceramic screw-in acetabular components. Between them are the interchangable heads with a 32-mm diameter (*left*) for the size I screw-in socket and cementable sockets (*right*) *with* 38-mm diameter for the Autophor sockets of sizes II–IV; each head size is available in 3 neck lengths

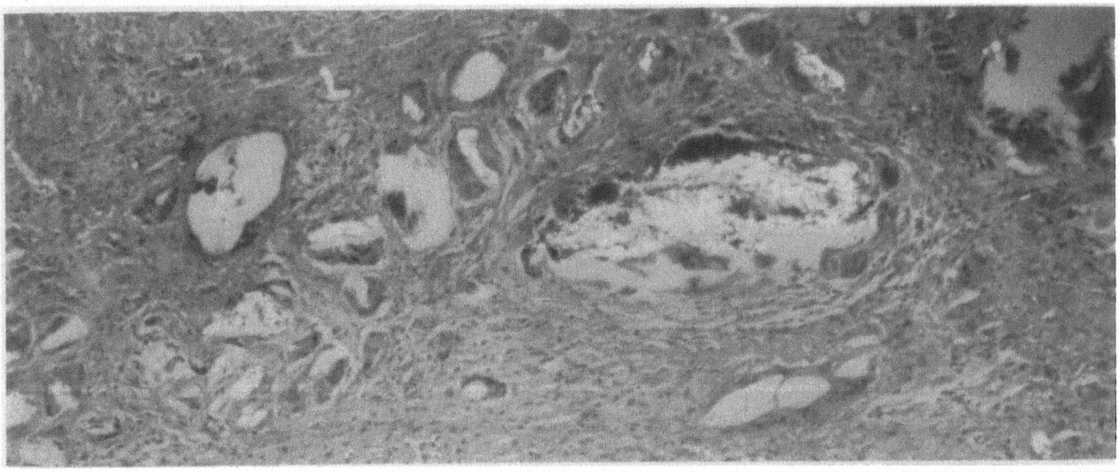
a

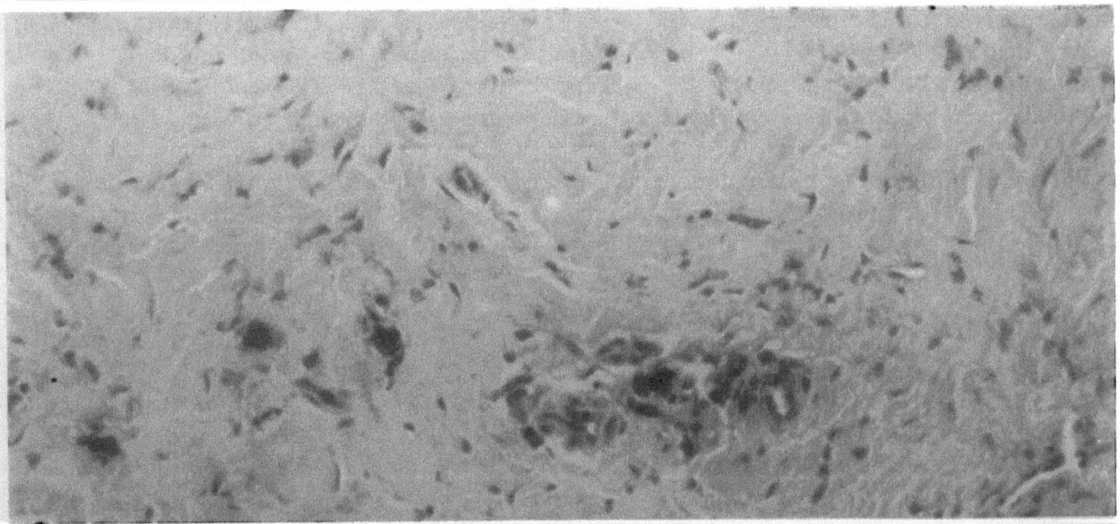
b

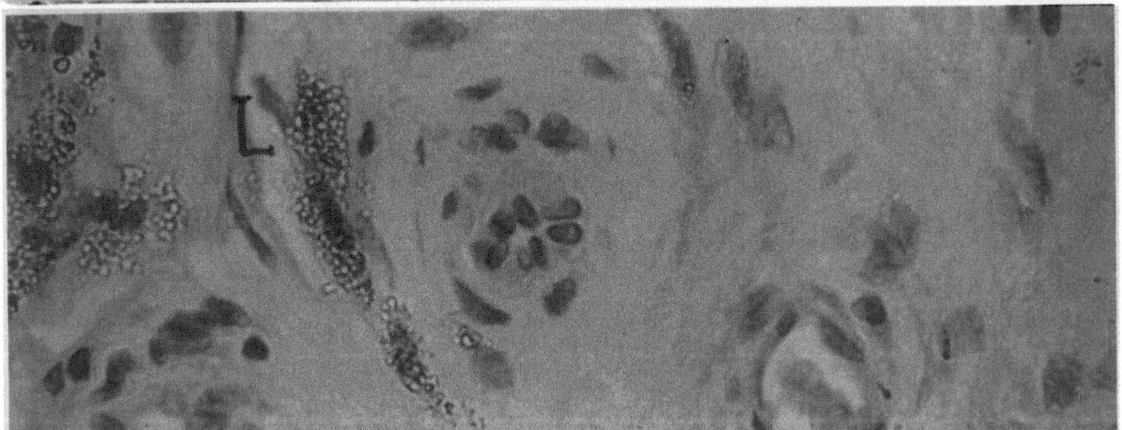

c

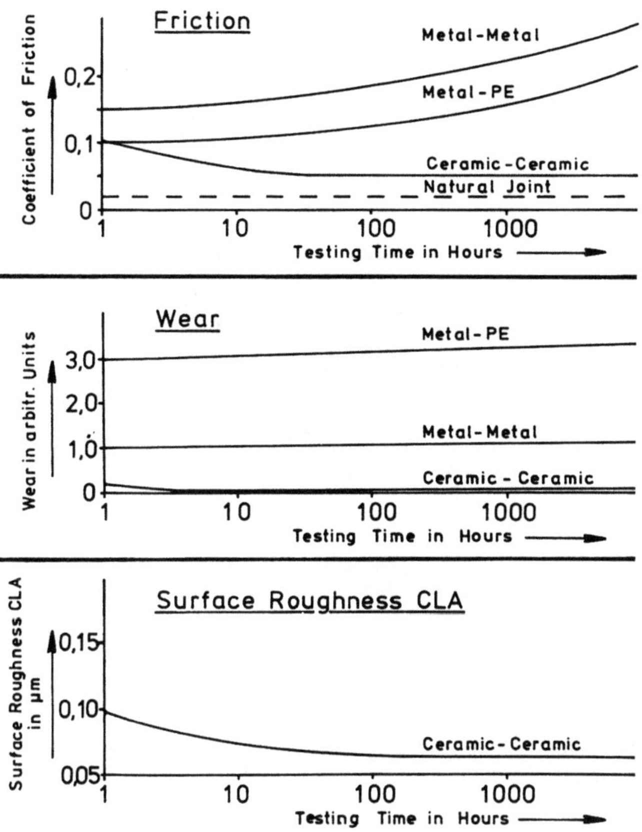

Fig. 6. Comparative simulator tests of various material combinations for hip prostheses (Dörre). The tests simulate several decades of actual service

self-anchoring bearing-rib stem or, conversely, a screw-in socket with a cemented stem, to create a "combined Autophor-Xenophor system." This option has proved especially useful in revisions of partially loosened prostheses.

Originally we limited the self-locking Autophor system to younger patients, who generally are considered to be poor candidates for standard cemented prostheses. Accordingly, most of our patients are middle-aged. However, we have also operated on adolescent patients, and increasingly we are implanting the system in patients over 60 years of age who are in good general health and have no osteoporosis. Since 1978 we have also used the Autophor system for the replacement of failed, cemented prostheses, even in older patients with unfavorable bone conditions. We reserve the cemented Xenophor prosthesis mainly for older patients, usually those over 60, who are in poor general health and have a short life expectancy and osteoporosis, in whom immediate stabilization is a more pressing concern than the longevity of the hip replacement.

Clinical Experience

The two pilot cases with a metal-on-polyethylne bearing-rib prosthesis in 1973 failed despite an initially good response. We began clinical use of the Autophor ceramic prosthesis in October, 1974, and since then we have garnered nearly 8 years of clinical experience with ceramic hip replacements, having passed the

Fig. 5. Histologic sections of capsular tissue: **a** With a conventional cemented metal-PE prosthesis, numerous refractive wear particles are visible in the tissue. There is a massive phagocytic reaction with the formation of foreign-body giant cells. **b** With a ceramic prosthesis, the capsular tissue is fully differentiated and contains few cells. Isolated macrophages containing minute ceramic particles are seen near the vessels (low-power objective). **c** Typical fine-grained wear debris. The particles are only a few microns in diameter and are easily ingested by macrophages. At *L* a wear particle is entering a lymph vessel for removal (high-power objective)

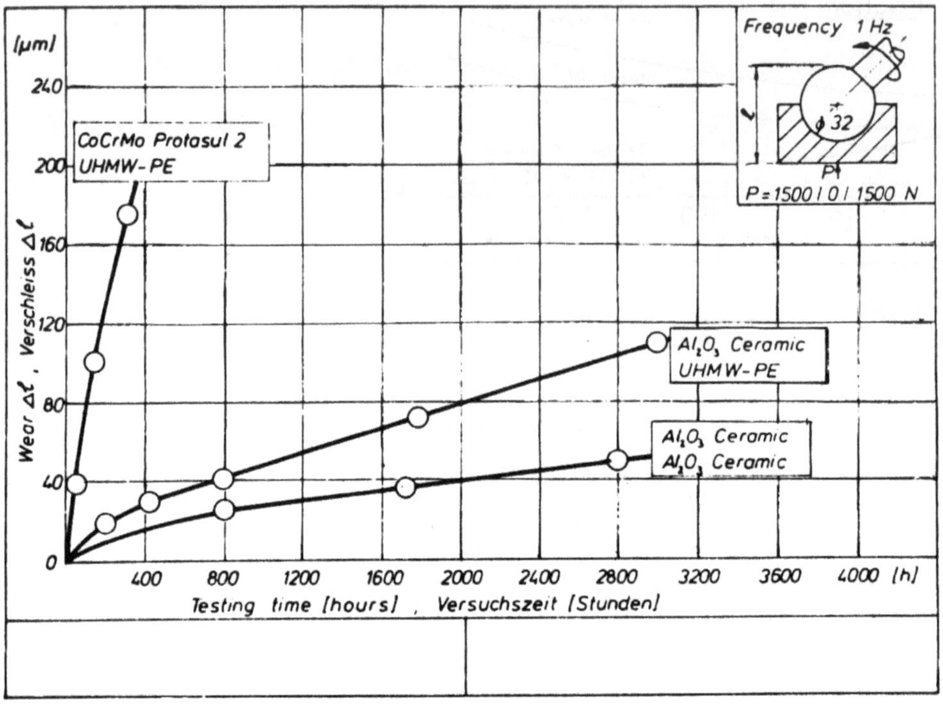

Fig. 7. Wear behavior of material combinations for hip prostheses in H_2O, simulator investigation (Semlitsch). Note rapid increase in polyethylene wear volume and relatively favorable behavior of the polyethylene-ceramic combination. The ceramic-ceramic design is optimum

1000-case mark on November 18, 1981. To date a total of about 1120 arthroplasties using ceramic components have been performed at our hospital (Autophor, Xenophor, and combinations). The last statistical review of our results was conducted at the end of 1981, based on a total of 962 total hip replacements with ceramic components. These consisted of 536 Autophor prostheses (55.7%), 374 Xenophor prostheses (389%), and 52 Autophor-Xenophor combinations (5.4%). All the Autophor prostheses were ceramic-on-ceramic; the Xenophor prostheses were about half ceramic-on-ceramic and half ceramic-on-polyethylene.

Our evaluation of results for the Autophor implantations was limited to the 432 prostheses that had been in place for at least 1 year, i.e., had been implanted by September of 1980, in order to obtain a fairly reliable "primary result." The 104 prostheses implanted after that time were disregarded.

Of the 432 cases evaluated, 415 were successfully followed. As this represents a rate of 96.1%, it may be considered highly representative. The remaining 17 cases (3.9%) were lost to follow-up.

The patients in our Autophor series included 12 adolescents (19 or younger) and many patients in their 30's, 40's and 50's. Only about 11% were older than 60. This contrasts sharply with series published for the Charnley-type cemented prosthesis and its modifications, which mainly included patients in the over-60 age group.

The arthroplasties were prompted by a wide variety of conditions. Most (31%) were performed for osteoarthritis of the hip secondary to dysplasia, including subluxations and luxations. There were many other forms of secondary osteoarthritis, most occurring as a sequel to epiphyseolysis, avascular necrosis of the femoral head, rheumatoid or infectious arthritis (including tuberculosis), or trauma (especially acetabular fractures). Idiopathic osteoarthritis was present in a few cases. In addition, 37 revisions were performed for failed cemented arthroplasties, mostly due to aseptic loosening; these were replaced with Autophor prostheses.

Due to the many cases of dysplasia and prior acetabular fractures, the anatomic conditions in the acetabular region were quite poor in a number of cases. Moreover, many hip joints showed unfavorable dislocations with limb shortening and severe contractures. Bony ankyloses and arthrodeses were present in a few cases, and these required alloplastic remobilization. Also, many patients had undergone prior operations (152 = 35.2%) that further complicated the situation. Most involved osteotomies, reductions of congenital or traumatic dislocations, and the aforementioned failed primary arthroplasties.

The main intraoperative complications, besides a few trivial trochanteric fractures, consisted of several femoral shaft fractures that mainly occurred during insertion of the curved type-I stem and during revisions in the face of very poor bone conditions. Also noteworthy are several nerve stretch injuries that occurred during the reduction of high, dysplastic hip joint dislocations, which is why we now defer this procedure for a second sitting (following primary distraction with a lenghtening apparatus).

Postoperative complications included 1 death (from liver atrophy) and 31 cases of clinically apparent thrombosis occasionally associated with pulmonary embolism, though the latter caused no deaths. There was a 1% incidence of early luxations.

Early reintervention was necessitated mainly by infection as well as by two cases of dislocation. In one of these the acetabular components had been implanted at an excessively "open" angle, while in the other the neck length of the femoral component was inadequate to produce sufficient muscular tension across the joint.

Most late reinterventions were prompted by aseptic loosenings. Four were necessitated by massive periarticular ossification, and several were done to remove internal fixation material (plate removal following a fracture, removal of troublesome cerclage wires from the greater trochanter).

Thirteen patients (3.1%) developed intractable, deep infections that necessitated removal of the prosthesis and resection (several of these

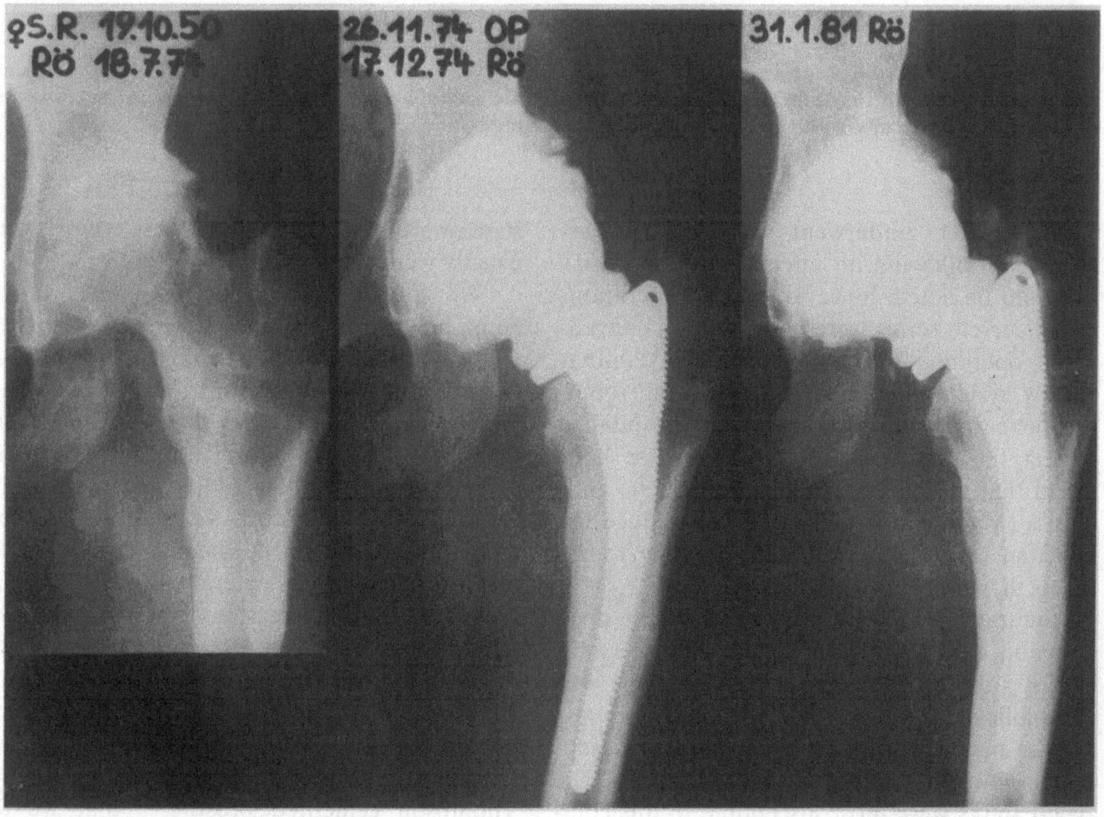

a **b** **c**

Fig. 8. Radiographic follow-up in a 23-year-old woman with severe osteoarthritis following an unsuccessful repositioning osteotomy (**a**). **b** Total hip arthroplasty with the type-I bearing-rib prosthesis. **c** 7 years later the system is still stable

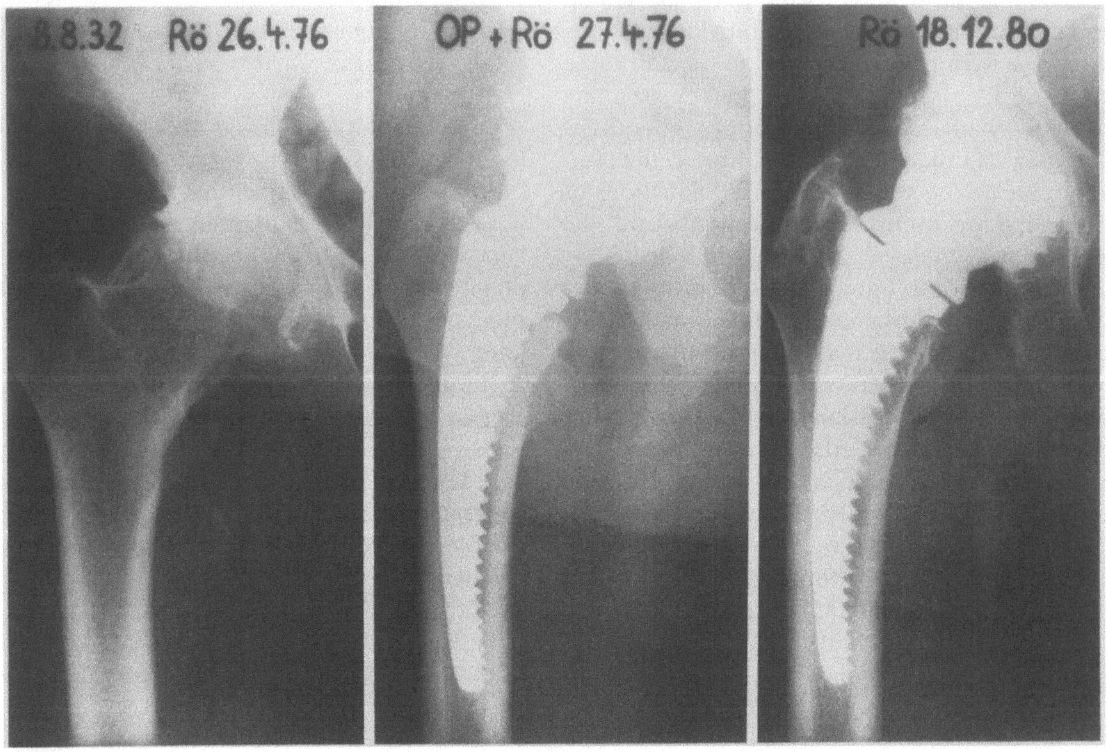

a b c

Fig. 9. Radiographic follow-up in a 43-year-old man with painful osteoarthritis of the hip **(a)**. **b** Uncemented total hip arthroplasty with the type-I prostheses. **c** 4½ years later the prosthesis is still well seated, and the socket and stem are well supported by surrounding bone

patients later underwent a revisional arthroplasty following an infection-free interval). It should be noted, however, that all operations in the current series were performed in conventional operating rooms that lacked a laminar airflow system. Two clean-air operating rooms are currently being installed at our hospital to correct this deficiency. In addition, we have found that a 3-day course of prophylactic antibiotics (Mandokef prophylaxis) can reduce the infection rate in conventional operating rooms to less than 1%.

Subtracting the 13 cases of intractable deep infection leaves 402 aseptic cases that were included in the follow-up (=96.9% of the 415 cases followed).

The major problem in these cases was aseptic loosening of the femoral endoprosthesis. The type-I stems were most susceptible to this complication. Generally, overt cases of aseptic loosening with severe complaints were managed by operative revision; loose type-I stems were replaced with either a cementable Xenophor stem or a type-II stem, while loose type-II stems usually were cemented.

We found that aseptic loosenings of the Autophor prosthesis tended to occur shortly after weight-bearing was resumed, requiring that the revision be done within the first two years. On the other hand, cases that showed no evidence of loosening during the first year of resumed weight-bearing tended to remain stable for the rest of the observation period. This contrasts markedly with the behavior of cemented arthroplasties, which generally are stable initially but have an increasing tendency to loosen with passage of time.

With the type-I stem, 108 follow-ups showed 21 cases of aseptic loosening (19.2%) that required revision. While this loosening rate was substantially lower than that of the Moore-Thompson cemented prostheses that we formerly used, we still considered it unacceptably high. This prompted us in late 1976 to abandon the type-I stem permanently in favor of the type-II stem.

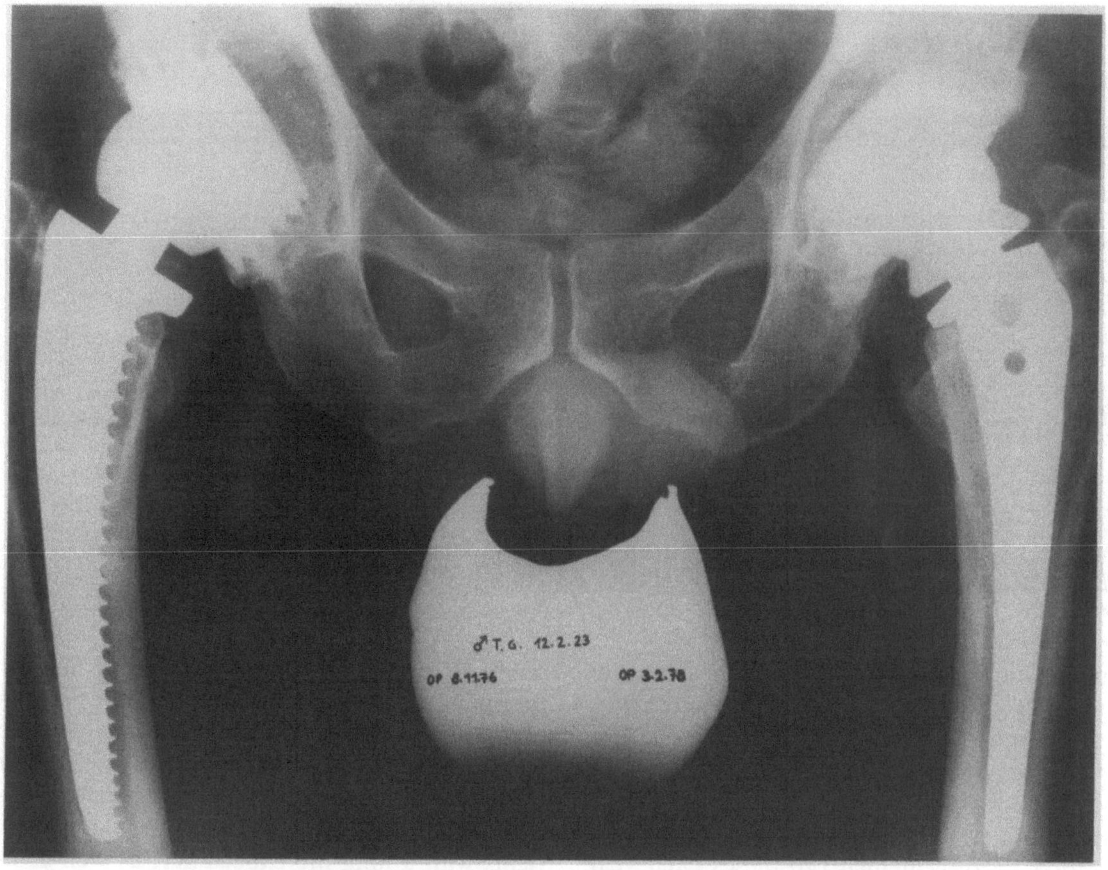

Fig. 10. Bilateral total hip arthroplasty. *Right:* Type-I bearing-rib prosthesis. Bone is visible in the hollows between the ribs. (Though the acetabular component was implanted at an excessively open angle, no wear is evident after 5 years.) *Left:* Arthroplasty with a type-II prosthesis after 3 years

In the 6 years since that time, use of the Type-II stem has greatly reduced the incidence of aseptic loosenings. Among the 307 aseptic cases reviewed to date, there have been only 12 aseptic loosenings (4.8%) necessitating revision.

The conical, screw-in acetabular prosthesis has proved extremely successful despite the deficient acetabula that were encountered in many patients. Only 4 aseptic loosenings occurred among the 415 aseptic cases reviewed (0.9%). Because all these loosenings occurred in patients who also had loose stems, the overall aseptic loosening rate since introduction of the type-II stem is only 4.8%.

Expressed differently, an aseptic stabilizing rate of 80.8% was achieved with the type-I stem, 95.2% with the type-II stem, and 99.1% with the screw-in acetabular component. Since we introduced the type-II stem in late 1976, we have achieved an overall stabilization rate of 95.2%.

Based upon 7 years' operating experience, we find that the Autophor system offers a 19:1 chance of stabilizing the uninfected hip. The risk of aseptic loosening, then, is 1:19 with this system.

As mentioned earlier, aseptic loosening of the autophor components usually occurs soon after the resumption of full weight-bearing. The main symptom is a femoral pain that radiates to the knee. There may also be an "adaptation" pain that occurs as the bony structures become adapted to the altered stress patterns. In these cases the patient should continue to use a cane or crutches until pain subsides, which may take up to a year or more. Loosening of the stem should be suspected if pain always occurs at the moment weight is borne and is elicited by the rotation test. Revision in such cases should not be delayed.

In contrast to cemented prostheses, the Autophor prostheses are characterized by an early risk of aseptic loosening with an appar-

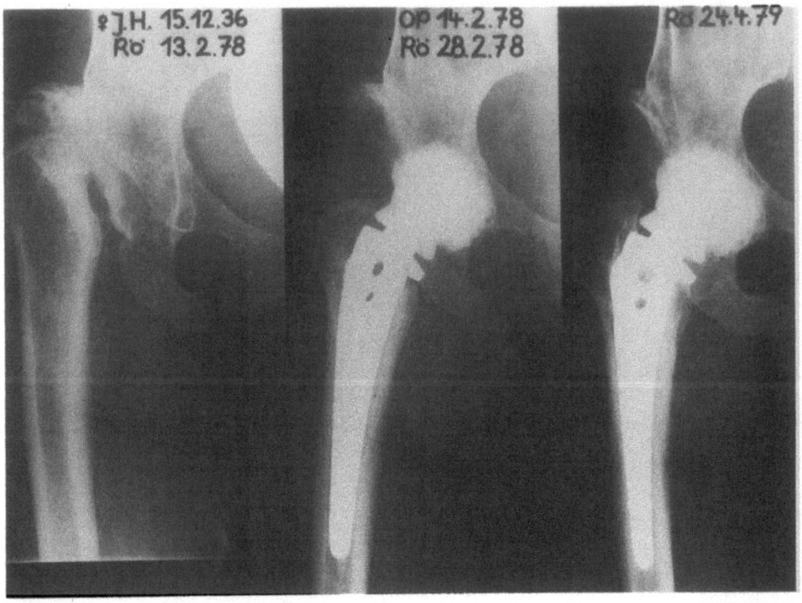

a b c

Fig. 11. Radiographic follow-up in a 46-year-old woman with severe osteoarthritis of the right hip complicated by dislocation and adduction contracture **(a)**. **b, c** Total arthroplasty with type-II bearing-rib prosthesis; a normal leg length is restored

ently low long-term risk. This is opposite to the initially good stability and increasing failure rate of cemented systems.

A variety of figures have been published on the failure rates of conventional cemented prostheses. Müller (1974) states that we lose an average of 1.5% of cemented prostheses each year. This corresponds roughly to Dobb's calculations for an improved Charnley prosthesis, which had a computer-projected mean lifetime (50% failure rate) of 34 years. A multicentric study conducted in the Federal Republic of Germany (Griss et al., 1981) indicated a 10-year failure rate of approximately 23% in a large patient population that mainly had cemented arthroplasties, though this rate was highly variable and tended to be lower in later years.

Comparing these data with the Autophor femoral component with a type-I stem, we find that short-term results are obviously poorer with the Authophor prosthesis. Even the type-II stem clearly has a higher loosening rate during the first 2 years than the cemented prostheses. When we examine the longer-term results, however, we find that after 4 to 5 years the results are statistically equal for the Autophor prosthesis and cemented prostheses, and that beyond that time the Autophor prosthesis is clearly superior to cemented systems. Of course it must be considered that the patient populations are not entirely comparable, since the Autophor series mainly included younger patients for whom a higher activity level may be presumed, as well as a number of older patients that had to undergo difficult revisions. On the whole, however, this comparative evaluation would seem to indicate that the Autophor system offers significant advantages in younger patients with a long life expectancy, as well as in revision arthroplasties for loose cemented prostheses in older patients.

The Autophor system offers additional advantages as well:

Joint mobility is significantly improved in most patients. While it was severely limited preoperatively in most cases, mobility in the most recent examinations was rated as excellent in 11.8% and good in 67.7% (total 79.5%). It was rated fair in 13.4% and poor in 7.1%. Most of the poor cases already had a severe restriction of joint motion preoperatively or developed periarticular ossifications postoperatively.

Radiographically, the periarticular ossifications were rated as mild in 5.1%, moderate in 2.1% and severe in 2.3% (total 9.5%). Thus, the ossification rate is no higher and the degree of ossification no more severe than we have experienced with cemented prostheses and are entirely comparable to favorable reports published by other authors.

The pain-free walking distance in our series was severely limited in most patients prior to operation. Only 2.6% could walk between 500 and 1000 meters, and only 1 patient (0.2%) could walk farther than 1000 m. At latest follow-up, however, 58.5% could walk farther than 1000 m without pain, and 17.7% could walk between 500 and 1000 m (total 76.2%). Thus, ¾ of the patients could negotiate ordinary walking distances. A limited pain-free walking distance between 100 and 500 m was reported by 15.3% of the patients, while 8.5% said they were unable to walk a significant distance without pain. It should be noted, however, that the "pain-free walking distance" does not represent an absolute limit, and that most patients said they were capable of walking considerably longer distances with some discomfort or with the aid of a cane.

Residual pain in our patients was partly the result of muscular fatigue, which was most commonly associated with hip dysplasia (dislocations, prior surgery), previous arthroplasties, hip resections, etc. Only a few patients complained of femoral pain, which may be interpreted either as muscle pain or, perhaps, as a sign of excessive loading of the bone. In no case was residual pain severe enough to warrant revision, however.

The Autophor arthroplasty was also highly successful from the standpoint of walking aids. Preoperatively, 10.5% of our patients needed 2 crutches and 35.6% needed 1 crutch or cane (total 46.1%); only 53.9% could walk without canes or crutches. At latest follow-up, none of our patients required 2 crutches; 3.2% continued to need a cane, and 22.9% occasionally used a cane for long walks. Overall, then, 73.9% of our patients required no walking aids whatsoever. (It should be noted that some of the walking aids were needed for pain on the opposite side, creating a situation that is difficult to analyze.)

The results of the operation were rated subjectively by the patients as "excellent" in 57.7% of cases and "good" in 15.9% (total 73.6%); 18.3% rated the result as "fair." Thus, the total rate of excellent to fair results was 91.9% according to the subjective rating. The remaining 8.1% gave a "poor" rating on account of restricted joint motion, muscular or femoral pain, or limping due to gluteal insufficiency (most frequent). However, these problems seem minor when viewed in relation to primary dislocations, severe post-traumatic lesions, joint stiffness (ankyloses and arthrodeses) and revision arthroplasties.

In the cases that required removal of the prosthesis because of infection, healing was appreciably more rapid than that following the removal of cemented prostheses – apparently because an uncemented prosthesis is inherently easier to remove than a cemented one and avoids the problem of cement residues that promote infection.

We are happy to report that in instances of infectious joint destruction or the direct revision of infected, cemented prostheses with an Autophor prosthesis, the great majority of cases went on to uneventful healing with no recurrence of infection (combined, of course, with removal of all infected and necrotic tissues and a prolonged, intensive course of antibiotics).

Moreover, the outcome of revisions with cemented prostheses for aseptic loosenings is satisfactory so far, although the long-term risks of cement remain a problem.

We do not believe that the cemented and uncemented methods of fixation should be viewed as competing techniques. Instead, we believe that each supplements the other, providing the orthopedic surgeon and his patients with a valuable alternative should one of the methods fail. Thus, bone cement can be resorted to in the event that an uncemented prosthesis loosens, while the cement-free technique provides a means of salvaging a failed cemented arthroplasty in the face of severe bone destruction. Among our own patients, we have seen many cases of severe bone destruction following primary arthroplasty with a polyester prosthesis (certain types of Weber-Huggler prosthesis, Müller prosthesis) that had been implanted in the early 1970s and later failed due to extensive foreign-body granulations.

Radiographic follow-ups of the operated hips clearly show adaptation of the bone to the new patterns of load distribution several months postoperatively. Adaptation to the ribbed prosthetic surfaces is particularly striking. As was demonstrated by the first Judet prostheses in 1956 and later by canine experiments during development of the bearing-rib prosthesis, a new layer of load-bearing bone forms at the ribbed surfaces of both the femoral and acetabular components. On x-ray this dense bone line is partially separated from the prosthetic surface by a thin radiolucent zone that consists histologically of connective tissue. This thin, interposed layer should not be interpreted as evidence of aseptic loosening, but rather as a kind of "expansion joint" which compensates for the different elastic properties of the bone and prosthesis. Similar expansion joints are commonly used in engineering to compensate for thermal or mechanical motion between different material layers. Loosening of the prosthesis should be suspected only if there is a radiolucent seam at least 1.5 mm thick that is associated with corresponding clinical symptoms.

The newly-formed load-bearing bone is seen especially well in the hollows of the socket threads and the bearing ribs of the type-I femoral stem. In the type-II stem, the recesses are hidden from view by the ridges that run along the edges of the stem. Nevertheless, the adaptation can still be observed on the outer surface of the type-II stem and below the collar.

In contrast to cemented prostheses, atrophy of the calcar as a result of "stress shielding" is extremely rare, and the loads imposed upon the calcar usually cause it to acquire a dense bone structure.

The formation of a bony "pedestal" below the distal end of the stem is also a result of stress transfer in that area and should not be considered evidence of loosening, as it may be for cemented prostheses. Also, there is often a visible thickening of the femoral cortex in the stem region, indicating a restoration of sound bone function.

Of particular importance is our finding that in all cases where the prostheses were positioned correctly at implantation, no head eccentricity developed at any time during the follow-up period that would indicate excessive wear, and no gaps appeared between the acetabular component and the inferior portion of the head like those described by Charnley (1979) for metal-polyethylene prostheses. Only in the rare cases where the acetabular component was excessively open, leading to excessive edge loading and recurrent subluxations, did gaps appear between the head and socket in the inferior portion of the joint. The fault lay not in the components themselves, but in the faulty implantation technique.

In 40 cases where the prostheses had to be removed due to infection or aseptic loosening, we were able to perform laboratory wear measurements on the retrieved prosthetic material. Measurements with a precision spherometer showed a very low degree of wear in most cases. Two cases (with Xenophor prostheses) were excluded from measurements due to fracture of the ceramic. In another 5 cases, the degree of wear exceeded the 200-μm measuring range of the instrument. Radiographic findings in these cases showed that this was probably due to excessive obliquity of the acetabular component leading to an unusual degree of edge wear. In the remaining 33 cases with a well-positioned socket, the wear rate after an average of 21 months was 2.6 μm/year for the socket and 5.4 μm/year for the head (average values). This linear wear is only about 1/40 to 1/80 of the wear reported for the Charnley prostheses and their modifications. Thus, both clinical experience and laboratory measurements confirm the low wear rate of the aluminum oxide ceramic (assuming a correct technique) that was demonstrated in the earlier simulator experiments of Dörre et al. (1975).

The revision arthroplasties also enabled us to obtain tissue samples, especially from the joint capsule, for histologic studies of wear debris and associated tissue reactions. We found that the wear of the ceramic-ceramic combination was generally quite low, and that the debris consisted essentially of minute particles with a size range of about 1–2 μm. Only in the rare cases where there was excessive obliquity of the acetabular component leading to recurrent subluxations and edge wear could larger particles up to about 15 μm in diameter be found (Harms and Mäusle, 1980). Apparently the fine wear debris is readily engulfed by macrophages and removed via the blood and lymph, creating a phagocytic cleansing mechanism that prevents an excessive accumulation of foreign material. Most notably, we observed no toxic or necrotic effects in the tissue cells. The debris-filled macrophages showed no degenerative changes, and no inflammatory or giant cells could be seen. In this respect the ceramic differs markedly from metal-polyethylene prostheses. Many of the wear particles from these prostheses are too large to be phagocytized and removed, and so they remain in the tissue, becoming engulfed by giant cells and finally exerting a necrotizing effect that transforms the entire capsule into a foreign-body granulation tissue. Apparently the ceramic prosthesis, with its low rate of wear and its small, easily-phagocytized wear particles, creates a compensated situation in which a balance is struck between the production and removal of wear debris. With the conventional metal-polyethylene prostheses, on the other hand, it is only a matter of time before tissue decompensation occurs.

Prosthetic fractures in our series were extremely rare: we found only 1 fracture in a type-I stem (made from the old cobalt-chromium alloy) and none in the type-II stems constructed of Endocast alloy. Similarly, we observed no ceramic fractures in any of the 415 Autophor cases included in our statistical review. Only at the beginning of this year did we see a ceramic head fracture in an Autophor prosthesis (too late for inclusion in the present evaluation) following an injury. The situation was quickly remedied by replacing the head.

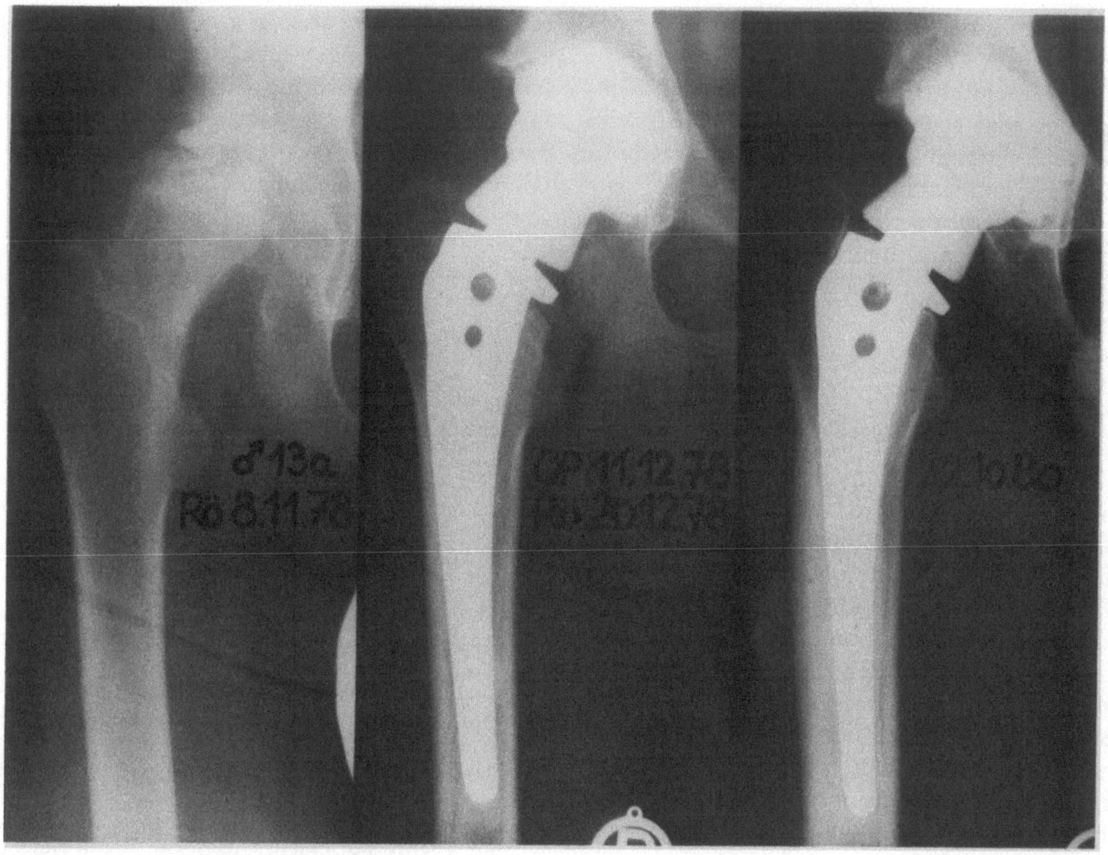

a b c

Fig. 12. Severe femoral head necrosis secondary to traumatic epiphyseal separation in a 13-year-old boy **(a)**. **b, c** Good bony adaptation following total hip arthroplasty with the bearing-rib prosthesis (youngest patient in series)

To date we have observed 4 fractures of ceramic-ceramic Xenophor prostheses involving the head, socket or both, but we have seen no fractures in Xenophor prostheses with a ceramic-polyethylene combination. Apparently the ceramic-ceramic combination is vulnerable to shock loading associated with trauma or subluxations. However, the overall incidence of ceramic fractures in our series is only about 0.4% and thus is substantially lower than the incidence of cement breakage in conventional cemented arthroplasties, in which the cement in effect represents an extra prosthetic component.

In view of the relatively low wear rate of the ceramic-polyethylene combination in simulator tests, and on the basis of clinical observations, we believe that the combination of a ceramic head and polyethylene socket is best for the Xenophor prosthesis. Because the Xenophor system is basically indicated for older patients, and given the low wear rate of the ceramic-polyethylene combination compared to metal-polyethylene, it is reasonable to assume that no significant wear problems will arise during the patient's lifetime. Whereas the metal-polyethylene combination has a useful life of about 10–15 years from the standpoint of wear, we have found that the ceramic-polyethylene combination has an average useful life of about 30 years before wear and associated foreign-body reactions become a problem. This should be more than adequate for patients over the age of 60, and the improved shock absorption of the ceramic-PE system should eliminate the problem of ceramic breakage. However, in younger patients with a presumed life expectancy of more than 30 years, and especially in patients below the age of 40, we still recommend the ceramic-ceramic combination in a cement-free design, i.e., the standard Autophor system, as it is the only system that can ensure adequate wear resistance for the life of the patient.

We should also point out that the self-locking cone that connects the ceramic head with the metal femoral stem performed flawlessly in our series, and that no loosening occurred.

In recent years we have been working on further refinements aimed mainly at improving the stability of our total hip systems. We hope to accomplish this by adding microstructural features to our model-II stem. In the new-generation self-locking prostheses of Judet ("porometal" prosthesis) and Lord ("madreporic" prosthesis), it has been shown that microirregularities on the prosthetic surface are conducive to bone ingrowth. In the Judet prosthesis this is accomplished through porosity, and in the Lord prosthesis through the presence of spherules. Recent reports of Judet (1975) and Lord on their stabilization rates coincide closely with those of our Autophor prostheses, which so far have employed only macroscopic surface features. We believe that by combining our coarse surface relief with microstructural features, mainly in the form of minute surface projections, we will be able to further increase our stabilization rates. Animal experiments in this area (Harms and Mittelmeier, 1980) are very promising, and we hope that the new design will be available for clinical use in the near future. It should be stressed, however, that the Autophor prosthesis already has reached a highly successful level of development.

Summary

The return to the self-anchoring principle with the second generation of cement-free prostheses employing the surface-enlargement principle has provided a highly successful alternative to cement fixation and the problems that it entails. Combining this principle with the use of highly wear-resistant aluminum oxide ceramic has substantially broadened our operative capabilities. In particular, the Autophor system enables total hip replacements to be done in younger patients who previously were poor candidates for such procedures. We also recommend it as a means of salvaging failed cemented arthroplasties, even in older patients. Of course success cannot be guaranteed in any operation, but our data indicate that the chance of a good long-term result is statistically very high, and it is hoped that future experience will bear this out. It is doubtful that the implant system represents an "ultimate solution" in its present form, but it certainty represents a notable milestone and a sound basis for further development.

References

1. Bentler H, Lehmann M, Strähli G (1974) Verschleißverhalten medizinaltechnischer Werkstoffe, Sulzer Technische Rundschau
2. Biehl G, Harms J, Mäusle E (1975) Tierexperimentelle und histopathologische Untersuchungen über die Anpassungsvorgänge des Knochens nach der Implantation von „Tragrippen-Endoprothesen". Arch Orthop Unfallchir 81:105
3. Boutin P (1972) Arthroplastie totale de la hanche par prothèse en alumine frittée. Rev Chir Orthop 58:229
4. Charnley J (1974) Clinical and laboratory observations on the rate of wear of different plastic materials in the sockets of artificial hip joints. 55th Scientific Meeting: "Materials for use in medicine and bilogy", Cambridge
5. Charnley J (1979) Low friction arthroplasty of the hip. Theory and practice. Springer, Berlin Heidelberg New York
6. Diehl K, Harms J (1976) Beanspruchung und Umbau bei der Alloarthroplastik des coxalen Femurendes des Hundes mit einer selbsthaftenden Tragrippenprothese. Arch orthop Unfall-Chir 84:89–104
7. Diehl K, Harms J (1976b) Über die Aussagekraft tierexperimenteller Ergebnisse mit Hüftendoprothesen. Z Orthop 114:17–25
8. Dörre E, Beutler H, Geduldig D (1975) Anforderungen an oxidkeramische Werkstoffe als Biomaterial für künstliche Gelenke. Arch Orthop Unfallchir 83:269
9. Dörre E, Geduldig D, Happel M, Lade R, Prüssner P. Willert HG, Zichner L (1976) Animal studies on bone ingrowth kinetics of ceramic material under dynamic stress. J Biomed Mater Res 10:493–502
10. Griss P, Krempien B, Andrian-Werburg H v, Heimke G, Fleiner R (1973) Experimentelle Untersuchung zur Gewebeverträglichkeit oxidkeramischer (Al_2O_3) Abriebteilen. Arch Orthop Unfallchir 76:270
11. Groher W (1980) Erfahrungen mit der Keramik-Tragrippen-Hüftprothese nach Mittelmeier. Med Orthop Techn 100:30
12. Harms J, Mäusle E (1980) Biokompatibilität von Implantaten in der Orthopädie. Hefte Unfallheilkd 144:1–118
13. Harms J, Mittelmeier M (1980) Statistische Auswertung von 4 Jahren klinischer Prüfung der

Hüft-Alloplastik mit Keramik-Tragrippen-Endoprothesen. Med Orthop Techn 100:25–29
14. Judet R (1975) Totale Hüftendoprothesen aus Porometall ohne Zementverankerung. Z Orthop 113:828–829
15. Mittelmeier H (1974) Zementlose Verankerung von Endoprothesen nach dem Tragrippenprinzip. Z Orthop 112:27
16. Mittelmeier H (1975) Selbsthaftende Keramik-Metall-Verbund-Endoprothesen („Tragrippen-Prothese"). Med Orthop Techn 95:152–159
17. Mittelmeier H (1976) Anchoring hip endoprosthesis without bone cement. In: Schaldach M, Hohmann D (eds) Engineering in medicine, vol 2. Advances in artificial hip and knee joint technology. Springer, Berlin Heidelberg New York, p 387
18. Mittelmeier H (1979) Keramik-Tragrippen-Prothesen ohne Zement (Kongreßbericht 1979). Langenbecks Arch Chir 349:315–319
19. Mittelmeier H (1980) Biomechanisch bedingte Grenzschichtreaktionen des Knochengewebes bei Verankerung von Endoprothesen. In: Jäger M, Hackenbroch MH, Refior HJ (Hrsg) Grenzschichtprobleme der Verankerung von Implantation unter besonderer Berücksichtigung von Endoprothesen. Thieme, Stuttgart
20. Mittelmeier H (1980) Sonderindikationen für zementfrei implantierbare Keramik-Tragrippen-Endoprothesen. Med Orthop Techn 100:32–35
21. Mittelmeier H (1980) Problemfälle bei der Hüftalloplastik mit Keramik-Tragrippenprothesen. Med Orthop Techn 100:36–38
22. Mittelmeier H (1980) 4 Jahre klinische Erfahrung mit Keramik-Tragrippen-Hüftprothesen. Med Orthop Techn 100:19
23. Mittelmeier H (1981) Implantate aus Aluminium-Oxyd-Keramik. Symp. über Biomaterialien. Schriftenreihe der Med Orthop Techn 5:76 (Gentner Verlag)
24. Mittelmeier H (im Druck) Alloarthroplastik des Hüftglenkes – derzeitiger Stand (Unter besonderer Berücksichtigung von Keramik-Endoprothesen). Therapie-Woche
25. Mittelmeier H, Harms J (1977) Die Anwendung von Keramik in der Gelenkersatz-Chirurgie. Med Orthop Techn 97:55–57
26. Mittelmeier H, Harms J (1979) Hüftalloplastik mit Keramik-Endoprothesen bei traumatischen Hüftschäden (Unter besonderer Berücksichtigung zementfrei implantierbarer „Autophor"-Tragrippen-Endoprothesen. Unfallheilkunde 82:67–75
27. Mittelmeier H, Harms J (1979) Derzeitiger Stand der zementfreien Verankerung von Keramik-Metall-Verbundprothesen. Z Orthop 117:478–481
28. Mittelmeier H, Harms J (1980) Pathologische Verankerungen an Implantatlager bei Endoprothetik mit Zementimplantation und Selbstverankerung. 16. Jahrestagung d. Dtsch. Ges. f. Plast. und Wiederherstellungschir., Düsseldorf 1978. Springer, Berlin Heidelberg New York, S 298
29. Mittelmeier H, Singer L (1956) Anatomische und histologische Untersuchungen von Arthroplastikgelenken mit Plexiglas-Endoprothesen. Arch Orthop Unfallchir 48:519
30. Mittelmeier H, Dawihl W, Dörre E, Altmeyer G, Hanser U (1979) Zur Tribologie von Hüftgelenksendoprothesen aus Aluminiumoxydkeramik. Med Orthop Techn 99:114
31. Mittelmeier H, Harms J, Mäusle E (1979) The biocompatibility of alumina ceramics. 10. Congr. of the European Federation of the Int. College of Surgeons, Milan 1977.
32. Mittelmeier H, Biehl G, Harms J (1980) Röntgenologische Anpassungsvorgänge des Prothesenlagers bei zementfreier Verankerung von Keramik-Tragrippen-Endoprothesen. In: Jäger M, Hackenbroch MH, Refior HJ (Hrsg) Grenzschichtprobleme der Verankerung von Implantaten unter besonderer Berücksichtigung von Endoprothesen. Thieme, Stuttgart
33. Mittelmeier H, Hanser U, Harms J (1980) Lösung des biochemischen und mechanischen Zementproblems mit Apatit-Carbonfaser-Zement? In: Jäger M, Hackenbroch MH, Refior HJ (Hrsg) Osteosynthese, Endoprothetik und Biomechanik der Gelenke. Thieme, Stuttgart, S 62–68
34. Mittelmeier H, Hanser U, Harms J (1980) Zur Lösung des Zementproblems mittels Apatit-Carbonfaser-Knochenzement. Z Orthop 118:658
35. Müller ME (1970) Total hip prosthesis. Clin Orthop 72:46
36. Müller ME (1974) Der derzeitige Stand der Totalendoprothese des Hüftgelenkes. Z Orthop 112:933
37. Rossak K, Brinkmann KE (1980) Erfahrungen mit dem Einsatz von Keramik-Totalprothesen zum Austausch ausgelockerter Totalendoprothesen des Hüftgelenkes. Med Orthop Techn 100:31–32
38. Salzer M, Zweymüller K, Locke H, Plenk H Jr, Punzet G (1975) Erste Erfahrungen mit einer Hüfttotalendoprothese aus Biokeramik. Med Orthop Techn 95:162–164
39. Salzer M, Zweymüller K, Locke H, Plenk H Jr, Punzet G (1975) Biokeramische Endoprothesen. Med Orthop Techn 95:40–45
40. Willert HG (1973) Tissue reactions around joint implants and bone cement. In: Chapchal G (ed) Arthroplasty of the hip. Thieme, Stuttgart
41. Willert HG, Puls P (1972) Die Reaktion des Knochens auf Knochenzement bei der Allo-Arthroplastik der Hüfte. Arch Orthop Unfallchir 72:33
42. Willert HG, Semlitsch M (1974) Kapselreaktionen bei Gelenkprothesen. Schweizerisch-Niederländische Orthopädie-Tagung, Lausanne
43. Willert HG, Semlitsch M (1976) Kunststoffe als Implantatwerkstoffe. Med Orthop Techn 4:94

A Screw-Anchored Intramedullary Hip Prosthesis

G. Bousquet and F. Bornand

During the period from 1974 to 1977, we observed several complications associated with the use of various types of uncemented prosthesis. In these systems the acetabular component was constructed either of polyethylene or a metal-plastic combination. The long femoral components were made of "porometal." The following complications were observed:

- Acetabulitis due to poor tolerance of the polyethylene in the cartilage bed.
- Acetabulitis due to friction of metal against cartilage.
- Femoral pain due to a poor stem-to-canal fit.
- Femoral pain based on a change of elasticity in the femur with an osteoperiosteal reaction.

To avoid these complications, we developed an intramedullary prosthesis in 1978 that employs the following principles:

1. Acetabular component:
   - optimum preservation of acetabular elasticity
   - optimum distribution of compressive stresses
   - minimum alteration of bone structure.
2. Femoral component:
   - high-shear-strength intramedullary stem
   - optimum, harmonious distribution of compressive forces along the femur
   - stability against rotation
   - preservation of femoral elasticity
   - chemical neutrality.

The Prosthesis

The prosthesis (Fig. 1) consists of a metal socket, which is driven into the acetabulum. Its outer surface is coated with Al_2O_3. Three elements make it possible to attach the socket in the proper orientation: the ilium, the ischium and the pubic bone.

The inferior rim of the socket was rounded to prevent contact between it and the femoral neck.

In the femoral component, the intramedullary stem is threaded externally and tapered slightly to minimize bone damage during insertion and ensure an optimum stem-to-canal match. This design enables the stem to gain attachment in the cortical bone while supporting "corticalization" of the cancellous bone.

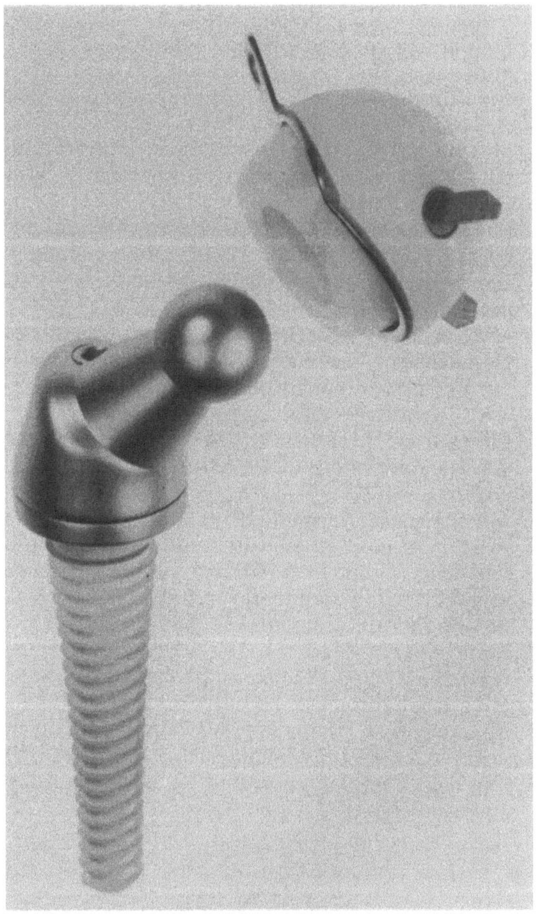

Fig. 1. Metal acetabular socket with rounded inferior rim

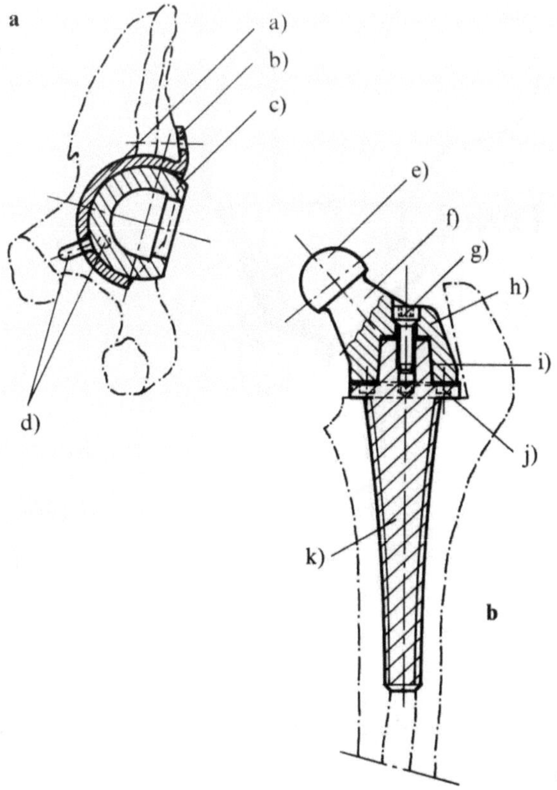

a) Metal backing
b) Fixation clip
c) Polyethylene socket
d) Screw for anchoring the socket to the ischium and pubis
e) Spherical prosthetic head (22 mm diam.)
f) Neck of prosthesis
g) Connecting bolt
h) Base of head-neck assembly
i) Conical mounting post
j) Buttress collar with 8 perforations
k) Special conical thread with Al_2O_3 coating

Fig. 2a, b. Prosthesis with polyethylene socket (RCM 1000)

The friction torque in such a system is 7 daN. The total contact area available for stress transfer to the bone is 3500 mm². Consequently, the pressure on the bone is equal to 0.3 daN/mm². The shear forces on the cancellous bone and cortex amount to 0.2 daN/mm².

The collar of the femoral prosthesis is oriented horizontally, thus permitting stress transfer to the cortex.

The head and neck assembly is a single piece that attaches to the proximal end of the intramedullary stem. The femoral head is 22 mm in diameter and comes in 3 different neck lengths.

The polyethylene socket (RCM 1000) consists of two spherical parts. This creates a dual articulation which enhances the mobility and stability of the device. The friction torque between the cup and 22-mm head is 0.3 daN. The friction between the outer socket and polyethylene cup is 2.5 times greater.

Most motion takes place between the head and cup. The metal is vacuum-cast Inox 22 CND 17-B.

A ceramic backing is available to ensure complete chemical inertness. This avoids the interposition of connective tissue between the bone and prosthesis while promoting corticalization of the bone. Implantations of Al_2O_3-coated prostheses in sheep are planned.

Figure 3 shows an electron microscopic view of the bone-ceramic interface taken at two different magnifications. The bone is on the left (O) and the ceramic on the right (C). The higher magnification reveals an osteoid border (BO) in immediate contact with the ceramic.

Insertion of the Prosthesis

1. We use the posterolateral approach of Koher-Gibson, which necessitates division of the external rotators. The femoral head is dislocated, and the femoral osteotomy is carried out.
2. The femoral osteotomy involves two cuts: the first perpendicular to the axis of the shaft and the second at right angles to the first, along the greater trochanter (Fig. 4).
3. The medullary canal is then prepared using a gouge, intramedullary reamer and tap (Fig. 5).

a

b

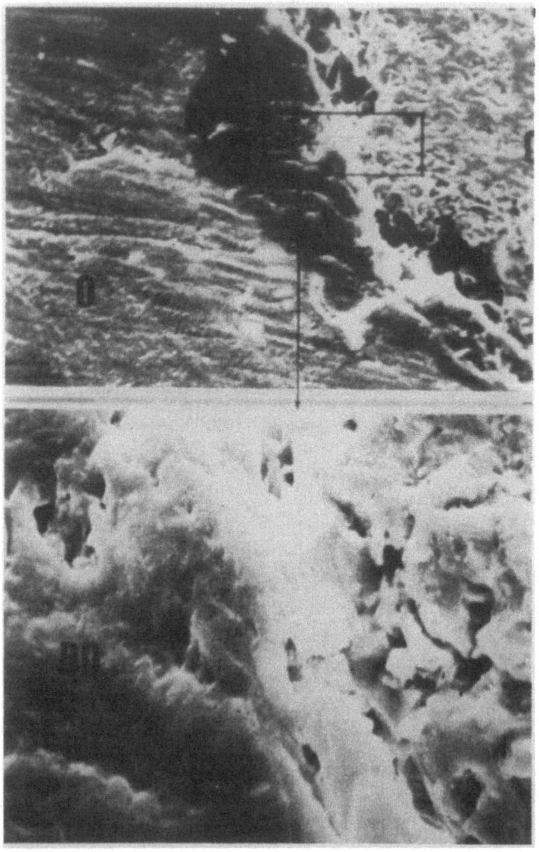

Fig. 3 a, b. Electron micrographs at 2 different magnifications showing region of contact between bone and ceramic. In **a** the bone is on the left (*O*) and the ceramic is on the right (*C*). The higher magnification in **b** shows the osteoid border (BO) in close contact with the ceramic

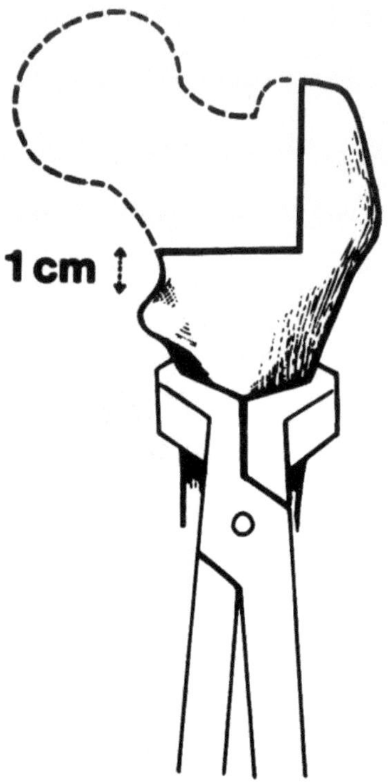

Fig. 4. Double osteotomy of the proximal femur

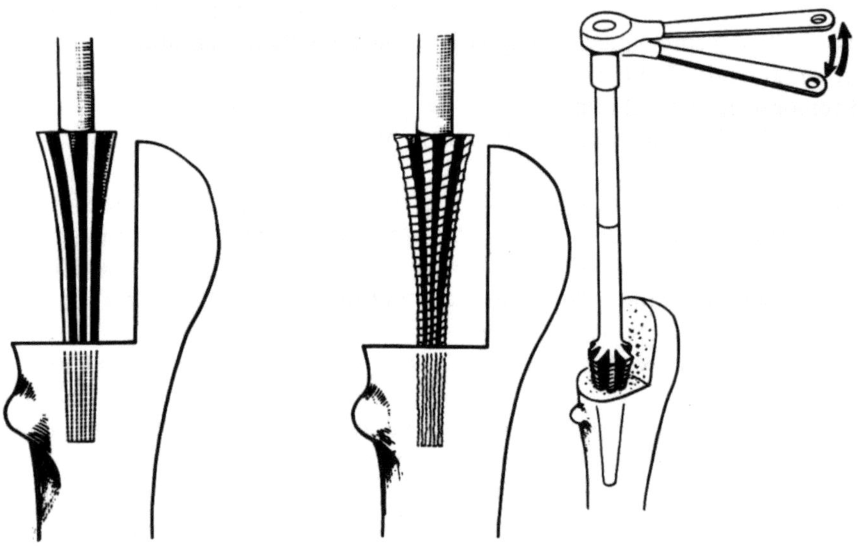

Fig. 5. Preparation of the medullar canal

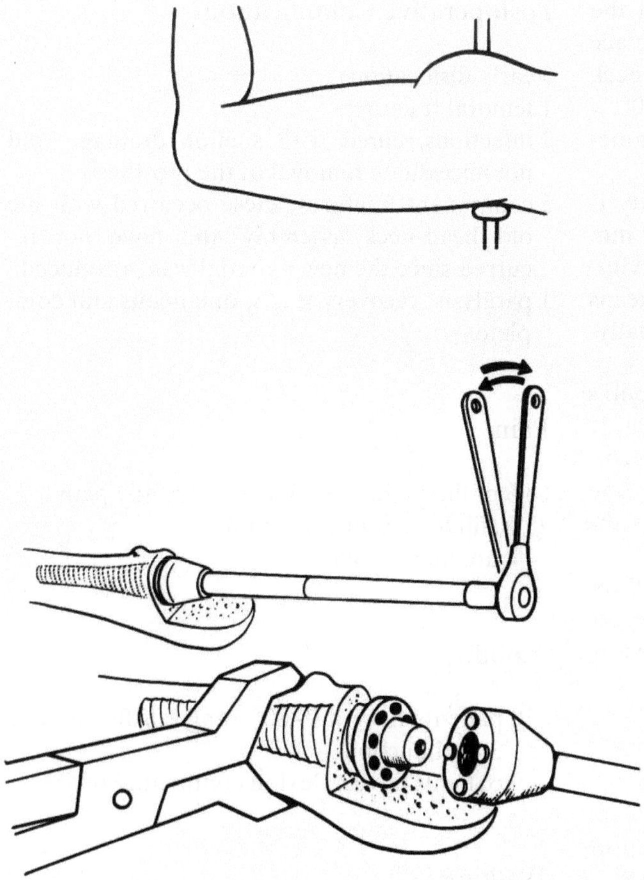

Fig. 6. Insertion of the intramedullary stem

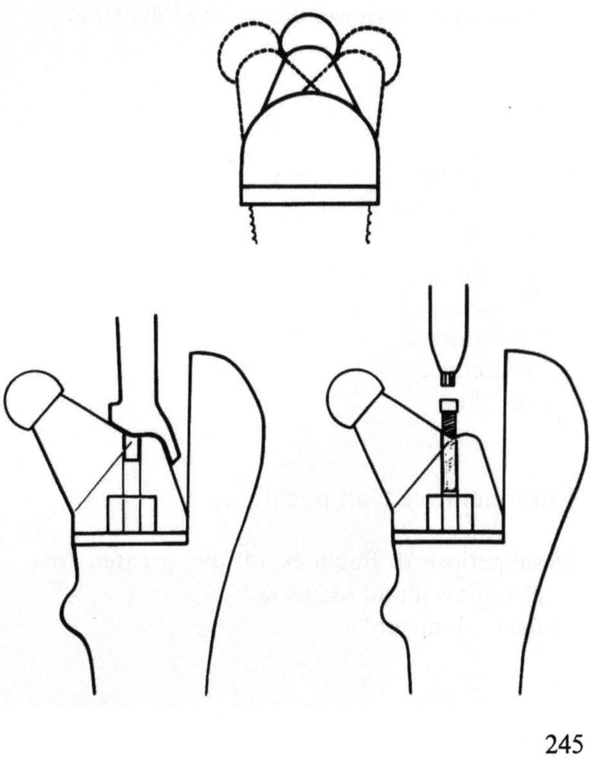

Fig. 7. The anchoring pegs are driven into the pubis and ilium, and then the head and neck assembly is mounted on the stem

4. After the canal has been threaded with the tap, the femoral stem is screwed into place with a special wrench (Fig. 6). The neck length is measured with the knee flexed 90°.
5. Next the acetabulum is reamed to the diameter of the acetabular prosthesis.
6. A trial prosthesis is inserted, and stability is tested. The trial prosthesis should be 2 mm larger than the diameter of the reamed cavity.
7. The socket is attached to the ilium by means of a screw passed through the cranially-directed eye in the socket.
8. The anchoring pegs are driven into the pubis and ilium. Then the head and neck assembly is mounted on the intramedullary stem in correct anteversion and secured with a bolt (Fig. 7). Reduction of the artificial hip is the final step.

Following the implantation, we insert three suction drains. Prophylactic antibiotics are not administered. Full weight bearing is allowed on the first postoperative day.

Results

To date we have implanted this prosthesis in more than 600 patients. We have followed 168 of them for periods ranging from 345 to 1110 days.

Mobility is comparable to that obtained with other types of prosthesis.

A statistical review indicates the following:

Etiology

136 osteoarthritis (primary)
6 congenital dislocations
6 arthritis
12 aseptic necrosis
3 acetabular fractures
2 arthrodeses
2 miscellaneous
1 revision

Intraoperative Complications

28 subperiosteal fractures of the greater trochanter, without sequelae
3 femoral fractures

Postoperative Complications

5 early dislocations
1 femoral fracture
2 infections, cured with suction drainage; did not necessitate removal of the prosthesis
5 component fractures; these occurred with the old head-neck assembly and have not recurred since the new material was introduced
1 paralysis; recovery was spontaneous and complete.

Pain

68% of the patients no longer have any pain.
28% still have transitory pain.
4% are unchanged.

Mobility

130 patients have a 0–80° range of flexion and 30° abduction.
9 patients have a flexion contracture of 5°.

Walking

36% can walk without impediment.
46% can walk over 4 km.

Revisions

9 patients had to undergo revisions:

- 5 due to component fractures. The broken component was replaced at revision.
- 2 due to infection (see above).
- 2 due to technical flaws. Reoperation became necessary during the first 3 months due to inadequate depth of insertion of the intramedullary stem.

Experimental and Clinical Experience with Carbon Hip Endoprostheses

H. Rettig and U. Weber

The burgeoning popularity of total hip replacements and the consequent rise in the incidence of failed arthroplasties has provided an impetus for the development of new prosthetic models and for the introduction of advanced biomaterials.

The causal significance of wear debris in the loosening of prostheses – a significance which Willert and others have pointed out – has prompted a search for prosthetic materials with more favorable wear resistance properties.

Carbon has long been used as an implant material in cardiovascular surgery. Its biocompatibility has been proven repeatedly in animal studies (Stanitzky and Moony) as well as in scores of subsequent human implantations.

The excellent gliding properties of graphite have long been recognized and exploited in technology, but the softness of the material has rendered it unsuitable for use in joints.

Under a research grant from the Ministry for Research and Technology of the Federal Republic of Germany, the firm Schunk Ebe of Heuchelheim was able to develop advanced carbons by means of carbide formers such as silicon. A wear resistance comparable to that of aluminum oxide ceramic was achieved. Fiber-reinforced carbon rods showed an excellent ultimate bending strength when subjected to cyclic loads. Their elastic modulus closely approaches that of bone.

Readiness to take, tissue compatibility, and kinetics of appositional bone growth were investigated both *in vitro* and *in vivo* at the Orthopedic Hospital of Giessen. It was found that these characteristics corresponded fully to the basic material graphite.

Since 1980, 17 patients have received surface-replacement prosthesis made of silicon-reinforced carbon. The biocompatibility and function of the arthroplasties have proved to be excellent in the initial phase.

Due to the rigorous standards imposed by the Federal Ministry on the physicotechnical properties of endoprosthetic stems, the first artificial joints made of carbon were implanted in the form of double-cup systems.

The double-cup or surface-replacement arthroplasty involves less bone resection and thus is more amenable to revision than conventional total hip replacements using intramedullary stems. However, the more difficult primary operative technique and probable restrictions of joint mobility postoperatively should not be underestimated. Investigations at our center (U. Weber) in cooperation with the Mathematical Institute of the Technical College of Darmstadt (Prof. Hotschek) have shown that the range of motion achieved with a double-cup arthroplasty can in no way match that of a standard endoprosthesis. The reason for this lies in the morphology of the joint, in which the gliding member is a hemisphere.

Positioning the femoral cup in alignment with the femoral neck, i.e. in varus, would permit a substantially greater range of motion. However, it would also increase the biomechanical risk of subsequent failure due to loosening of the cup or fracture of the femoral neck. Hence, the femoral cup is mounted in a valgus position in order to enhance mechanical stability, even though this necessarily reduces the available range of motion. We are aware of these critical problems of the double-cup arthroplasty as they relate to carbon double-cup systems as well, and we have taken them into consideration. In fact, they have limited the clinical indications to such a degree that only 17 patients have received silicon-reinforced carbon cups since November of 1980.

Since then, stems reinforced with carbon fibers have been developed to the point where, in simulator tests, they are able to withstand both static and cyclic loads with 1½ times the stability of steel. Thus, animal experiments with stem prostheses can be continued in the near future with the implantation of standard-design carbon prostheses having stems and articulating parts constructed of the same basic material. In addition, the excellent appositional bone growth kinetics that have been demonstrated in animal studies and push-out tests prove the feasibility of the cementless implantation of these prosthetic models.

References

Stanitzky CL Moony (1973) Osseus attachment to vitreus carbons, J Biomed Mater Res Symp 4:97–108

Weber U (1976) Biocompatibilität von Kohlenstoffen. Vortrag BMFT, Bonn

Weber U (1981) Kohlenstoffe als Implantatwerkstoffe in der Hüftgelenkendoprothetik. Thieme, Stuttgart

Willert HG, Buchhorn U (1981) Aussagewert biologischer Tests im Rahmen der Überprüfung von Biomaterialien, Symposion über Biomaterialien 1950 Gießen. Gentner, Stuttgart (Schriftenreihe der med. orthopädischen Technik Band V)

Results of Animal Studies on the Use of Carbon Fiber-Reinforced Plastic Prostheses

J. Harms, H. Mittelmeier and E. Mäusle

In recent years there has been a marked trend toward the use of self-locking implants in endoprosthetics, i.e., types of prosthesis that gain attachment to the bone without the aid of cement.

In the case of femoral endoprostheses, a preference has emerged in favor of long, straight stems having various types of "ingrowth" surface structures.

As for the acetabular component, the conical, screw-type prosthesis first described by Mittelmeier in 1973 appears to be gaining wide acceptance. Various materials have been tried for the prosthesis, ranging from all-polyethylene and metal-backed polyethylene cups to components made of Al_2O_3 ceramic.

In the past we have tended to favor the alumina ceramic owing to its excellent tribologic properties. In more than 1000 implantations of the uncemented sockets, the incidence of aseptic loosening was well below 0.5%.

Excessive wear or fracture of the acetabular prosthesis is a danger only if it is implanted at an excessively vertical or open angle. However, because errors of this type are not avoidable in all instances, we began looking for a material that would be largely immune to such complications. We wanted a material whose strength and wear resistance were comparable to Al_2O_3 ceramic, but which had an "isoelastic" behavior approximating that of bone.

Working with the firm Bosch, we developed a carbon fiber-reinforced triacine resin and conducted experiments to test its serviceability as an endoprosthetic material. While these experiments are still far from complete, we believe that the preliminary results are interesting enough to report at the present time.

Mechanical Properties

From a mechanical standpoint, the new material has demonstrated several intriguing properties:

Bending Strength

The bending strength of the material can be varied between 250 and 1000 N/mm^2, depending on the length and direction of the reinforcing fibers. This range is comparable to that of metallic materials.

Elastic Modulus

The E modulus can be varied between 20,000 and 100,000 N/mm^2 and thus can be closely matched to that of the host bone. It should be remembered, of course, that the bending strength and E modulus cannot be varied independently of each other.

Edge-Fiber Elongation

The edge-fiber elongation, which serves as an index of stress-strain behavior, is between 1 and 1.5%, regardless of fiber length and direction, and approximates that of bone.

Tribologic Properties

The material is very similar to polyethylene in terms of its friction properties. It appears to be more favorable than polyethylene in terms of wear behavior owing to its superior creep properties. However, the results in this area are not 100% reliable, and further experimental work is needed.

Biocompatibility

In preliminary experiments, the biocompatibility of the polymer was tested at the Batelle Institute in Frankfurt:

Subcutaneous Implantations in Animals

Long-term studies following subcutaneous implantations of specimens in animals showed no toxic effects on the tissues. Examination of the connective-tissue membrane surrounding the specimens revealed carbon-fiber and matrix particles from the specimen surface deposited among the collagen fiber bundles. This debris elicited no apparent tissue reaction.

Intra-articular Injections of Triacine Particles

Triacine particles injected intra-articularly were found within the synovial membrane after 6 weeks and caused no adverse response.

Osteocompatibility

In terms of compatibility with the host bone, the carbon fiber-reinforced triacine resin proved superior to polyethylene. For the most part, direct contact was observed between the uncoated portions of the specimens and the newly-formed surrounding bone. Polyethylene specimens, by contrast, were invariably separated from the bone by intervening connective tissue.

Pull-Out Test (Spector)

In the pull-out test, the carbon fiber-reinforced triacine resin showed a markedly better adhesion in the femoral shaft than polyethylene. This adhesion was found to increase continuously with implantation time.

Summarizing the results of the Batelle study, it may be said that the newly-developed fiber composite TCF appears exceptionally well suited for the fabrication of skeletal endoprostheses. Its favorable biocompatibility is attributed to its excellent overall stability, especially with regard to the thermal release of monomers and oligomers.

One year ago we began testing the new material as an acetabular implant in experimental animals under weight-bearing conditions. The test implants were miniaturized versions of the conical, screw-in design developed by Mittelmeier. The acetabulum was prepared and a thread cut in the bone to receive the component, which was screwed into the pelvis until stable.

The femoral components consisted of a metal-alloy intramedullary stem combined with an Al_2O_3 head, which articulated with the triacine resin socket.

In all cases it was possible to achieve a stable primary seating of the acetabular component. This enabled the animals to start full weight-bearing 3–4 days postoperatively, which was continued until the animals were killed. So far only 3 of 15 animals have been killed after periods of 9 and 12 months.

Radiographic Findings

Radiographs indicate a very good adaptation of the bone to the carbon fiber-reinforced triacine socket. No bone resorption has yet been observed at the implant-bone interface. It appears, in fact, that the bone density around the implant has increased with implantation time. This would agree with the findings of the Batelle Institute that, given favorable biomechanical conditions, the prosthesis can become integrated into a newly-formed, fully-differentiated bone bed.

Postmortem Findings

Necropsy revealed a relatively thin, newly-formed joint capsule which showed a slight, dark discoloration at the caudal acetabular border. No significant intracapsular effusion was apparent. The acetabular prosthesis was found to be absolutely stable and showed no evidence of the "pump" phenomenon that is usually seen with loose prostheses.

Histology of the Joint Capsule

Histologic examination of the hip joint capsule showed excellent tissue compatibility for both the carbon fibers and the triacine resin. Only a mild cellular reaction was noted in the vicinity of visible triacine particles and the carbon fibers. This is identical to the reaction that the Batelle Institute observed following the direct intra-articular injection of TCF particles. There was no sign of the large histiocytes that are often found in great numbers around polyethylene wear debris.

Bone reactions at the implant boundary have not yet been investigated. However, based on clinical and radiologic findings and on earlier studies with other materials, we have every confidence that an intimate bone-implant interlock will be discovered.

Owing to the favorable results of preliminary research, we have implanted a screw-type acetabular component made of the new material in two human patients. Because studies on wear behavior are not yet complete, however, we fitted each socket with a polyethylene insert.

We hope that the new prosthetic material will provide a viable alternative to metals and ceramics. Experimental results to date are highly encouraging, although a number of problems remain to be solved.

Regeneration of the Femoral Shaft following Revision Arthroplasties with Uncemented Plastic Prostheses

B. Störmer and G. Hierholzer

Introduction

The clinical problems associated with single or multiple revisions of total hip arthroplasties are well known. The main difficulty in such cases is a deterioration of femoral and acetabular bone stock. In patients with extensive cortical bone destruction whose revisions are done with conventional cemented devices, the "crutch-stick" prosthesis and acetabular roof shell of Mueller or acetabular support shell of Burch/Schneider generally are the only systems worthy of consideration. Unfortunately, the long-term success rate of revision arthroplasty is quite poor when conventional prostheses are used. Accordingly, we rarely use total hip arthroplasty as a means of treating hip disease in younger and middle-aged individuals. However, a revision arthroplasty is the only option available in patients who have had prior total hip arthroplasties and show clinical and radiologic evidence of loosening.

Clinical Problems

For loose total hip prostheses associated with advanced osteolysis of the acetabulum and proximal femur, Harris [1] and Sarmiento [6] recommend a long-stem femoral prosthesis combined with extensive homologous bone grafting. Banked bone from the femoral head and neck provides the best source of graft material. We believe that the "isoelastic" uncemented plastic prosthesis described by Mathys [4] and developed clinically by Morscher [5] has morphological, mechanical and physico-chemical properties that could solve many of the clinical problems associated with revision total hip arthroplasties.

The uncemented plastic prosthesis, supplemented by extensive grafting with autologous cancellous and corticocancellous bone, presumably would create conditions more favorable for bony regeneration than would revision with a cemented prosthesis. This line of reasoning, together with the results of preliminary clinical studies, has prompted us to continue clinical testing of the system. We justify this on the grounds that revisions with cemented prostheses do not produce satisfactory long-term results. In using the uncemented plastic prosthesis, our main technical objective is to create the strongest possible anchorage in the deficient proximal femur so that the necessary biomechanical interactions can take place between the implant and the bone. Similar considerations apply to anchorage of the plastic acetabular prosthesis in the osteolytic acetabular roof. Often this goal cannot be achieved through operative technique alone, and supplementary bone grafting becomes necessary as a means of obtaining a sufficient bone bed.

Illustrative Case

The case in question involves a man, now 36 years old, who in 1964 sustained multiple skeletal injuries, including a femoral neck fracture, during a job-related accident. Initially the fracture was treated conservatively, but 6 months later it had to be fixed internally with a nail and plate. Avascular necrosis of the femoral head developed subsequent to the operation, and a Moore prosthesis was inserted one year later. In 1972 this prosthesis was removed and a total endoprosthesis was inserted. In 1979 a re-revision with a long-stem prosthesis had to be performed because of loosening. Shortly thereafter the loosening recurred, accompanied by massive osteolysis of the proximal femur and acetabular roof. Then, in 1981, a third revision was performed using an uncemented prosthesis. Extensive cancellous bone grafting of the acetabular bed was also done at that time, and cor-

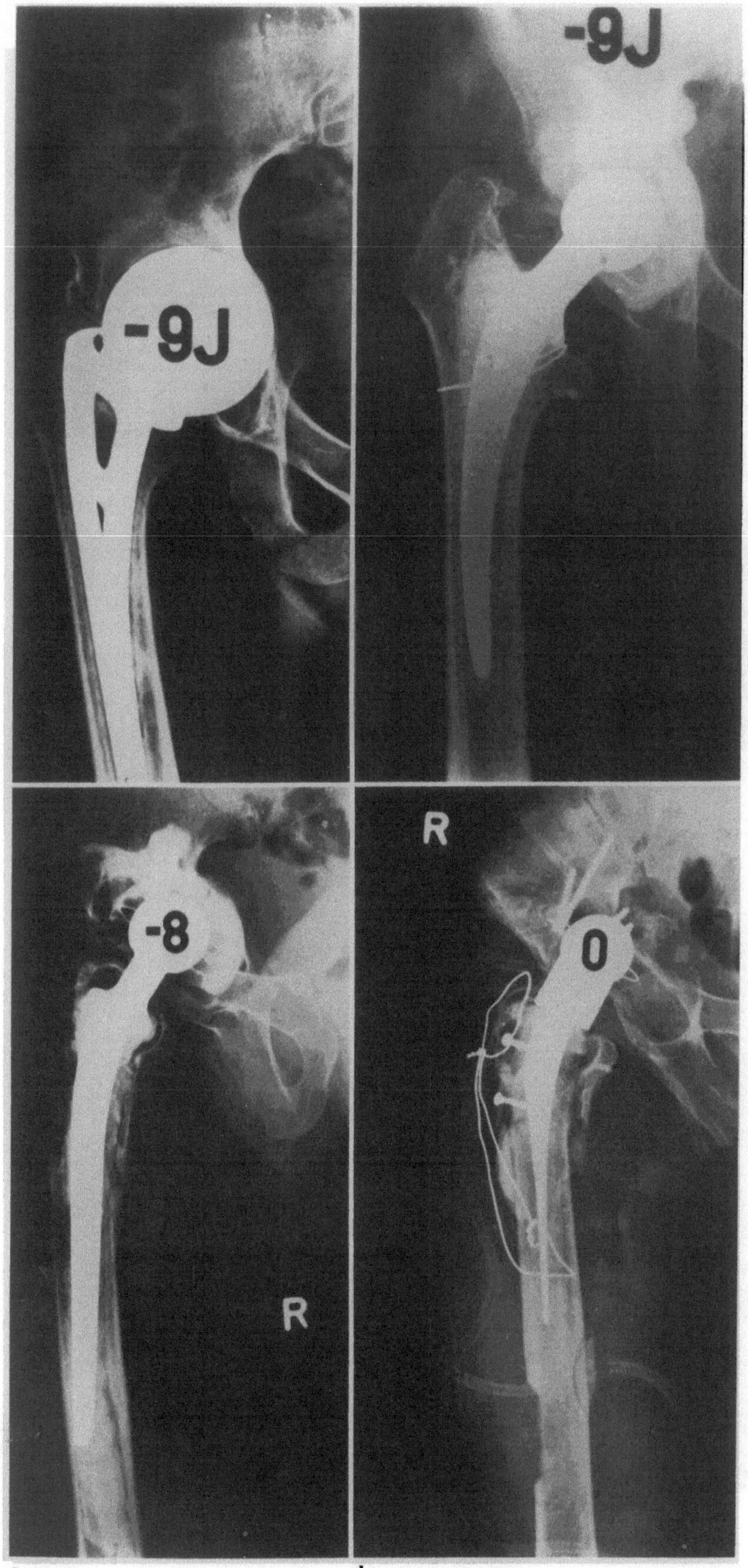

a b c d

Fig. 1 a–l. A 36-year-old man sustained a femoral neck fracture that was fixed internally with a nail and plate. Femoral head necrosis developed, and initially a Moore prosthesis was inserted **(a)**. A first revision was performed due to loosening **(b)**, and 7 years later a second revision was done with a long-stem endoprosthesis **(c)**. In 1981 the latter was removed due to a grade-3 instability in the shaft region and migration of the acetabular component into the pelvis; it was replaced with an uncemented plastic prosthesis **(d)**. Cancellous autografting of the acetabulum was also necessary at that time, and the femoral shaft was augmented with 2 corticocancellous grafts. Follow-up films show good bony union in the acetabulum and reconstructed femur **(e–h)**. The functional result is also good **(i–l)**

Fig. 1 e–h

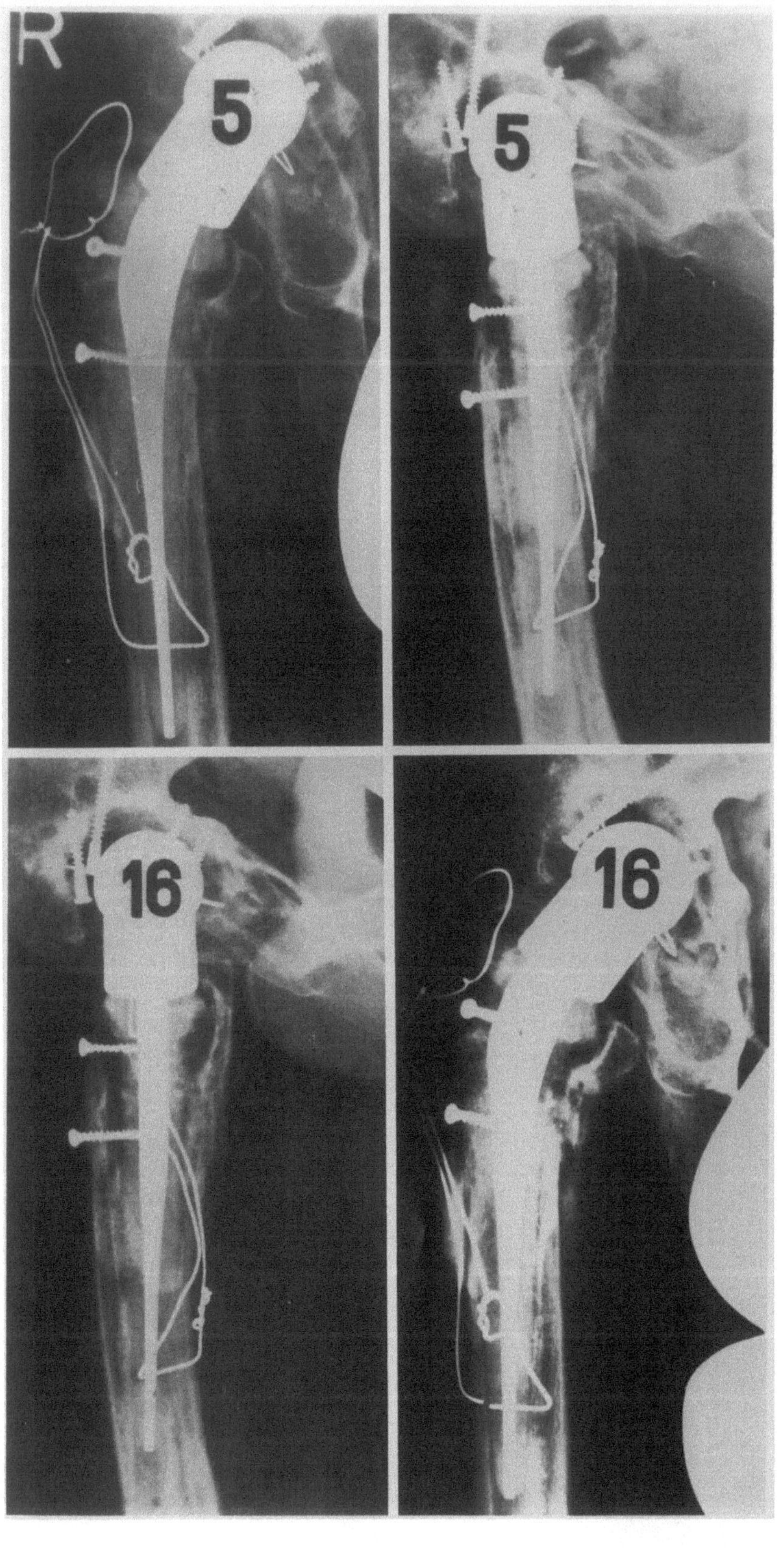

e f
g h

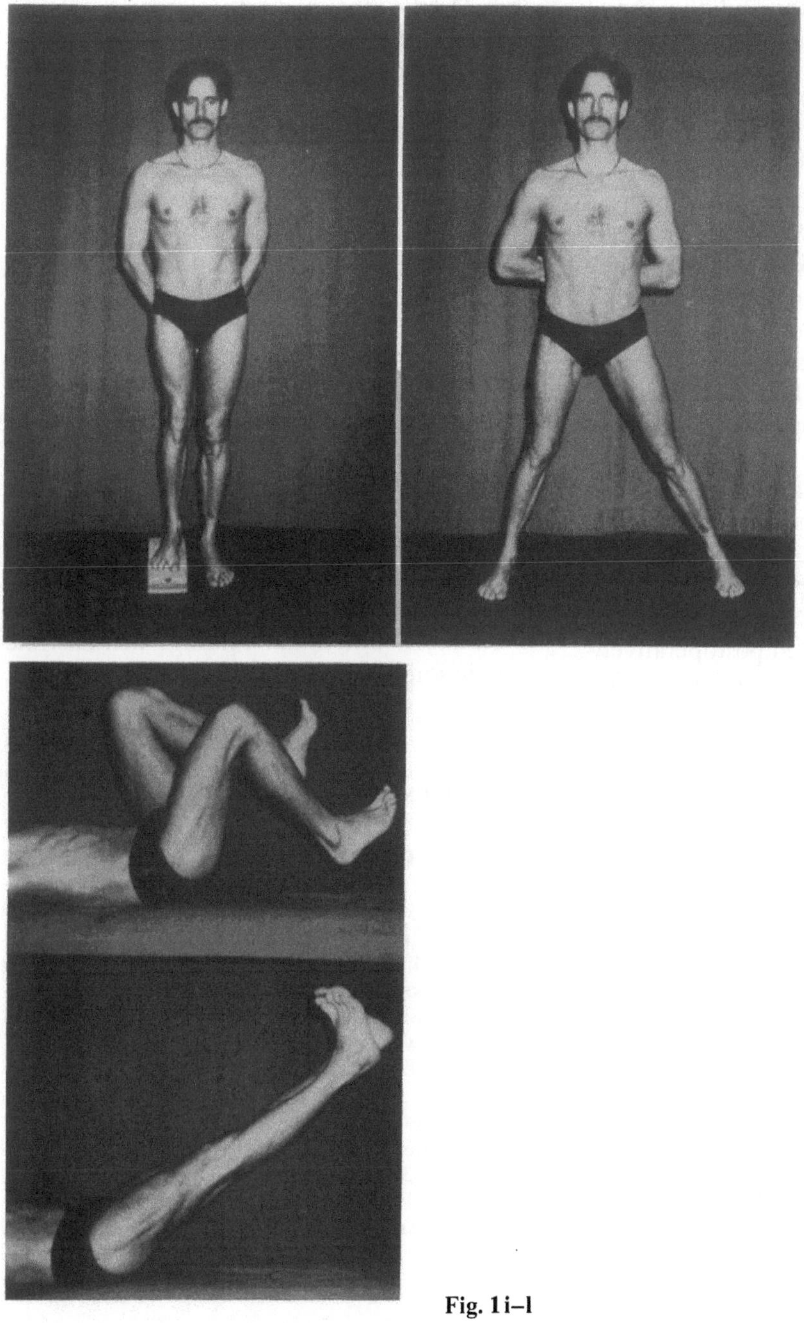

i k l

Fig. 1i–l

ticocancellous grafts were used to augment the proximal femur. Today the patient is free of discomfort and has almost complete mobility in the operated hip; 3 cm of length was lost in the operated limb (Fig. 1).

To date we have performed 12 revision arthroplasties with the "isoelastic" plastic prosthesis using the technique and indications described. The longest follow-up is 16 months. Thus, we are dealing with preliminary results relating to a specific clinical problem, and our main purpose in presenting them is to stimulate further study and discussion.

Discussion

When the bone undergoes elastic deformation following a total hip arthroplasty, a reversible displacement occurs at the interface between the more or less rigid implant and the bone. This is what is meant by "relative motion" [7]. Because this deformation is always present to some degree, an "elastic" implant is better able to follow the bone than a "rigid" one, and this serves to minimize relative motion.

Isoelasticity offers a means of avoiding potentially disruptive changes from tension to compression, in which the contact surface becomes unloaded and then loaded in the opposite direction [7]. If the proximal femoral shaft is already damaged as a result of osteolysis, reconstructive measures become especially important. The object of reconstruction is to create the largest possible contact area between the plastic and the bone, and thus maximize the surface area available for stress transfer. In areas where primary contact cannot be achieved due to deficiences of existing bone stock, autografting must be employed. This will enable secondary contact to be established postoperatively during the course of bone remodeling. The straight stem of the isoelastic prosthesis more closely approximates the axis of the shaft than does a curved prosthetic stem and helps to minimize shear forces and relative motion. The neck-stem angle, which has been modified to 144°, lessens stress on the medial cortex in the calcar area while improving stress transfer to the more distal portions of the shaft. The long-term mechanical effects of this valgus orientation on the acetabulum and the knee joint remain to be seen and merit close observation. Atraumatic preparation of the shaft, cementless insertion of the prosthetic stem, and supplementary autologous bone grafting contribute significantly to revascularization and thus to bony regeneration of the graft bed. The question of the primary biocompatibility of incompletely-polymerized monomers has been answered by the studies of Kallenberger [2] and other authors. There is as yet no conclusive evidence that the fully-polymerized cement has a long-term toxic effect on tissues. On the other hand, the danger of loosening associated with the phenomenon of "cement aging" is well documented.

Neither of these dangers is a problem with the uncemented "isoelastic" prosthesis, whose surface, according to tissue culture studies, is largely bioinert [3].

Summary

Prompted by the problems associated with the revision of failed total hip arthroplasties, we attempted to determine whether results could be improved by use of the "isoelastic" uncemented plastic prosthesis. Points of surgical technique, biomechanical factors, and the special morphologic problems associated with advanced osteolysis are discussed. Long-term results are not yet available, but initial findings demonstrate the basic soundness of the therapeutic concept.

References

1. Harris WH (1981) Allografting and total hip replacement. XV. World Congress of SICOT, Rio de Janeiro 1981
2. Kallenberger A (1982) Untersuchungen zur Zellkompatibilität von Knochenzementen. Symposion Hüftgelenksendoprothetik, Berlin 1982
3. Kinzl L, Burri C, Mohr W, Paulini K, Wolter D (1976) Gewebeverträglichkeit der Polymere, Polyäthylen, Polyester und Polyacetylharz. Z Orthop 114:777
4. Mathys R (1973) Stand der Verwendung von Kunststoffen für künstliche Gelenke. Aktuel Traumatol 4:253
5. Morscher E (1979) Isoelastische Prothesen. Langenbecks Arch Chir 349:321
6. Sarmiento A (1981) Lysis of the femoral neck. XV. World Congress of SICOT, Rio de Janeiro 1981.
7. Schneider R (1982) Die Totalprothese der Hüfte. Aktuel Probl Chir Orthop 24:1–299

Six Years' Experience in Revision Total Hip Arthroplasties with Uncemented Ceramic Prostheses

K. E. Brinkmann and J. Harms

The loosening of prosthetic components is a pressing problem in total hip arthroplasty. The reimplantation of loose total prostheses is extremely difficult. Metal sheaths, supporting rings and specially-shaped prosthetic devices have been developed in an effort to improve the attachment of revisionary prostheses. It is common for loosening to occur shortly after revisions due to the bone damage caused by removal of the primary prosthesis. Complete removal of the prosthesis followed by a Girdlestone resection is no longer regarded as an acceptable option in most patients and should at most be considered only in elderly patients with septic complications. Younger patients, who generally are still active professionally, will seldom tolerate the loss of stability and noticeable limb shortening associated with complete removal of the prosthesis.

Encouraged by our positive experience with self-retaining ceramic acetabular prostheses, we first undertook the revision of failed THAs with ceramic sockets in February, 1976, at the suggestion of Rossak. We dispensed with the use of bone cement in these operations (Rossak and Brinkmann, 1977). By May of 1982 we had performed similar revisions in more than 200 patients.

Surgical Technique

The hip joint may be approached through either an anterior or posterior incision, depending on the need to reconstruct portions of the bony acetabulum.

After removal of the loose prosthesis, all regenerated capsular tissue is excised, and the former implant bed is freed of granulation tissue and residual cement. The freshened acetabular recess is packed with a mixture of autologous and banked cancellous bone. Defects in the floor or wall of the acetabulum are repaired with blocks of corticocancellous bone taken from the tibia or iliac crest. The self-retaining ceramic acetabular component may be screwed into the reconstructed bone bed, or it may be held in place by means of bolts or simple elastic tension. The loose femoral stem is removed together with its cement mantle and, in younger patients, is replaced with a self-retaining stem about which autogenous cancellous bone is packed. In older patients, conventional cement fixation of the stem is used so that a more rapid mobilization can be achieved.

Postoperatively, a regimen of partial or non-weight bearing on the operated hip is maintained for 6–8 weeks. Our original rule of strict immobilization in a full-length hip spica has been modified to meet individual needs. If the primary stability of the ceramic acetabular component is good, we either immobilize the hip for 3 weeks in a half-length spica, or we dispense with plaster fixation altogether. Patients should use axillary crutches for an additional 6–8 weeks to limit the load on the operated hip. Full weight-bearing is deferred until radiographs indicate bony integration of the prosthesis.

Statistical Review

During the period from February 1976 to May 1982, we revised failed THAs in 245 patients (142 women, 103 men) using the technique and apparatus described. A Lindenhof ceramic prosthesis was implanted in 129 of these patients, and a Mittelmeier socket in 116. An "Autophor" femoral endoprosthesis was inserted in 34 patients. In 46 patients the revision was bilateral.

At the time of the revision the patients ranged in age from 39 to 82 years (average, 55). Loosenings had been confirmed on the basis of clinical findings, radiographs and bone scans.

Complications

The complications in our series included 5 deep infections, which necessitated complete removal of the prosthesis. In 18 patients we observed secondary migrations of the ceramic acetabular component due to various causes. In 8 cases this necessitated a re-revision, and in 3 of these cases the prosthesis had to be removed without replacement. In 6 other patients the prosthesis became stably integrated following an initial slight migration or tilting of the component. Transitory peroneal nerve palsy developed in 8 cases, and femoral nerve palsy in 2 cases. This regressed completely in 6 of the patients, but a mild residual palsy persisted in the remaining 4. We attribute these complications to intraoperative stretch of the femoral or sciatic nerve.

As we have gained experience, modified our surgical approach and operative technique, and relied more on the use of autologous cancellous bone and fibrin adhesive, we have been able to reduce significantly the incidence of such complications as secondary loosening and nerve stretch.

Results

One hundred patients out of the 245 in our series have been followed for a period of 4 years. More than 150 have been followed for at least 2 years. These follow-ups have shown that, with very few exceptions, the self-retaining ceramic acetabular prostheses have become solidly integrated into the host bone. In most of our patients the primary bone bed had to be augmented, and in some cases this was done entirely with banked bone.

The range of motion of the operated hips, especially in rotation and abduction, was markedly restricted during the first postoperative year. The degree of the restriction depended upon preexisting joint contractures, migration of the prosthetic components, the length of time the joint was immobilized in plaster, and the age of the patient. As time passed and more weight was borne on the hip, the patients regained and in many cases even surpassed their preoperative range of motion.

In subjective terms, the patients were highly satisfied with the operative outcome. Only a few of the patients in the series from February 1976 to December 1979 still used a cane, and only one still used an axillary crutch.

Our results to date indicate that the use of ceramic acetabular prostheses and self-retaining endoprosthetic stems for revision arthroplasties can restore stability to the operated hip on a long-term basis. Clinical findings and radiographic follow-ups show that, even in the face of extensive preexisting bone damage, the ceramic prosthesis can be securely and permanently anchored with the aid of autologous cancellous bone and allografts. Complications can be avoided through improvements of surgical technique and especially by the use of autologous cancellous bone from the posterior iliac crest.

We believe that the procedure described offers a solution to the problem of the failed total hip arthroplasty, even in cases that appear to be unsalvageable.

References

Boutin P (1974) Les prothéses totales de la hanche en alumine. L'ancrage direct sans ciment dans 50 cas. Rev Chir Orthop 60:233

Eichler J (1973) Ein Vorschlag zur operativen Behandlung der Protrusio acetabuli. Arch Orthop Unfallchir 75:76

Griss P, Heimke G, Silber R, Krempien B, Hachner K, Merkle B (1975) Erste Erfahrungen mit der Keramik-Metallverbundprothese. Med Orthop Techn 6:159–162

Mittelmeier H (1974) Zementlose Verankerung von Endoprothesen nach dem Tragrippenprinzip. Z Orthop 112:27

Plaue R, Städtler J (1975) Infizierte Hüftendoprothesen – ein aktuelles Problem. Z Orthop 113:965–973

Rossak K, Brinkmann KE (1977) Erfahrungen mit dem Einsatz von Keramik-Totalendoprothesen zum Austausch ausgelockerter Totalprothesen des Hüftgelenkes. Z Orthop 115:290–299

Weber BG, Stühmer G, Semlitsch M (1974) Erfahrungen mit dem Kunststoff Polyester als Komponente der Rotationstotalprothese des Hüftgelenkes. Z Orthop 112/5:1106

Witt AN, Hackenbroch MG (1976) Therapeutische Möglichkeiten bei gelockerten Hüfttotalprothesen. Z Orthop 114:330–341

Revision Arthroplasties with the Isoelastic Total Hip Replacement

W. Dick, H. Jenny and E. Morscher

Introduction

The incidence of revision arthroplasties for loose total hip replacements is on the rise. The ratio of primary total hip arthroplasties to revision arthroplasties at our hospital is presently about 4:1. Expressed in numbers, this means that revision total hip arthroplasties are being performed at the rate of about 80 per year. Projections based upon a mathematical model indicate that the revision rate at our hospital will double during the next 8 years. Thus, if present trends continue, by 1990 one revision will be performed for every two primary arthroplasties.

In the first section below, we shall discuss the use of cementless plastic acetabular cups for revisional replacements. In a second section we will examine the issue of cementless femoral components as it relates to revision arthroplasties.

Replacement of the Acetabular Component

Aseptic loosening of the acetabular cup poses a major threat .to the long evity of hip arthroplasties, particularly because it is often associated with substantial losses of pelvic bone stock. These defects may involve the roof of the acetabulum, the floor, and the anterior and posterior pillars, and can seriously hamper attempts at revision. The extent of the defects is often surprising at diagnosis, but their occurrence can be explained: The patient feels well for several years after the arthroplasty and stops coming in for routine checks. Wear gradually sets in and at first is associated with minimal discomfort. Meanwhile the patient has become older and has been constantly and imperceptibly reducing his level of activity and the demands placed upon the hip joint. Still, the prosthesis, once loosened, leads to a mechanical destruction of the acetabular bone, combined with osteolytic destruction caused by aggressive frictional granulation tissue. At first the destruction is slow, but it becomes progressively more rapid until the patient finally presents for examination. Occasionally, the patient will come in only after the acetabulum has completely penetrated into the lesser pelvis.

There is general agreement as to the goal of treatment in such situations: Implant a new prosthesis having the same longevity as the average primary arthroplasty. The means to this end are varied, and the technical appliances, such as acetabular cups, wire mesh, fixation screws, etc. are known. However, it is increasingly being recognizd that a biologic reconstruction of the deficient acetabulum is superior to prosthetic replacement alone [3, 5]. Successful combinations of bone grafts and traditional cemented cup systems have been described [1, 3, 4, 5, 6, 10, 13]. Thus, the goal of treatment can be expanded to include correction of the acetabular deficiency through bony reconstruction in order to provide bone stock comparable to that available for a primary arthroplasty.

Cementless prosthetic systems would appear to be very well suited for use in conjunction with bone grafts, for they avoid the difficult problems of primary fixation and the entry of cement into the grafted bone [2, 9, 11, 12]. In addition, because these systems entail minimal loss of bone stock while avoiding additional damage to the acetabular socket, whose vitality may already be compromised, they are also advantageous in cases where the acetabular deficiency is too small to warrant grafting, and only a larger acetabular cup is needed. The same applies to revisions for a failed femoral component in which it is necessary to replace an acetabular cup that is heavily worn but is still firmly attached to the bone.

Method

While *autologous* cancellous bone from the head and neck of the femur is available for the grafting of defects associated with protrusio acetabuli and hip dysplasia, and is suitable for use with all acetabular prosthetic systems [1, 4, 6, 10, 13], this bone cannot be obtained from the same access used for revision arthroplasties. The removal of autologous bone from the posterior aspect of the wing of the ilium necessitates repositioning of the patient, a prolongation of operating time, additional blood loss, and turbulence in the operating room. Moreover, bone may not be available in sufficient quantities. We generally use *homologous* cancellous bone, therefore, which is either taken from the neck and head of the femur during primary arthroplasties in the form of chips or blocks, or is obtained from upper tibial osteotomies. After a culture has been taken, the graft material is deep-frozen at −20 °C for 3 months without additives before we approve it for use. No tissue matching or blood typing is done.

Technique

After the old cement is removed, the acetabular cavity is freed of connective tissue, which usually separates easily, and is well freshened with a curette. The extent of the curettage will be limited by any medial wall defects that may be present. Smooth, white sclerotic zones and ridges, which are often encountered, are perforated with a drill and 2-mm bit. Two grafting techniques have proved satisfactory: Either small cancellous bone chips are stacked together and packed into the acetabular cavity using the prosthetic cap as a pestle, or larger blocks are laid into the defects and shaped as needed with a cutting drill. Cementless polyethylene cups [7, 8] are available in 2-mm increments up to an outside diameter of 64 mm. After the graft has been applied, the anchor holes are drilled to receive the pegs of the cup. Generally, it is possible to bury one peg, or at least its tip, in autochthonous bone and not just in the graft. The cup is inserted and secured with screws. If the anterior and posterior screw holes overlie a defect, the screws may be inserted through the wide rim of the cup at any point desired. We expect the graft to undergo some degree of compaction and shrinkage under stress, causing retraction of the cup with consequent fracture of the screws. With this in mind, the screws are designed so that they will fracture at the 3rd thread from the end to prevent the head from slipping back into the joint.

Postoperative Care

Postoperative care is always the same: The patient is mobilized immediately on two crutches and puts no weight on the operated limb, although foot exercises are performed. The patient is discharged after 2–3 weeks (or 6 weeks at the latest). Full weight-bearing is permitted after 8–12 weeks (14 weeks at the latest).

Clinical Material and Results

We reviewed 50 consecutive revision arthroplasties using an uncemented cup. The average observation period was 12 months (6–24 months). Forty-six revisions were performed for failed cemented cups, 1 revision for an infected, uncemented polyethylene cup, 1 revision for an uncemented ceramic cup, and 2 revisions for acetabular floor penetration by a femoral-head prosthesis.

In 12 cases the new cup could be implanted without bone grafting, and in 38 cases acetabular deficiencies were sufficient to warrant cancellous grafting. Homologous bone was used in 35 cases, autologous bone in 2 cases, and a combination of both in 1 case. The volume of graft material required for a given case was derived from 1–4 donors; the thickness of the graft layer ranged from 3 to 20 mm.

No complications arose during implantation of the acetabular component. Two femoral shaft penetrations occurred during stem implantations. Postoperatively, no incompatibility reactions or infections have yet been observed.

Forty-eight of the 50 patients walk without crutches and without complaints, and radiographs show union of the graft and incorporation of the acetabular prosthesis. The initially amorphous graft material appears to have undergone a vital remodeling under physiologic

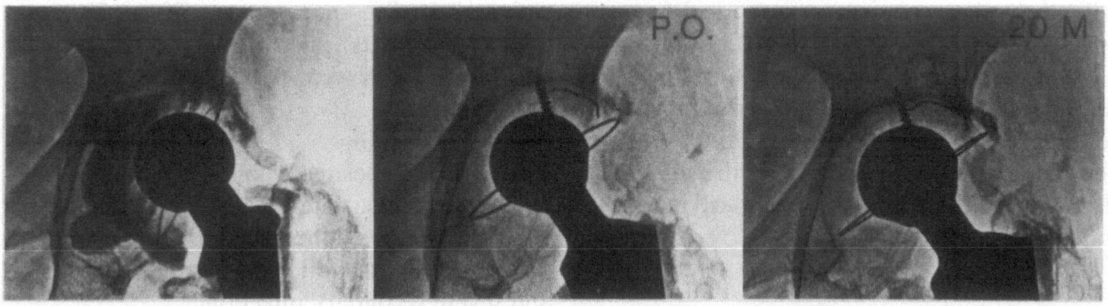

a b c

Fig. 1 a–c. 69-year-old woman (S.E.). **a** Loose acetabular cup with presence of large defect. **b** Total hip revision, defect repaired with homologous cancellous bone. **c** 20 months after revision the initially amorphous graft has undergone vital remodeling under loading and has developed a directional trabecular structure; a "neocortex" has also formed around the cup

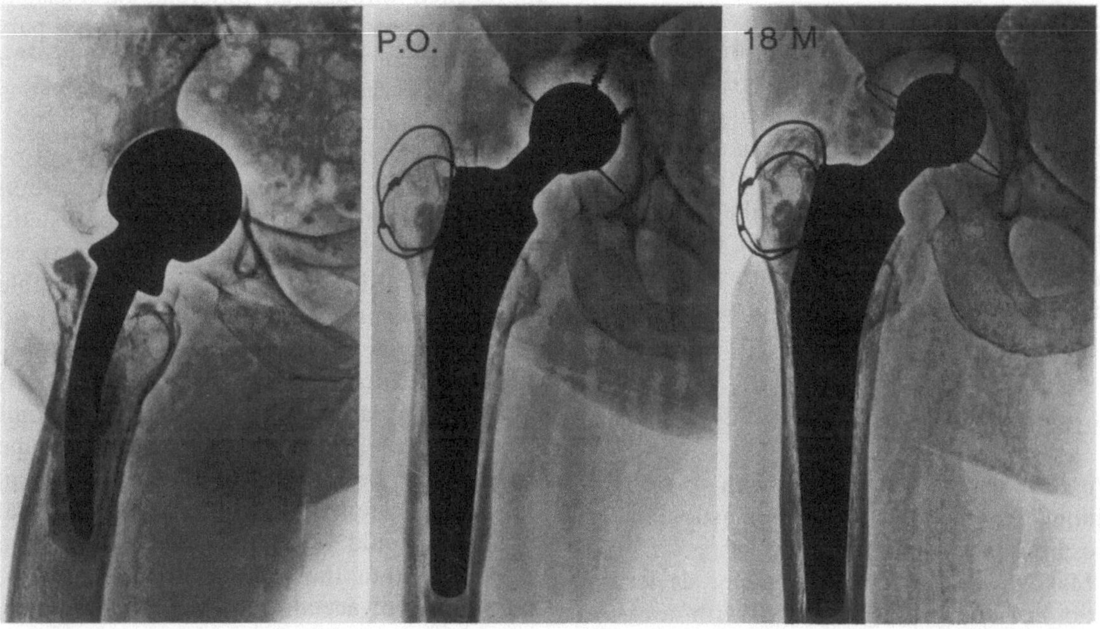

a b c

Fig. 2 a–c. 63-year-old woman (S.R.). **a** Central migration of a prosthetic femoral head. **b** Total hip revision, defect in acetabular floor repaired with homologous cancellous bone. **c** 18 months after revision a stress-resistant sclerotic layer has formed around the acetabular cup; the acetabular floor graft has undergone slight compaction and is fully consolidated

loads, acquiring a directional, stable trabecular structure. In addition, a new, dense, stress-resistant layer, or "neocortex," has formed around the cup and its cranial anchoring pegs, both within the grafted bone and in its interfacial zone with the autochthonous pelvic bone (Figs. 1 and 2). Apparently, the grafts have united with no appreciable volume reduction, for the screw fractures expected to result from compaction of the cancellous bone have failed to occur in the great majority of cases. Among the 48 patients, we noted 1 fractured screw and 1 bent screw with subsequent consolidation of the bone around the cup.

In 2 cases we rated the result as poor due to renewed medial migration, tilting, and failure to develop the stable bony structure and "neocortex" around the cup that we demand for a good result. One of these 2 patients (both females) can bear weight unassisted and without pain, while the other requires a cane and reports moderate complaints and restricted motion.

Analyzing these 2 cases, we find that the major fault probably lay in inserting the cup too deeply, creating a protrusio situation: The inlet plane was not lateralized to the anatomic site by a sufficient amount of underlying bone stock.

Replacement of the Femoral Component

As with the acetabulum, a deficiency of bone stock in the proximal femoral shaft can be a great problem in revision arthroplasties. All too often the operator is faced with enormous, grotesquely-shaped bone cavities that must somehow be prepared to accept the new prosthetic components. The idea of resolving such situations without the disadvantages attendant upon the use of bone cement is an obvious one. Revision without cement offers a means of avoiding additional damage to the bone stock, which already is marginal both qualitatively and quantitatively. A reconstruction of the bone around the stem of the prosthesis is the surgical goal.

Indications

We consider the following criteria to be indications for the use of an isoelastic femoral prosthesis in revision arthroplasties:

1. Massive destruction and patchy devitalization of the proximal femur with areas of severe osteolysis.
2. The presence of an unusually broad proximal medullary cavity with a thin cortex that would require large amounts of bone cement to be applied around the new prosthesis.
3. Younger patients in whom a regeneration of the damaged bony encasement can be hoped for, so that it will be possible to do any future revisions without extensive bone defects.

Patient Population

During the period from December 1980 to the spring of 1982, a total of 10 revisions were performed at our clinic using the isoelastic femoral prosthesis. There were 6 female and 4 male patients ranging in age from 50 to 79 years (average, 70 years).

The revisions were prompted by the following situations:

5 aseptic loosenings,
3 loosenings associated with low-grade infection,
1 loosening associated with frank osteitis involving extensive bone destruction,
1 Girdlestone hip following a total hip revision and severe secondary infection.

Technique

The patient is placed in the supine position with the hip slightly elevated. The hip joint is approached through an anterolateral incision made through the old scars. The proximal part of the incision should be placed such that the iliac crest is accessible for obtaining autologous cancellous bone.

After removal of the loosened femoral prosthesis, all the bone cement and granulation tissue must be removed from the femoral shaft. The medullary cavity is reamed out to expose as much viable internal bone surface as possible in the proximal femur, taking care not to weaken unduly the diaphyseal bone, and especially the lateral cortex, which already is thinned and damaged. After reaming is completed, a special instrument set is used to shape the proximal end of the femoral shaft to accept the isoelastic femoral prosthesis. The femoral prosthesis should have a full, snug seating when introduced into the femoral shaft. Gaps between the polyacetal stem and the bone are packed with autologous cancellous bone. Bony apposition is especially important in the collar area of the prosthesis. Any large bone defects in the proximal femoral shaft must be repaired with autologous bone grafts.

The neck length of the prosthesis (28 mm, 34 mm, 40 mm, 44 mm) is of course matched to individual circumstances. The greater trochanter, which is detached for the implantation, is reattached using conventional means.

Results

An initial follow-up of 10 patients examined a short time after operation indicates the following:

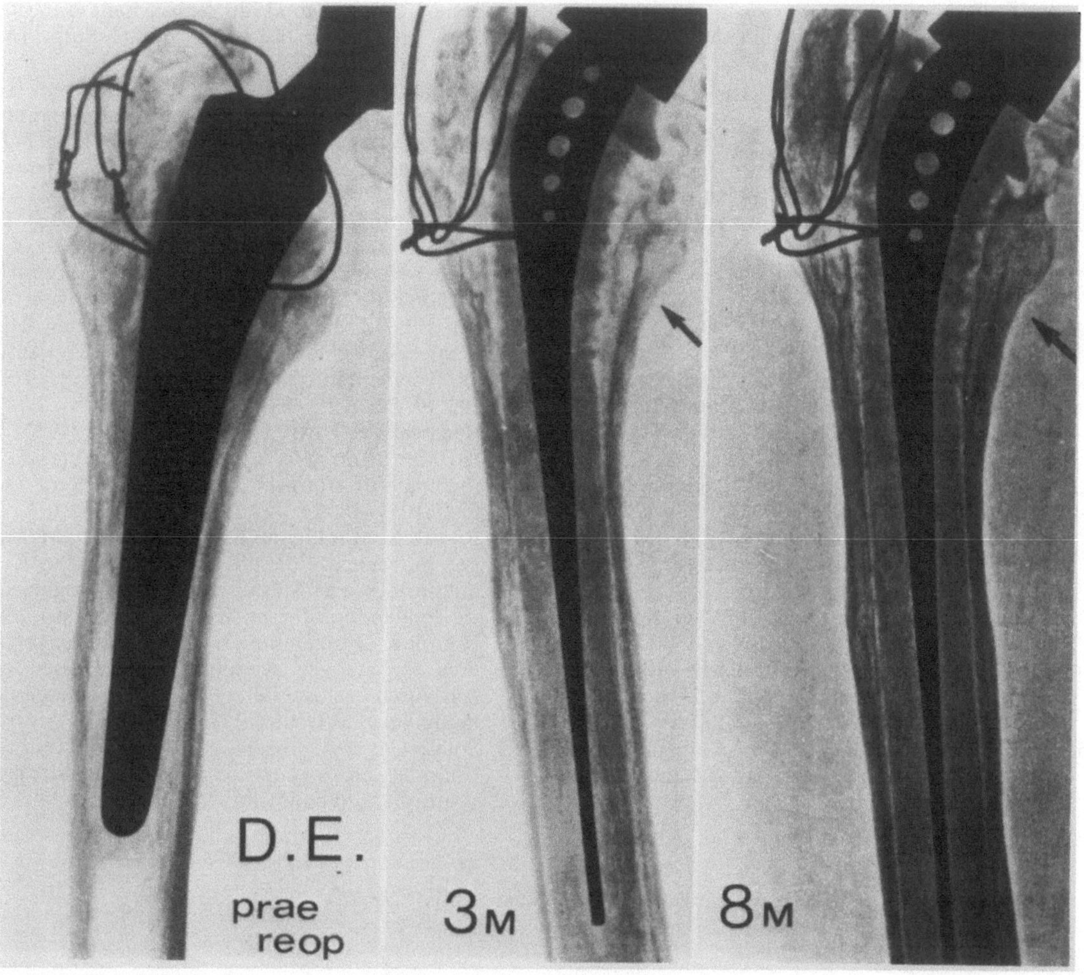

a b c

Fig. 3a–c. 73-year-old woman (D.E.). **a** Loose stem and suspected low-grade infection. **b** Femoral prosthesis replaced and bony sheath reconstructed with homologous cancellous bone, chiefly on the medial side (*arrow*). **c** 8 months after revision, graft is well incorporated (*arrow*)

All 10 patients are again able to walk without mechanical aids.

Residual complaints in the operated hip are entirely comparable to those of patients whose revisions were done with a cemented stem.

The same may be said of the mobility of the operated hip.

The patients whose revisions were occasioned by a low-grade infection show no signs that would indicate a flare-up of infection.

A fistula still exists in the patient whose revision was originally prompted by extensive osteitis. However, repeated contrast studies have shown a marked reduction in the size of the fistulous tract system in the femoral shaft, which was very extensive preoperatively.

Radiographs in practically all patients indicate that a more or less pronounced settling of the isoelastic prosthesis has occurred within the medullary cavity, and that the stem is wedged firmly in place by surrounding bone. Signs of a normalization and regeneration of the bony canal itself, which was severely damaged preoperatively, are also evident in the radiographs (Fig. 3).

It is not yet possible to make a definitive assessment, of course, because long-term results are not yet available. However, it is already apparent that the isoelastic femoral prosthesis made of polyacetal resin offers an alternative to conventional cemented prostheses in many candidates for revision arthroplasty, with these advantages:

1. No additional damage to bone stock from cement.
2. Possibility of reconstructing a bony sheath around the prosthesis.
3. Creation of a "third line of defense" in younger patients so that a 2nd revision might be performed at a later date.

References

1. Bereiter H, Morscher E (1982) Spongiosaplastik des Pfannenbodens beim totalprothetischen Ersatz der Protrusionshüfte. Beitr Orthop Traumatol 29:408–416
2. Dick W, Morscher E (1982) Homologe Spongiosa als Werkstoff bei Problemfällen der Hüftchirurgie. In: Hackenbroch M, Refior J, Jäger M (Hrsg) Osteogenese und Knochenwachstum. Thieme, Stuttgart New York, S 226–230
3. Harris WH (1982) Allografting in total hip arthroplasty. Clin Orthop 162:150–164
4. Heywood AWB (1980) Arthroplasty with a solid bone graft for protrusio acetabuli. J Bone Joint Surg [Br] 62/3:332–336
5. Marti R, Besselaar PP (1981) Spanplastiken bei primärer Totalprothese und Totalprothesenwechsel. Z Orthop 119:711–714
6. McCollum DE, Nunley JA, Harrelson JM (1980) Bone-grafting in total hip replacement for acetabular protrusion. J Bone Joint Surg [Am] 62/7:1065–1073
7. Morscher E, Dick W (1983) Cementless fixation of "Isoelastic" hip endoprostheses manufactured in plastic materials. Clin Orthop 176:77–87
8. Morscher E, Dick W, Bombelli R (1982) Cementless fixation of the acetabular component in total hip arthroplasty. In: Winter GD, Gibbons DF, Plenk H Jr (eds) Biomaterials, 1980. Wiley, Chichester New York Brisbane Toronto Singapore
9. Parhofer R, Mönch W (1982) Erfahrungen über den Ersatz einzementierter, gelockerter Hüft-Totalendoprothesen durch zementlos implantierte Totalendoprothesen. Med Orthop Techn 102:49–52
10. Ranawat CS, Lawrence DD, Inglis AE (1980) Total hip arthroplasty in protrusio acetabuli of rheumatoid arthritis. J Bone Joint Surg [Am] 62/7:1059–1065
11. Rossak K, Brinkmann KE (1977) Erste Erfahrungen mit einer zementlos zu verankernden Keramikprothese zur Austauschoperation ausgelockerter Totalendoprothesen. Z Orthop 115:290–299
12. Rossak K, Brinkmann KE (1979) Erfahrungen mit dem Einsatz von Keramik-Totalprothesen zum Austausch gelockerter Totalendoprothesen des Hüftglenkes. Z Orthop 117:485–488
13. Sotelo-Garza A, Charnley J (1978) The results of Charnley arthroplasty of the hip performed for protrusio acetabuli. Clin Orthop 132:12–18

3½ Years' Results of Lord Primary Total Hip Arthroplasties and 1½ Years' Experience with Revision Arthroplasties for Loose Cemented Prostheses

O. Stampfel, W. Pommer, R. Trauner and V. Santner

During the period from October 1978 through May 1982, a total of 171 Lord-type intramedullary stems were implanted at our center (Table 1). The first 5 stems implanted were combined with cemented Müller acetabular components. In 10 cases we used a ceramic head manufactured by another firm that appeared to fit well on the conical neck of the Lord stem. In one patient a ceramic head fractured during a fall, whereupon we learned that a slight lack of congruity existed between the conical recess in the head and the conical neck of the stem. Afterward we began using metal heads exclusively. The remaining 9 ceramic heads that were implanted are still functioning well after 3 years. In 1979 we abandoned the cemented socket in favor of a screw-in metal ring with a polyethylene insert, combining this component with a Lord stem and metal head. The available acetabular and stem sizes have proved adequate for the great majority of primary arthroplasties. A larger stem would be required only for very wide medullary cavities, which mainly are encountered during revision arthroplasties. An acetabular component larger than the largest size now available (62 mm) also would be advantageous for revisional surgery.

A miniature acetabular component is currently available for extreme cases (dysplasia), as is a 22-mm head that is compatible with all stem sizes. We could have used these components on one occasion, and we did in fact use them in one patient.

Table 1. Implanted Lord Prostheses

1978	3
1979	18
1980	34
1981	68
1982	48
	171
Primary operations:	148
Revisions	23

Indications

Initially we decided to reserve uncemented prostheses for exceptional cases and to implant them only in biologically younger patients. The first 32 patients ranged in age from 37 to 73, with an average age of 60.

While the indications in the younger age group continue to be very strictly limited, we no longer feel that age alone is a contraindication for uncemented total hip arthroplasty. Limits are set, of course, by the presence and degree of senile osteoporosis and by the size of the medullary cavity (or, equivalently, by the lack of a sufficiently large stem).

In the younger age group, we feel that an uncemented THA is indicated in patients with constant, severe hip pain who are not good candidates for a double-cup arthroplasty. However, when deciding between a double-cup arthroplasty and an uncemented THA, it is necessary to consider factors other than just the age of the patient. The primary disorder and the patient's general condition (biological age) must be taken into account, and the options must be presented to the patient so that an informed decision can be made.

Surgical Technique and Special Problems

Acetabular Component: The essential difference between implanting a cemented acetabular component and an uncemented component that screws into place is that the uncemented socket requires a straight, direct approach to the acetabulum. It is not possible to work "around the corner" as it is with a cemented prosthesis. If surgical access is not adequate, it is likely that the cup will be positioned in excessive anteversion, thus increasing the risk of dislocation. In addition, the borders of the acetabulum must be accurately exposed by careful removal of the capsule and the labrum acetabulare. Because the Lord reamer is not front-cutting, a different reamer must be used for initial cartilage removal from the shallow acetabulum. The acetabulum must be adequately deepened with reamers or gouges, as needed, and the Lord reamer repeatedly inserted into the acetabular recess to ensure adequate medialization of the component. If the cup is screwed in before the acetabulum has been adequately deepened, it may be extremely difficult to remove despite its superficial seating. The component is ideally positioned when it projects slightly beyond the superior and anterior borders of the acetabulum and is flush with the posterior border. In the protrusio hip, the cartilage is carefully removed from all parts of the acetabulum (including the floor), and the largest possible Lord reamer is used to shape the acetabulum so as to prevent medial displacement of the metal ring and thus avoid pressure on the acetabular floor.

Experience has shown that a thread-cutting instrument is unnecessary. The metal ring has a high, sharp thread which exerts a good self-tapping action during insertion.

If, during preparation of the acetabulum, it is noted that little or no cortical bone is present and the bone is somewhat porous, primary looseness of the prosthesis can be corrected by going to the next larger component size without first using the corresponding-size reamer.

Femoral Component: Due to the marked valgus orientation of the Lord stem, the skin incision is placed less cranioanteriorally than usual. The gluteal muscles are notched anteriorally. The cranioposterior portion of the femoral neck with the greater trochanter and trochanteric fossa must be well visualized. The small lateral rotators (especially the pyriform and obturator muscles) are released at their insertions, at which point the proximal femur should be well exposed within the operative field.

The horizontal saw cut should be made just proximal to the lesser trochanter so that the prosthetic neck will not be too short. The vertical cut should be placed well laterally to ensure that the greater trochanter will not fracture

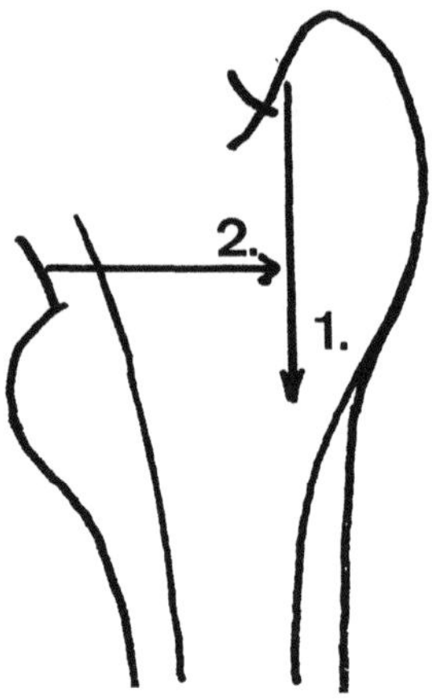

Fig. 1. Cuts comprising the femoral neck resection

when the stem is driven into the femural shaft (the stem will have a somewhat more valgus orientation than the corresponding rasp). To avoid sawing in the direction of a possible fracture line, it is better to make the vertical cut before the horizontal cut (Fig. 1).

The goal is to obtain a maximum contact area between the prosthetic stem and the interior cortex. This is achieved by using the largest rasp possible. If it is difficult to drive the rasp into the femur, then the medullary canal must be widened further with an intramedullary reamer. The prosthetic stems are slightly larger than the corresponding rasps and reamers, and so excessive force during insertion can cause the femoral shaft to crack or fracture. However, it is better to take this risk than to dispense with reaming and insert a stem that is too small. This leads to pain in the lateral thigh on weight-bearing, which may gradually subside as a result of appositional bone growth around the stem, or may progress to loosening.

In one-third of cases we ream the medullary cavity before inserting the stem. We had two complete shaft fractures and one fissure fracture in the first 32 operations of the present series, as opposed to two complete fractures and two fissure fractures in the remaining 139.

We did not treat apical fractures of the greater trochanter, but complete avulsions of the trochanter were repaired with Kirschner wires and tension bands. Complete shaft fractures were treated with screws, plates and 3–4 months of non-weight bearing, and fissure fractures with cerclage wiring and 6–8 weeks of non-weight bearing. These procedures had no apparent effect on the anchorage of the prosthesis.

When proper attention is given to these intraoperative difficulties and adjunctive procedures, which are common in any uncemented arthroplasty, complications should not be a significant problem.

Postoperative Management

Initially we favored non-weight bearing for 6–8 weeks postoperatively, but later we could see no justification for it. However, some therapeutic exercises, such as straight leg raising, subject the hip joint to very large and potentially damaging forces. We allow the patient to stand between the 1st and 3rd postoperative day. Gymnastic exercises, sustained walking and stair-climbing are encouraged as pain subsides. The resumption of weight-bearing should be delayed only after certain unstable revision operations.

Postoperative Complications

Postoperative complications in the present series are summarized in Table 2.

One 67-year-old man suffered a dislocation during a fall at home 4 weeks after surgery. He went to bed at once because of the pain but was not hospitalized until 4 days later. When reduction was attempted under general anesthesia, a massive, fatal pulmonary embolism occurred.

A 48-year-old man experienced recurrent dislocations due to malposition of the acetabular component, and so a revision was performed. Painful calcifications began to form within a few months, and at reexploration after 1 year both the acetabular component and stem were found to be completely loose. Granulation tissue was found between the metal and the bone, but no pus; no pathogenic organisms could be demonstrated. Each bone bed was freshened, and larger-size components were inserted. So far (6 months postoperatively) signs of slight calcification are apparent, but there is no evidence of loosening, and the patient has only very mild complaints.

In one 57-year-old woman (chronic polyarthritis, diabetes), signs of a purulent infection appeared 6 weeks postoperatively. Following copious drainage, the joint was irrigated twice daily with beta-isodone solution, and 3 smears in 2 weeks were negative. In the 4th smear, *Staphylococcus aureus* were found. The infection did not improve, but by 3 months after the first operation the femoral prosthesis was securely fixed to the bone. A 10-cm-long window had to be cut in the anterolateral cortex before the stem could be removed by retrograde impaction. Firmly-adherent bone was found among the spherules at several sites on the surface of the stem.

Of the 21 patients with radiologic signs of heavy calcification, 12 have restricted motion and other complaints, but none is yet ready for revisional surgery.

Table 2. Postoperative Complications (n = 148, Without Revisions)

Dislocation with subsequent fatal pulmonary embolism	1
Infection	1
Dislocation plus loosening	1
Calcification	32
– heavy	21
– light	11
Deep venous thrombosis	2
Nerve lesions	0

Results of Follow-Up

The first 32 patients (18 men, 14 women) were followed closely for a period of 2 years after their surgery (24–44 months postoperatively). As reported above, the average age was 60. Average length of hospitalization was 14 days (8–22 days). Severe osteoarthritis of the hip was the most frequent primary disorder (Table 3).

The functional ratings for the operated hips according to the d'Aubigné scale are presented in Table 4.

Table 3. Primary Disorders (n = 32)

Osteoarthritis	22
Femoral head necrosis	2
PCP (chronic polyarthritis)	3
Congenital dislocation	1
Post-trauma	2
Status after double-cup arthrp.	2

Table 4. Hip Function According to d'Aubigne Scale

	Preoperative	Postoperative
0	–	–
1	3	–
2	22	–
3	7	2
4	–	3
5	–	9
6	–	18
	32	32

Table 5. Results

Excellent	(6)	18	84%
Good	(5)	9	
Fair	(4)	3	
Poor	(3)	2	

Results were inconsistent in terms of reliance on walking aids. Thus, many patients continue to use crutches either because of anxiety or other complaints (2 have diseased contralateral hips, 1 has severe lumbar lesions). Two patients had fair hip function and intermittent complaints but did not use walking aids (Table 5).

Subjectively, 28 patients are satisfied with their result and 4 are dissatisfied, although the latter have shown both objective and subjective improvement over their preoperative status. One patient has complained of a general ache in the operated limb, but her complaints cannot be localized or objectified.

Radiologic Changes

Radiographs show calcifications in 8 patients. In 6 patients the changes have the same localization, extending posteriorally in a convex arc from the greater trochanter to the pelvis. These changes cannot always be correlated with complaints, however.

1. *Reactions in the Acetabulum:* Bone is diffusely apposed to the superior, major weight-bearing area of the metal cup; there is no lucency between the implant and bone, and no residual acetabular cortex is visible there (Fig. 2). In the inferior portion of the cup, where less weight is borne, the cortical bone frequently is preserved. In one protrusio hip we packed the floor of the acetabulum with cancellous bone to eliminate voids. In another case apposition occurred spontaneously, without bone grafting (Fig. 3). The important thing in such cases is to select a sufficiently large acetabular prosthesis and to remove all cartilage from the non-weight-bearing area of the protrusio with a small reamer in order to freshen the cortex.

2. *Reactions in the Femur:* If sufficient contact has been established in the medullary cavity between the prosthetic stem and the cortex, reactions are minimal (Fig. 2). X-rays sometimes show a small degree of cortical resorption in the calcar area or a rounding of the horizontal cut surface over the lesser trochanter. In one case we observed a distal "plugging" of the medullary cavity around the stem tip, and in another we witnessed a slight cortical hypertrophy in that area. In prostheses that lacked a diffuse seating, we observed the changes illustrated in Fig. 4. These changes could not be correlated with specific clinical symptoms, however.

Encouraged by the good clinical results of primary hip arthroplasties, we attempted to use uncemented prostheses for the revision of failed cemented arthroplasties (Table 6). We felt that such prostheses could be of particular value in difficult cases. The first patients to undergo the revisions had primary cemented prostheses which loosened within 2–4 years after insertion. The cemented, long-term prostheses that were inserted to replace the failed prostheses also be-

Table 6. Revision Arthroplasties (n=23, since Jan. 1981)

Acetabular component alone	2
Femoral component alone	1
Bilateral	5
After 2 cemented arthroplasties	5

Fig. 3. a Osteoarthritis with protrusio in a 57-year-old woman. **b** Lord prosthesis implanted without bone grafting of the acetabular floor. **c** 1 year post-implantation. The bone is closely apposed to the stable acetabular component, which bears weight only on the surfaces of its threads

limited motion in a 62-year-old man. **b** Lord prosthesis immediately after implantation. **c** 1 year post-implantation. **d** 40 months post-implantation. The acetabular component is ideally seated and is surrounded by homogenous appositional bone; the femoral stem shows an excellent, diffuse seating within the canal

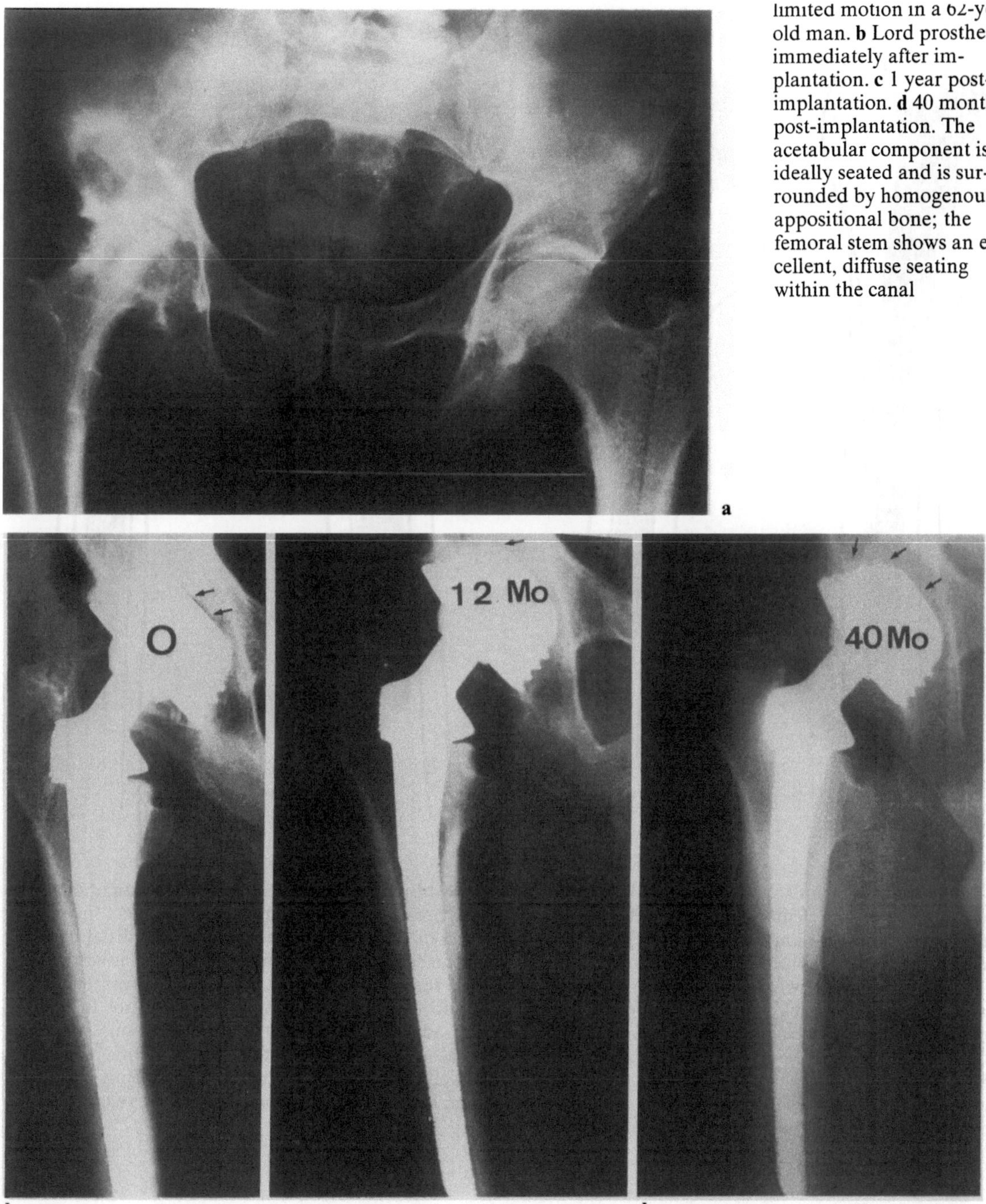

a

b c d

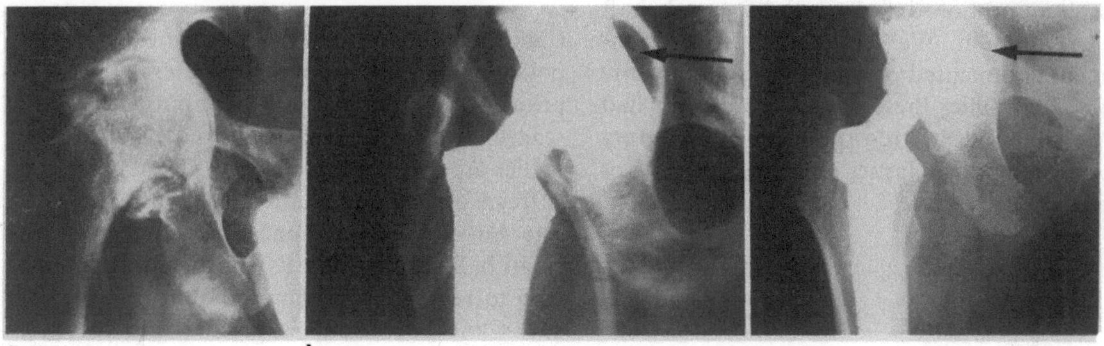

a b c

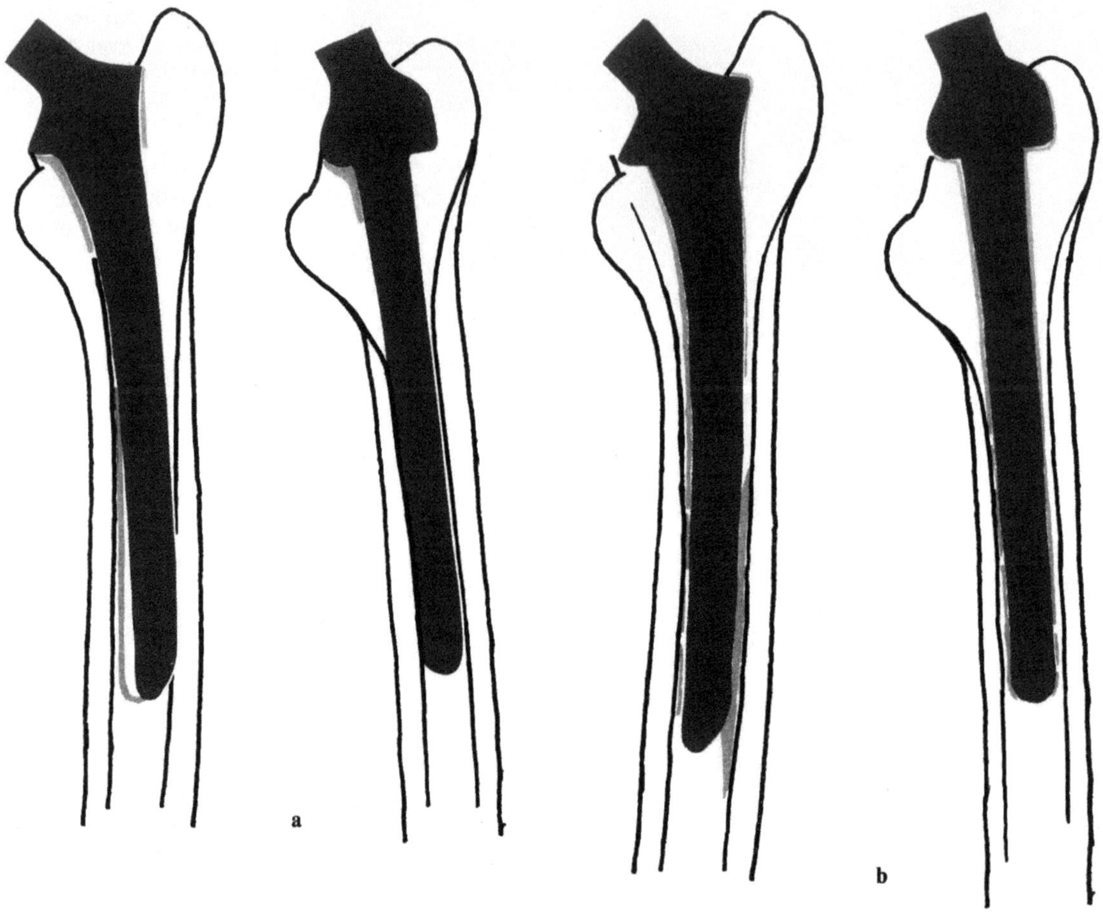

a b

Fig. 4 a–f. Bone reactions associated with an imperfect seating of the femoral component (after at least 2 years, implantation). *Light shading:* cortical bone resorbed and replaced by cancellous tissue. *Heavy shading:* dense, newly-formed cortical bone. *Intramedullary lines:* lucencies up to 3 mm wide. New bone does not appear during the first year and usually begins to form between 18 and 24 months postoperatively. **a** No loosening (firm axial seating); medial lucency; seating did not change with time. **b** Primary seating not firm; lucency close to bone; patient complained of pain for 1 year. **c** Primary seating not firm in all areas; solid circumferential contact in midportion of stem; lucency not apposed to distal end of stem; no complaints. **d** Primary seating relatively firm; diffuse remodeling of the cortex to the prosthetic surface? no complaints. **e** Primary seating not firm; lucency adjacent to proximal part of stem; massive cortical hypertrophy at stem tip. **f** Primary seating relatively firm; massive cortical hypertrophy distally; patient had intermittent complaints for 1 year

came loose within 1–2 years, associated with massive resorption defects in the femoral shaft and acetabulum. We felt that a properly-implanted, uncemented prosthesis offered the only hope of salvaging these cases, because we had never witnessed any resorption in our primary uncemented arthroplasties – only remodeling or appositional growth.

Surgical Technique

Cancellous bone is always taken in the largest possible quantities from the ipsilateral iliac crest prior to the hip surgery. It is important that all scar tissue be carefully removed. The muscle bellies are dissected free, and the acetabular bed is freed of all granulation tissue with a curette. The smooth cortical bone is freshened with a small ball reamer over its entire surface, taking care to remove a minimal amount of bone tissue. Cancellous bone is grafted into the ace-

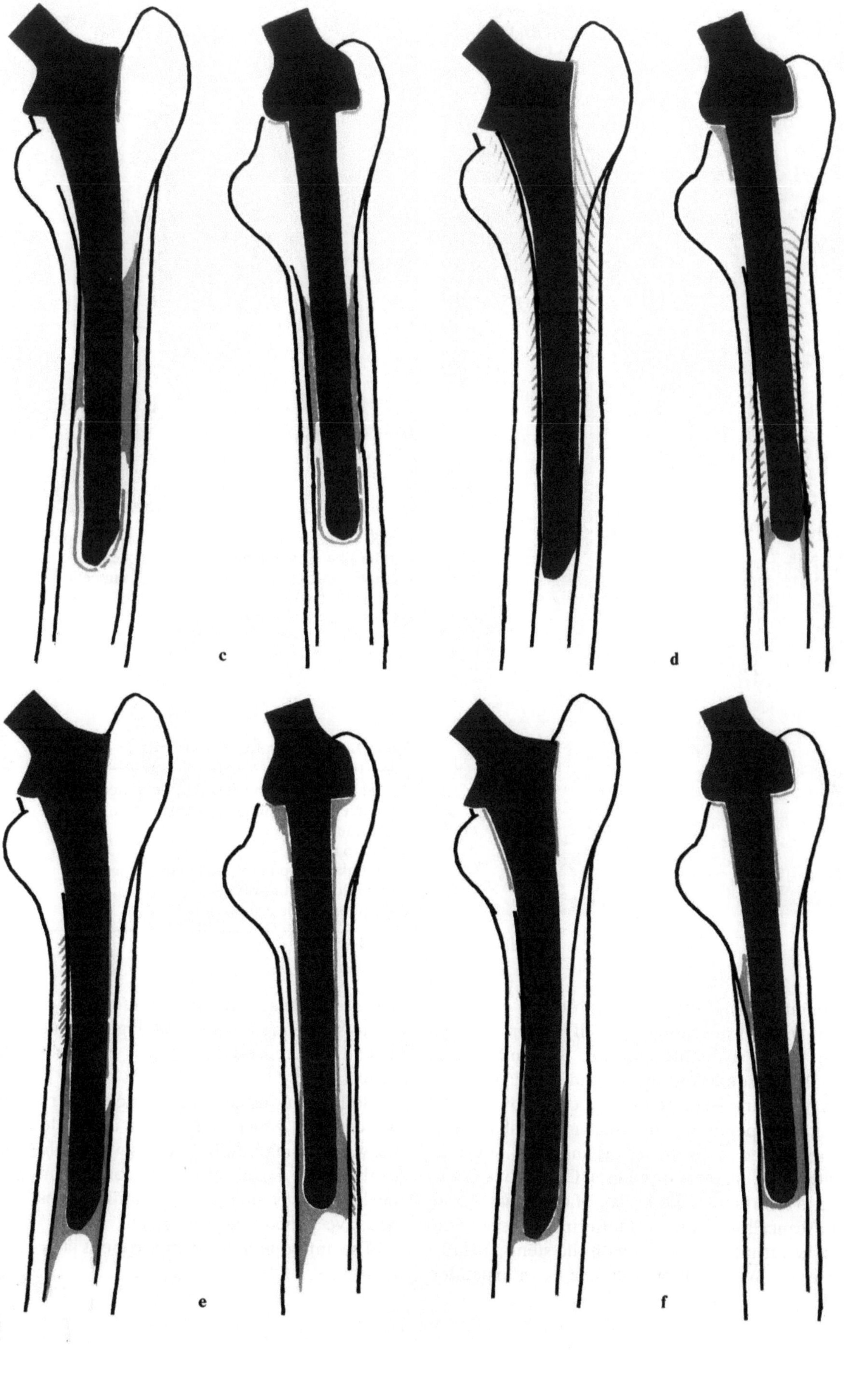
c
d
e
f

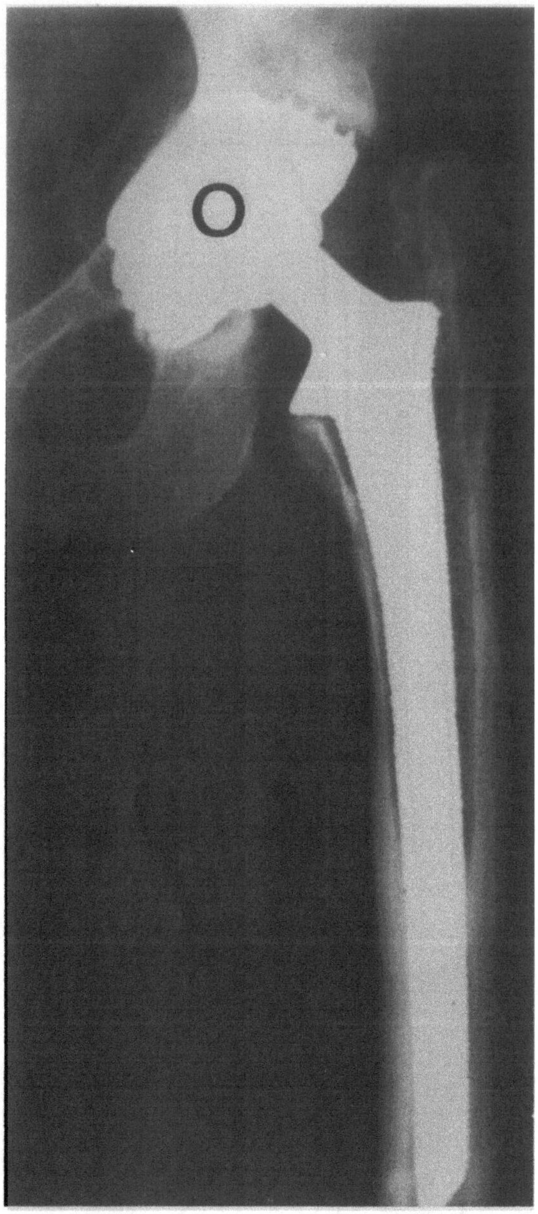

a

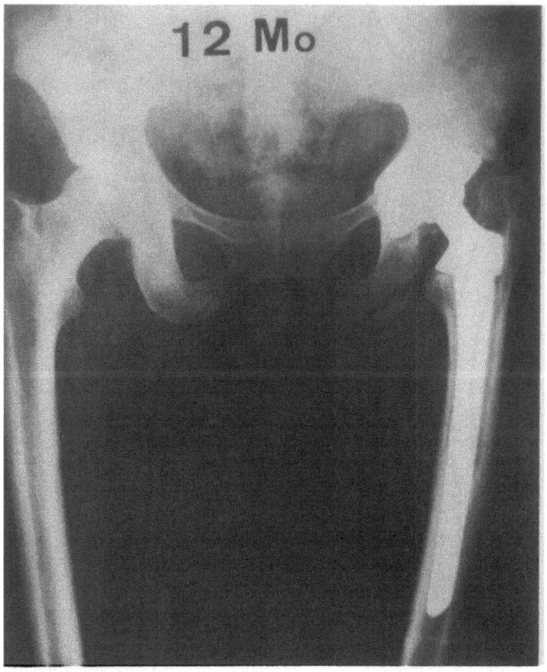

b

Fig. 5. a Status after revision of a cemented prosthesis that had been reattached and again became loose. Immediate postoperative radiograph; cancellous bone grafting. **b** 1-year radiograph shows good bony apposition with no migration

Table 7. Intraoperative Complications (n = 23)

Apical avulsion of the greater trochanter	2
Total avulsion of the greater trochanter	3
Shaft fracture	1
Stem too small	2
Acetabular component unstable (revised at same sitting)	1
Postoperative dislocation	2

tabulum only if the largest prosthetic cup cannot gain a firm seating by itself. Unfortunately, the largest available cup size (62 mm) is too small in some instances, and even the intramedullary stem is often too narrow in revisional operations. In the femoral shaft, the smooth bed is freshened as much as possible with drills, reamers or gouges. Cancellous grafting is always utilized. In half of cases, we mixed the cancellous bone with fibrin adhesive and packed it into the cavity with the stem partially inserted. We use fibrin adhesive as an expander of the graft material (on several occasions we had to supplement with homologous bone) and to bind free cancellous bone in the absence of cortical bone.

Besides the usual complications, there were two cases in which the largest available stem size was too small. In both cases we matched the firmly-seated Lord acetabular component with the largest uncemented Zweymüller prosthesis that gave a good stem-to-canal fit.

The intraoperative complications are listed in Table 7.

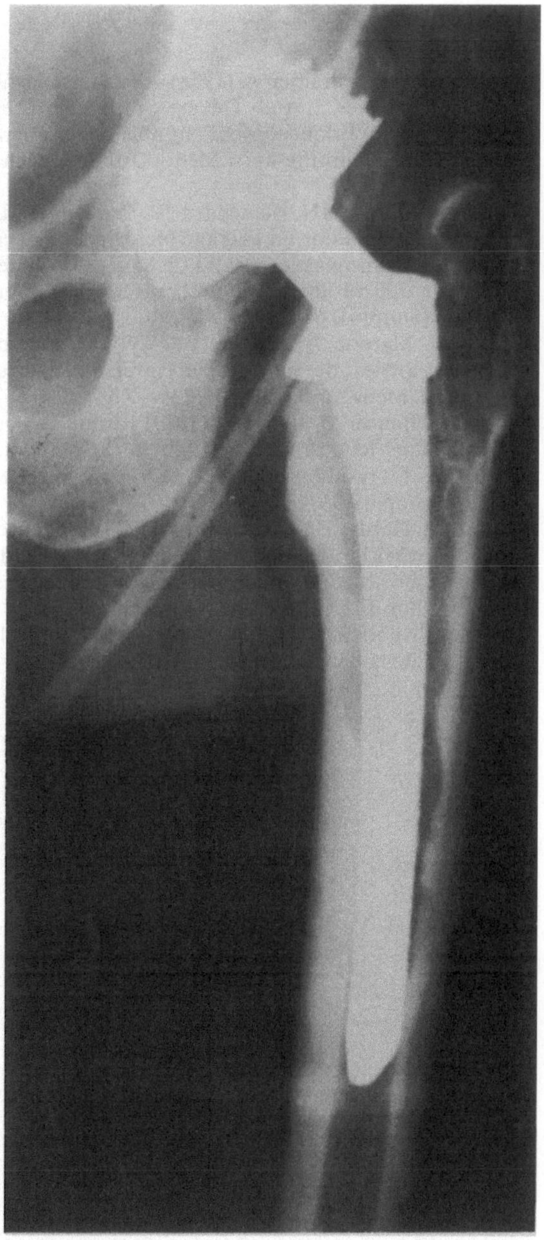

a

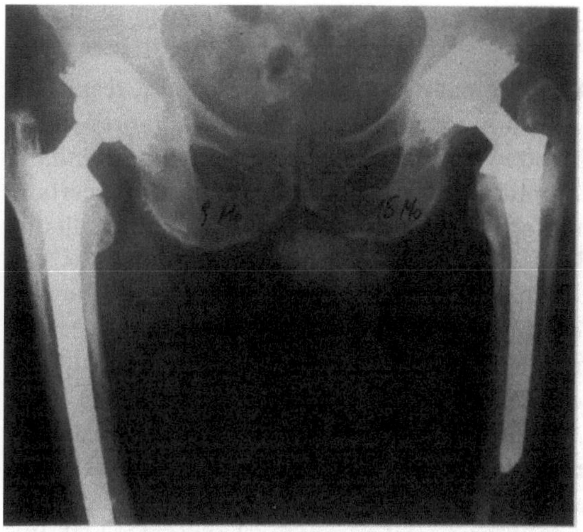

b

Fig. 6. Status after revision of a loose cemented prosthesis in the left hip. **a** At 15 months postoperatively, seating is good and there is good bony apposition. **b** 9 months postoperatively, also after revision

Table 8. Late Complications (n = 23)

Infection	0
Loosening	1 (?)
Calcification	2

Table 9. Preliminary Results (n = 23)

Excellent	5	48% (Excellent + Good)
Good	6	
Fair	9	
Poor	3	

Postoperative Management

In contrast to primary arthroplasties with the Lord prosthesis, weight-bearing following revision arthroplasties is contingent upon the stability achieved and on bone stock. In the majority of cases (70%) we had to enforce 6–12 weeks of non-weight bearing.

The 1½-year length of follow-up does not yet permit a definitive assessment of the results (Tables 8 and 9). However, several operations performed more than a year ago show excellent reactions of the old bone tissue and of the grafted cancellous bone (Figs. 5 and 6).

We feel that the results to date justify our continued use of the apparatus and techniques described. While it is still too early to draw final conclusions on the optimum prosthetic system for revision THA, we are convinced that the future of this type of surgery lies in the uncemented prosthesis combined with cancellous auto- or allografting.

Summary

A preliminary report is made on the results of 171 Lord total hip prostheses implanted from October 1978 through May 1982, and attendant complications are detailed. Aside from certain intraoperative technical problems, the results to date are highly encouraging.

The first 32 patients were closely followed for at least 2 years after their operations (24–44 months); 84% of the results were rated as good to excellent by the d'Aubigné scale [7].

In a series of 23 revision arthroplasties started in January 1981, loose cemented prostheses were replaced with uncemented implants (revisions were total except for 2 cases in which the acetabular components alone were replaced). Cancellous bone grafting was used in all cases, especially as a means of femoral augmentation. The lack of large-size acetabular components and intramedullary stems was a problem in several instances.

Without making a definitive evaluation, it may be stated that the results of both primary and revisionary arthroplasties have been highly encouraging.

References

1. Huggler AH, Schreiber A (1978) Alloarthroplastik des Hüftgelenkes, 2. Aufl. Thieme, Stuttgart, S 122
2. Lord G (1980) Erfahrungsbericht über 400 zementlose Hüfttotalprothesen. Med Orthop Techn 1:39–43
3. Lord G, Marotte JH, Blanchard JP, Guillamon JL, Gory M (1978) Pour un ancrage biologique sans ciment des arthroplasties totales de hanche. Premier bilan de 200 prothèses madréporiques. Rev Chir Orthop [Suppl II] 64:5
4. Lord G, Marotte JH, Bancel P (1979) 300 arthroplasties totales de hanche par implants madréporiques. Mem Acad Chir 105:236–240
5. Lord G, Bancel M, Bancel P (1979) Risque de corrosion dans les prothèses métalliques. Comparaison entre les prothèses lisses et madréporiques. Rev Chir Orthop 65:317–326
6. Lord G, Hardy JJ, Kummer FJ (1979) An uncemented total hip replacement. Experimental study and review of 300 madreporique arthroplasties. Clin Orthop 141:2–16
7. Merle d'Aubigné R (1970) Cotation chiffrée de la fonction de la hanche. Rev Chir Orthop 56:481

Experience with Revision Arthroplasties for Failed Cemented Total Hip Replacements Using Uncemented Lord and PM Prostheses

R. Parhofer and W. Mönch

Since December, 1979, we have not used cement in our revisions of failed total hip arthroplasties. To date, 67 revision arthroplasties have been performed in 63 patients (Table 1). Fifty-nine of these were first revisions, and 8 were re-revisions. The patients averaged 68.2 years of age. Fig. 1 shows the increase in the number of revisions performed by us in recent years as well as the types of prostheses used. Initially we used Lord prostheses. For various reasons we abandoned their use, however, first in primary arthroplasties and later in revisions as well. Lately we have been using PM prostheses exclusively. Most of the revisions had become necessary after a period of 6–10 years. In all but 3 cases we replaced both the femoral and acetabular components of the failed THA.

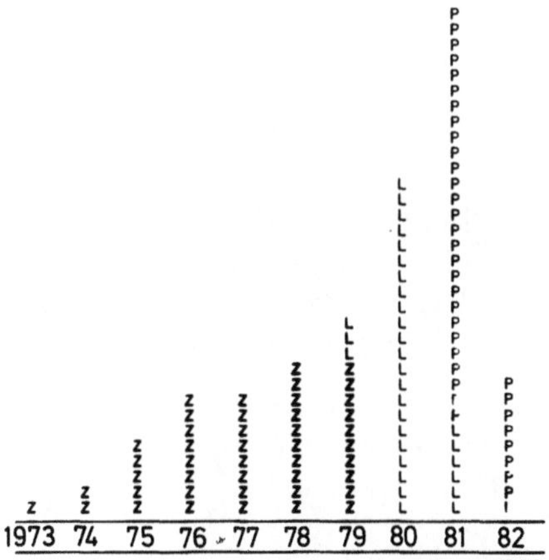

Fig. 1. Number of revision arthroplasties performed on a yearly basis. *Z* Revision done with cemented components; *L* revision with uncemented Lord prosthesis (How Medica); *P* revision with uncemented PM prosthesis (Aesculap Instruments)

Today we attempt to use the smallest acetabular component possible, in both primary and revisionary operations. Reconstruction of the acetabulum, which is carefully freed of all residual cement and granulation cysts, is undertaken with a large autograft taken from the contralateral iliac crest. We try to place two grafts, each as large as possible, on two opposite sides of the acetabulum. The grafts are held tightly against the borders of the acetabulum by the screw thread of the conical cup and give the prosthesis a firm seating within the acetabular recess. Additional bone is packed around the acetabular rim and within its floor. In most cases the acetabular floor is badly damaged, and often it must be deepened somewhat to provide better purchase for the screw threads of the prosthesis.

In revision arthroplasties we generally do not use a thread-cutting instrument in the bony acetabulum, but insert the definitive self-tapping prosthesis directly to obtain a solid primary seating.

Based on our experience with 368 prostheses implanted without cement, 248 of which were PM prostheses, we devote much attention to the seating of the femoral endoprosthesis, both in primary arthroplasties and in revisions. Only an accurate stem placement with broad contact between the stem surface and cortex can ensure a

Table 1. Revision Arthroplasties Performed at our Hospital

Number of revisions performed	First revision	Second revision	Average age of patients
♂ 21	18	3	70.7
♀ 46	41	5	67.0
♂ + ♀ 67	59	8	68.2

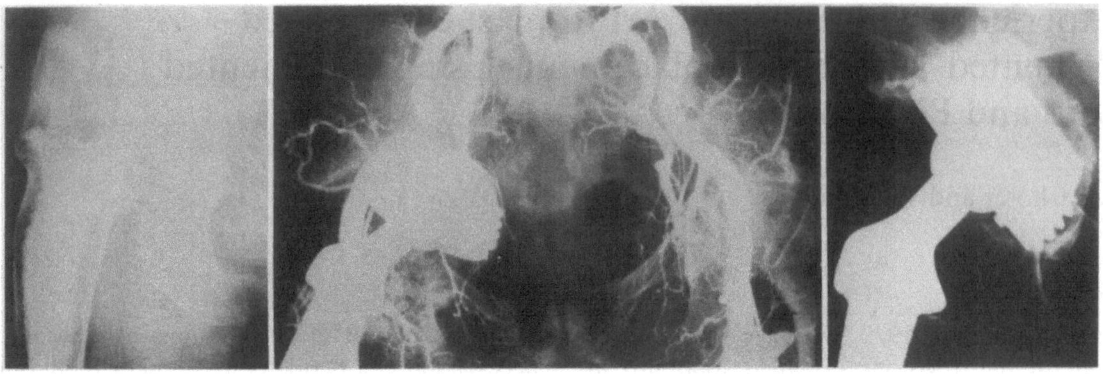

a b c

Fig. 2. **a** 80-year-old woman who underwent a primary arthroplasty 4 years ago and had a first revision 6 months later due to infection. **b** Check angiogram showing migration of the acetabular component into the pelvis. **c** Fifteen months after re-revision

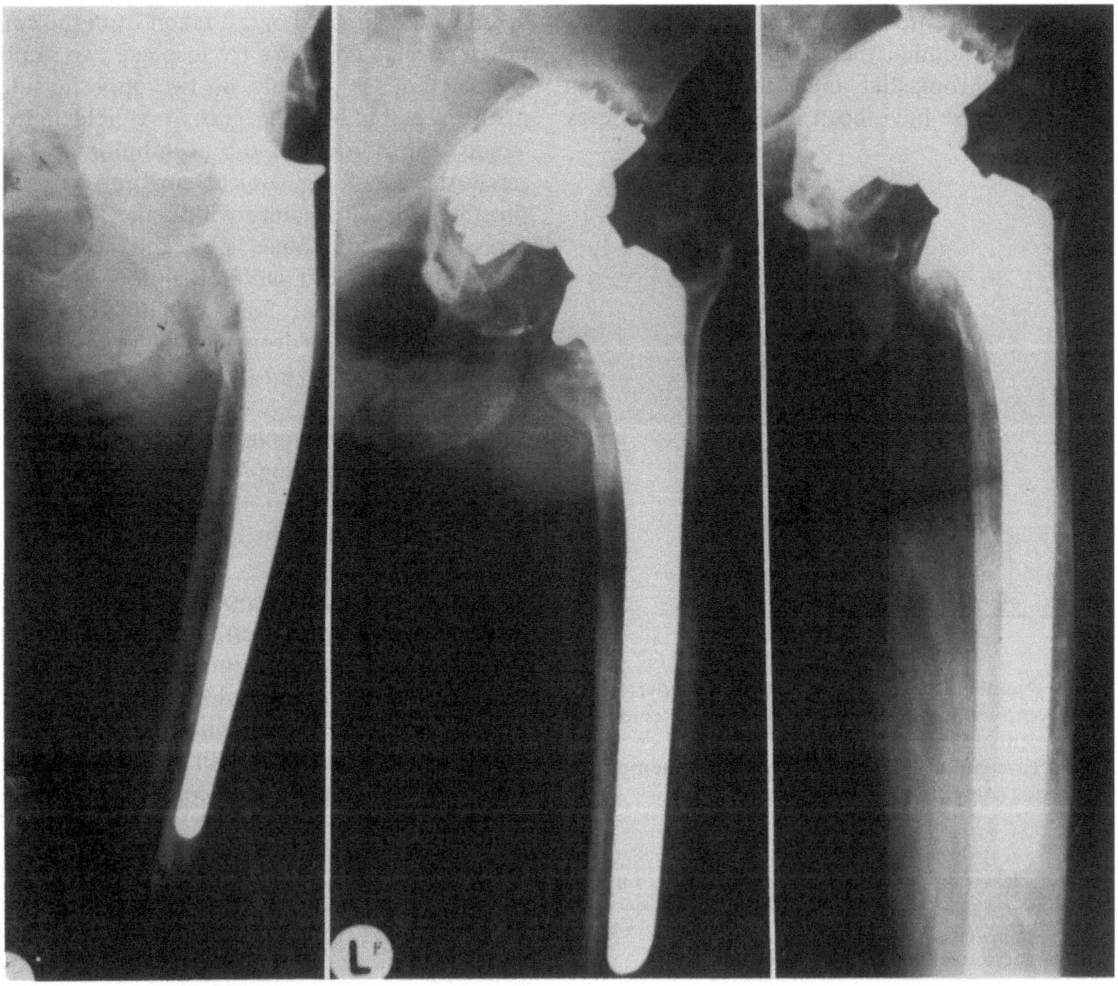

a b c

Fig. 3. 70-year-old woman who underwent primary arthroplasty 9.5 years ago. **a** Massive acetabular destruction (October 1981). **b** December 1981, 4 weeks after revision. **c** Five months after revision; there has been rapid union of the grafted bone

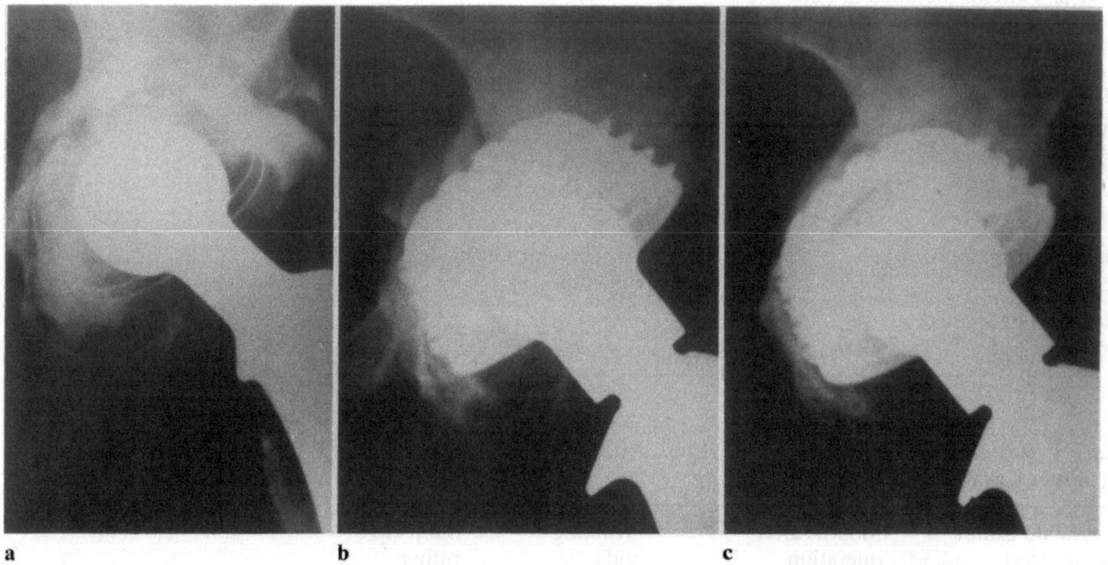

Fig. 4. 80-year-old woman who underwent primary arthroplasty 9 years ago. **a** There is damage to all portions of the acetabulum. **b** Four weeks after operation. **c** Six months later. There is slight subsidence of the femoral stem with consolidation of the calcar. The films show that rapid bony integration is possible even with severe preexisting bone damage

satisfactory result. We take particular care to avoid a varus placement of the stem. When a proper stem seating is obtained, we often observe a very good stimulation of bone formation in the calcar area.

The Lord Prosthesis

An illustrative case for the Lord THR involves an 80-year-old woman who underwent a primary total hip arthroplasty 4 years ago and 6 months later had to have a first revision due to infection (Fig. 2a). Three and a half years later the patient was presented to us with severe suppurating fistulae. Following initial treatment by suction irrigation in early December, 1980, we inserted a Lord prosthesis but refrained from bone grafting, reasoning that the grafts would be lost should the infection recur. The acetabular prosthesis migrated into the pelvis under the slightest load, as indicated by the angiogram in Fig. 2b.

In late January, 1981, the patient underwent a re-revision. Extensive autografting with iliac bone was done at that time, since no new signs of infection had appeared. Fig. 2c shows the integration of the prosthesis 15 months later. The leg is again capable of bearing weight.

The PM Prosthesis

The surprisingly rapid regeneration of the often badly-damaged bone and the rapid integration of the PM prosthesis by consolidation of the grafted bone are illustrated by the serial radiographs in Figs. 3 and 4, which were made only a few months postoperatively.

Results of Follow-Up

A survey of the patients included in our follow-up is presented in Table 2. By the end of last year we had performed 58 revision arthroplasties in 55 patients. Forty-two of these patients presented for their follow-up examinations. In 8 cases we had to obtain follow-up data by telephone, part of which was supplied by family physicians. Two patients have died, one from causes unrelated to the operation. One patient was excluded from follow-up due to recurrent infection, and two patients failed to present for the examination.

The patients included in the follow-up had had their operation an average of 16 months before the examination (Table 3). Eleven patients

Table 2. Patients Included in Follow-Up

Summoned for follow-up:	55 patients with	58 revisions
Presented for follow-up:	42 patients with	44 revisions
Data obtained by telephone:	8 patients with	9 revisions
Died:	2 patients – 1 from stroke 28 days postoperatively, 1 from liver disease several months postoperatively	
Excluded from follow-up:	1 patient who underwent Girdlestone due to recurrence of infection	
Could not be located for follow-up:	2 patients	

Table 3. Results of Follow-Ups of Revision Arthroplasties (50 Patients, 53 Operations; Status as of June, 1982)

Follow-up examinations (incl. 8 by telephone)	Months after operation	Walking aids	Subjective rating
50	16.6	0=11 1=26 2= 3	+ =41 (+)= 6 0 = 3

required no walking aids, 36 used a cane, and 3 used 2 canes. Forty-one patients (82%) were totally satisfied with the result; 12% were partially satisfied, and 3 patients (6%) were dissatisfied. One of these, who had a loose intramedullary stem associated with a chronic periprosthetic infection, has since been reoperated.

In summary, the following points should be noted:

1. A failed total hip arthroplasty can be revised without cement even in elderly patients and in the face of severe damage to bone stock.
2. We always revise both the acetabular and femoral components of a failed THA.
3. Regeneration of the often badly-damaged bone is very rapid when autografting is employed, and bony integration of the uncemented prosthesis is surprisingly rapid and good.

Revision Arthroplasty with the Screw-Anchored Intramedullary Hip Prosthesis

G. Bousquet and F. Bornand

We do not consider it logical to perform a revision arthroplasty using the same technique that led to failure of the original prosthesis. We therefore suggest an uncemented, screw-anchored prosthesis as a means of revising failed arthroplasties.

Indications for Revision

Among our patients, we consider the following to be indications for a revision arthroplasty:
- severe pain in the area of the prosthesis
- septic temperature elevations
- ESR between 20 and 60
- radiologic evidence of prosthetic loosening
- positive bone scan.

Bone scanning, or scintigraphy, is a useful tool for assessing the status of an endoprosthesis. Normally the procedure shows a high uptake of radioisotope over a 6-month period. After that time, any diffuse uptake is considered a pathologic sign. A localized uptake points to an abnormality in the periprosthetic area. This finding is not specific, however, and it is not possible to differentiate between loosening and infection by this technique.

Loose Prostheses

We distinguish between three main forms of prosthetic loosening:

1. *Lytic forms* (with radiolucent seams) are difficult to revise because the cortical bone is greatly weakened. The seams are filled with connective tissue. Histologic examination reveals granulomas with polyethylene and methylmethacrylate debris. If all cement is removed, good-quality new bone can be expected to form around the screw-anchored prosthesis.
2. In the *hypertrophic form,* the quality of the bone stock is not impaired, and revision is less difficult.
3. In the *mixed lytic-hypertrophic form,* revision is somewhat tedious because femoral fractures can easily occur at the junctions between resistant and weakened areas.

Basic Principles of Revision Arthroplasty

Our objective is to achieve a restoration of bone stock on both the femoral and acetabular sides of the arthroplasty.

On the femoral side, the following steps are necessary: The cement must be completely removed with suitable gouges and with the aid of a small tap that enables fragmentation of the cement. Due to the high risk of splitting or fracturing the femur, especially in the lytic and mixed forms, we place cerclage wires around the femoral shaft before attempting to remove the cement. Before cutting the thread for the intramedullary stem, we immobilize the femur with two forceps. After tapping is complete, the bony wall is closely inspected. If it appears to be too thin, it is augmented by packing bone grafts into the medullary cavity. The outer cortex is also augmented if deficient.

The same principles are followed on the acetabular side, where bone grafting is mandatory (Figs. 1 and 2).

Timing the Revision of a Loose Prosthesis

The prime concern is to avoid the extensive destruction of bone stock. Hence, the revision should be done as soon as osteolysis is demon-

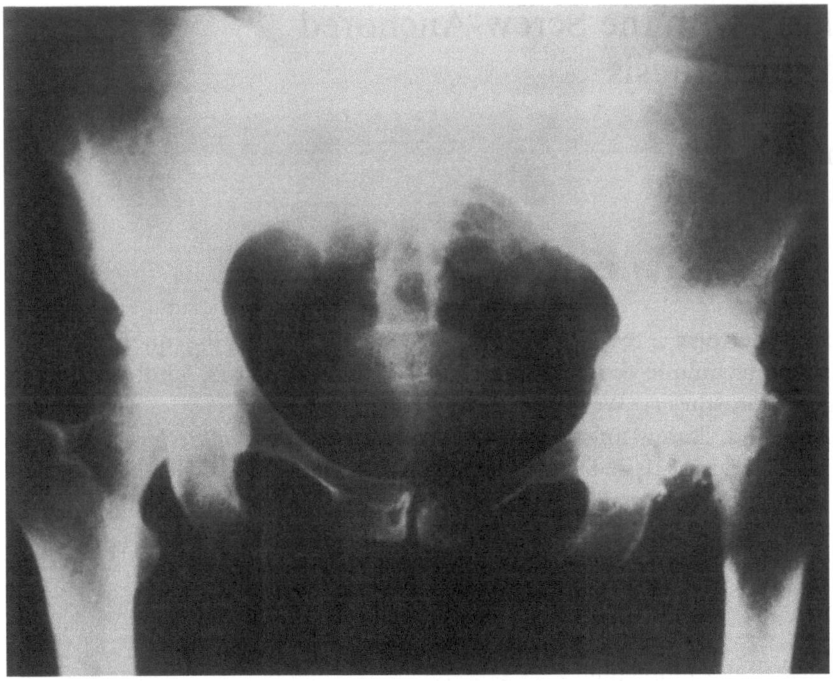

Fig. 1. Wagner double-cup arthroplasty with protrusio

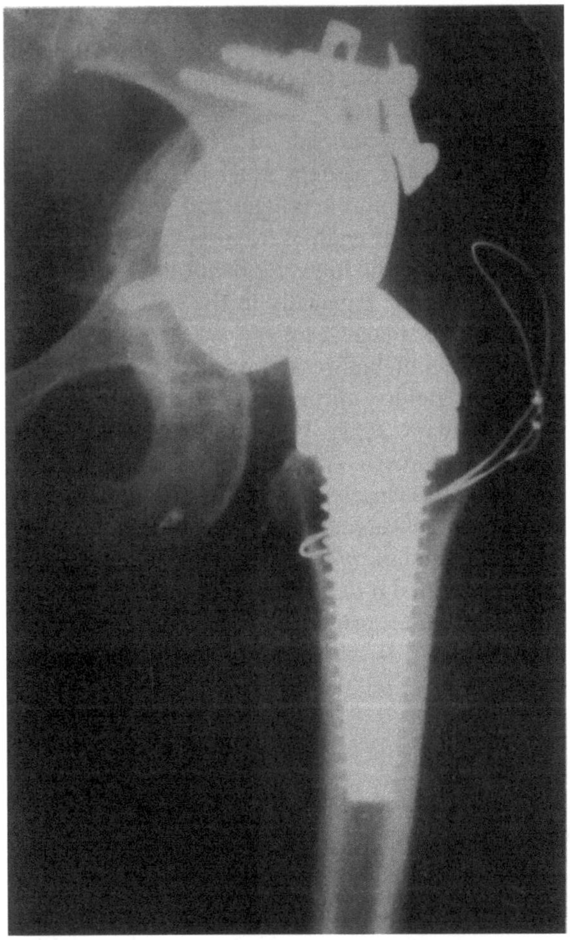

Fig. 2. Bone stock augmented with grafts, and arthroplasty revised with uncemented prosthesis

strated. Delays will only lessen the chance of a successful reimplantation. This is our basic philosophy.

Infected Prostheses

To date we have revised 10 infected prostheses with more than 1 year of follow-up. The revisionary prostheses were inserted an average of 8 months after removal of the infected implant.

Our procedure for the revision of septic arthroplasties is as follows:

- The prosthesis and all infected tissues are removed.
- A chain of gentamicin-impregnated beads is implanted in the surgical wound, provided sensitivity tests indicate susceptibility.
- If the organisms are not susceptible to gentamicin, we close the wound over suction drains and maintain suction irrigation for about 3 weeks; the drains are not removed until 3 negative cultures are obtained.
- The hip is kept in continuous traction during this period.
- Mobilization is started on a protective apparatus so that hip mobility will be preserved.
- Antibiotics are administered until the ESR has returned to normal.
- The revisionary prosthesis is inserted only after a constant ESR has been obtained.

Among the cases that have been revised to date using this technique, there have been no failures in more than a year of follow-up.

Results of Revisions of Loose Prostheses

We have performed 70 revisions of loose prostheses. Nineteen have been followed for more than a year.

Seven of these show very good results with excellent bone regeneration. One result is rated as fair. So far no infections have occurred.

We believe that the method described is an effective means of preserving bony stock and promoting bone regeneration through corticalization of the cancellous bone.

Subject Index

R. Bombelli

Osteoarthritis of the Hip

Classification and Pathogenesis
The Role of Osteotomy as a Consequent Therapy

With a Foreword by M. E. Müller

2nd revised and enlarged edition. 1983. 374 figures (partly in colour). XVII, 386 pages
ISBN 3-540-11422-X

Renato Bombelli, Professor of Orthopedics at the Universit of Milan, has treated more than 1 500 cases of primary and secondary osteoarthritis of the hip in the last 20 years. This book is the result of his clinical, radiological and surgical observations in the course of this distinguished career. In it Professor Bombelli details the biomechanics of the normal and diseased hip and shows that the natural healing proces can be accelerated through changes induced by surgery on the forces acting on the hip.

Bombelli's intertrochanteric osteotomy subjects the superi capsule of the hip to tension to induce osteophyte formatio along the superior lip of the acetabulum, forming a physiological "shelf" and thereby increasing the weight-bearing area of the hip. His procedure is shown to produce excelle results, particularly in young adults.

For this second, revised and enlarged edition, Professor Bombelli has further refined his classification of osteoarthritis of the hip, his theory of hip biomechanics, and the indications for osteotomy. He has also included updated clinic statistics which lend credence to his conclusion that, whereas the best hip replacement has an unknown but certainly finite life, a hip healed after osteotomy will often last lifetime.

Springer-Verlag
Berlin
Heidelberg
New York
Tokyo

MIX
Papier aus verantwortungsvollen Quellen
Paper from responsible sources
FSC® C105338

If you have any concerns about our products,
you can contact us on
ProductSafety@springernature.com

In case Publisher is established outside the EU,
the EU authorized representative is:
Springer Nature Customer Service Center GmbH
Europaplatz 3, 69115 Heidelberg, Germany

Printed by Libri Plureos GmbH
in Hamburg, Germany